THE RAYS

THE RAYS

A HISTORY OF RADIOLOGY IN THE UNITED STATES AND CANADA

Ruth and Edward Brecher

ROBERT E. KRIEGER PUBLISHING COMPANY
HUNTINGTON, NEW YORK

TO

The Gas-Tube Gang

Preface

The history of radiology in North America has been 73 years in the making and 10 years in the writing, with some of the same people involved in both phases. As detailed in this volume, the tremendous advances in radiation science and in the medical specialty of radiology have occurred within the lifespan of a man.

Professor Wilhelm Conrad Roentgen's discovery of the X ray at the end of 1895 was a predictable result of the Victorian era of science. Investigations of the properties of electricity, of vacuums, and of the foundations of modern physics led a whole generation of investigators into a similar path of experimentation. It was Roentgen who first observed and understood. Scant months later, Henri Becquerel and after that the Curies found that radiation might also come from natural substances as well as from an electrical discharge.

Physicians in America were quick to perceive the possibilities for medical applications of the revealing ray. They were almost as quick to apply the effects of X rays on living tissue to the treatment of disease. While much of the scientific development of radiation continued in Europe, its practical applications seemed particularly suited to the inquiring minds of Americans.

The earliest X-ray sources were partially evacuated glass tubes which would not work unless a residue of gas remained inside. These tubes were balky and unpredictable because the properties of the residual gases changed when they were heated and varied from day to day as well as from minute to minute. Happily for the progress of radiology, these gas tubes were replaced by a new variety developed by Dr. William D. Coolidge and first announced in 1913. However, for almost two decades, the mark of a true pioneer of radiology was his mastery of the use of the cranky gas tubes.

Beginning in 1958, a group of veteran radiologists, some dating their careers to the first decade of this century, began to gather for reminiscences at the annual meeting of the Radiological Society of North America. Soon the group became known as the "Gas-Tube Gang." After several meetings, the Gang began to dwindle due to the deaths of members. Those remaining became aware that with their deaths, an irreplacable part of radiology would be lost unless efforts were made to preserve the record.

Thus, the Gas-Tube Gang gained a serious purpose. This was reflected in 1961 by its transformation into the National Council for Radiological Heritage. The preparation of a history was proposed, and the creation of a museum was discussed. During 1961 and 1962, the American College of Radiology began to assume a responsibility for the history effort, lending the services of its staff and providing a further focus for discussions.

It was decided that the College and the American College of Radiology Foundation should take some of the initiative in the arrangements for both parts of the project. At the College's 1963 meeting, the National Council for Radiological Heritage agreed to become part of the Foundation.

In contemplating the preparation of a history of radiology, it seemed to those involved that the story was vital and exciting enough to justify a proper telling. As a genre, medical histories have not been great literature because they often take the form of official recordings or else develop as the recollections of physicians.

The ACR Foundation and the Council agreed to avoid this by inviting a professional writer with recognized performance in science and medicine to undertake the manuscript with the support of the Foundation. At the 1963 ACR meeting, a committee was formed to select and work with an author. Its members were: Maxwell Poppel, M.D.; Edwin C. Ernst, Sr., M.D.; J. W. J. Carpender, M.D.; Benjamin Orndoff, M.D.; Kenneth L. Krabbenhoft, M.D.; and John H. Gilmore, M.D., chairman.

After interviewing several writers, the committee invited Ruth and Edward Brecher to write the history of radiology in North America. Their previous interest in and writings about radiology, plus their reputation for painstaking research and lucid exposition, convinced the committee that a readable as well as authoritative book would result. The agreement was simple. The Brechers agreed to write a book under their byline with the sponsorship of the Foundation. Their work was to be done with the advice of the committee and with the cooperation of the College and its staff, but the manuscript was to be their effort. This has been the situation. The work was supported by a contribution to the Foundation from the Mallinckrodt Pharmaceuticals Division of the Mallinckrodt Chemical Works in St. Louis.

The Brechers began their work in the summer of 1963. They found that the literature was abundant from the earliest days. Their work continued at a good pace and was nearing completion in the spring of 1965, when Ruth Brecher became seriously ill. It was largely put aside during the last 1½ years of her life and was completed after her death by

Ed Brecher. The ACR Foundation is pleased to have both their names affixed to the history.

It is appropriate that the Mallinckrodt Company provided the bulk of support for the preparation of this history. The late Edward Mallinckrodt, Sr., became involved with radiology only a few years after Roentgen's discovery when his company began to supply barium-based contrast media for gastrointestinal examinations. The company has remained an active supplier of radiological materials since that time.

Throughout their work, Ruth and Ed Brecher welcomed the participation of the members of this committee. Segments of their manuscript were reviewed by dozens of radiologists and other experts in the field. The College, the Foundation and the Council are grateful to all those who participated in the preparation of this history.

From the beginning, American radiology has been a dynamic, tempestuous part of medicine and the American scene. Here is its story.

JOHN H. GILMORE, M.D.

Introduction

by Edward M. Brecher

Before my late wife Ruth and I accepted the invitation of the American College of Radiology Foundation to write this book, we made a preliminary survey of the available source materials. Were they adequate for the task?

We were amazed and delighted by what we found. When Dr. Arthur Williams Wright of Yale, for example, exposed on January 27, 1896, what was in all probability the first North American X-ray plate, he promptly dashed off one report for the *Engineering and Mining Journal* and a fuller paper a few weeks later for the *American Journal of Science.* His precedent was followed through the years by almost everyone concerned with radiology. For any given discovery, we could find in the published scientific literature at least one and often several contemporary accounts by the men who knew the facts best—the discoverers themselves. As they neared the end of their careers, moreover, many of the leading figures in this history also published reminiscent papers on their work and the work of their colleagues. Thus, a voluminous record was accumulated which historians in other fields might well envy. We saw from the beginning that our problem would not be the securing of reliable source materials but rather the selection of the most relevant and most interesting from the embarrassment of riches which faced us.

We accordingly adopted, in consultation with the Committee on History of the American College of Radiology Foundation, several limitations for our book. First, we decided not to attempt the impossible— an *exhaustive* history. Merely to describe in passing all of the thousands of contributions to radiology since 1896 would have resulted in a dry-as-dust chronicle rather than the readable narrative history at which we aimed. Hence, readers will seek in vain for more than a bare listing of splenoportography, intraosseous venography, hysterosalpingography, and many other significant topics to which whole books might properly be devoted.

We resolved also to focus this book primarily on radiological *ideas* rather than on men, institutions, or devices. Even within the realm of ideas, we chose to present full accounts of a few dozen developmental sequences selected as illustrative and inherently fascinating, even though this required a ruthless sacrifice of detail on other topics to keep the over-all length of the book within bounds. In many chapters we also found it necessary to omit recent developments or cite them only briefly in order to save room for an adequate presentation of the pioneering stages.

The limitation of this history to the United States and Canada was a practical necessity which both Ruth and I deeply regretted. Indeed, we have occasionally overstepped the formal boundaries and have reported on European contributions when the temptation proved too strong to resist. Let us hope that as other countries explore their own radiological heritage, it will eventually become possible to prepare a worldwide narrative history in which American and Canadian contributions can be seen in fair prospective.

American readers, meanwhile, will find vast quantities of data on European as well as American radiology in two other historical works published while this history was in preparation. One is an invaluable two-volume source book, *Classic Descriptions in Diagnostic Roentgenology* (1964), edited by Dr. André J. Bruwer. An outstanding merit of the fat Bruwer volumes is the skillful translation into English of the full texts of major radiological papers originally published in a wide range of other languages. The other recent work is a richly illustrated compendium of data on many aspects of worldwide radiology, *The Trail of the Invisible Light* (1965), by Dr. E. R. N. Grigg. The appearance of these works buttressed our decision to make our own book a *narrative* history emphasizing the sweep of events from 1896 to date. While most of Ruth's and my text was drafted before these books became available, I am pleased to acknowledge their great helpfulness to me during the final revision of the manuscript.

Our other debts are so numerous that they cannot here be even listed in full. Let me cite a few outstanding examples.

Three members of the Gas-Tube Gang—Drs. Edwin C. Ernst, Sr., Benjamin Orndoff, and W. Walter Wasson—were alive when this book was begun; all three were helpful, and the deaths of Dr. Ernst and Dr. Wasson while the book was in preparation came as a personal loss. Dr. Ernst and Dr. Ornoff tirelessly searched their files and their recollections of more than 60 years for details we needed, and Dr. Ernst supplied us with a very useful collection of fugitive materials not readily available in libraries. Drs. Traian Leucutia and Howard P. Doub, editor and editor emeritus, respectively, of the two leading radiological journals, were also generous in many ways, as was Dr. Ross Golden. We owe a particular debt to the late Dr. Robert S. Stone, without whose help Part IV of this book would have been impoverished. Dr. Kenneth L. Krabbenhoft is responsible for much more than the Epilogue which bears his name, including much of the basic research underlying Chapter 21. Dr. Maxwell Poppel's encouragement and penetrating criticism were both very welcome. Our book owes much both to the earlier writings and to the critical comments of Dr. Edith H. Quimby. Mr. Robert O. Gorson went to great pains to assist us on several health physics points. Dr. Paul C. Hodges was helpful on several portions, and especially on Chapter 8. We have made use at several points of the pioneering studies of radiological history in Boston undertaken by Dr. Lloyd E. Hawes. The rich collections of the Yale Library of Medicine, and the unfailing courtesy of its staff, made this undertaking feasible.

Our debt is very great to Dr. John H. Gilmore, chairman of the Committee on History of the American College of Radiology Foundation, and to Mr. Otha Linton of the American College of Radiology staff, on whom we relied for many services and whose diplomatic skills smoothed our way at every stage. All six of the members of the Committee on History, including Dr. James W. J. Carpender, were helpful, and I am particularly grateful for their patience during Ruth's prolonged illness.

Finally, Ruth particularly requested that I acknowledge here her lifelong indebtedness to her teachers, the late Professor Frederick J. Manning of Swarthmore and Professor Samuel Eliot Morison of Harvard, as well as my similar debt to the late Alexander Meiklejohn of the University of Wisconsin Experimental College, Professor Brand Blanshard of Swarthmore and Yale, and Max Lowenthal, Esq., of the New York bar.

Yelping Hill
West Cornwall, Connecticut
June 1969

Contents

PART IV. RADIOLOGY IN THE NUCLEAR ERA

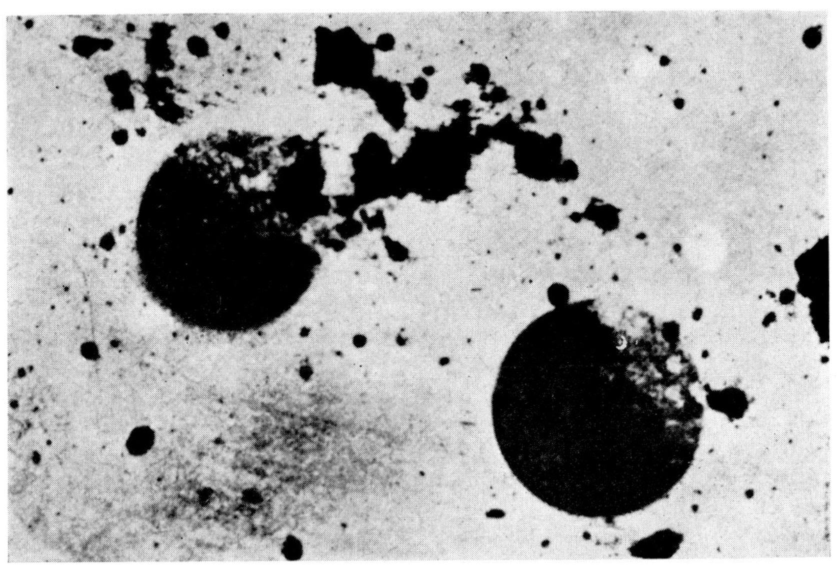

PLATE I. Professor Goodspeed in Philadelphia accidentally made this Roentgen ray picture on February 22, 1890, but failed to realize its importance. From American Institute of Radiology (George Eastman House, Inc., Rochester, New York). See page 3.

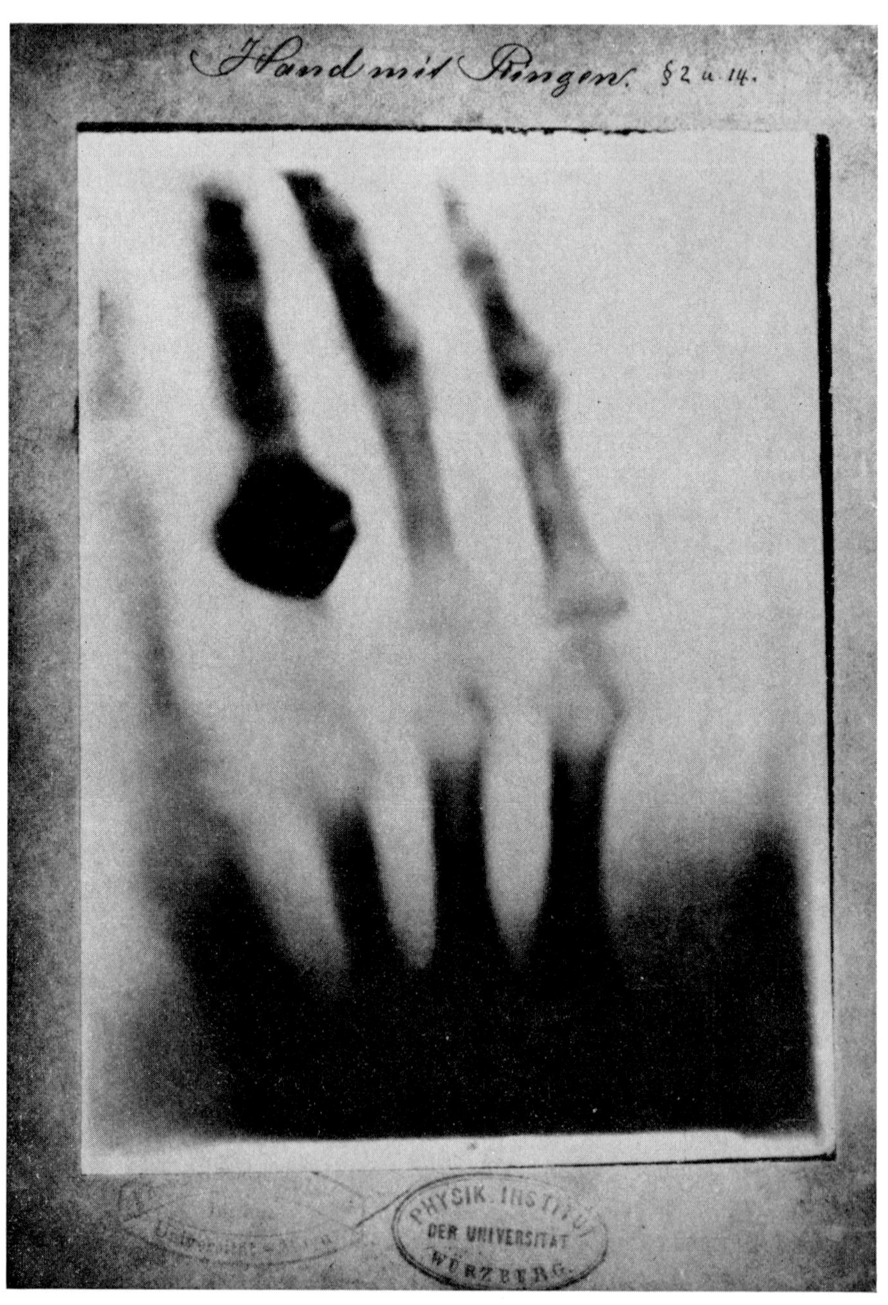

PLATE II. Early X-ray image of a hand with a ring, made by Professor Roentgen. The hand may have been Frau Roentgen's.

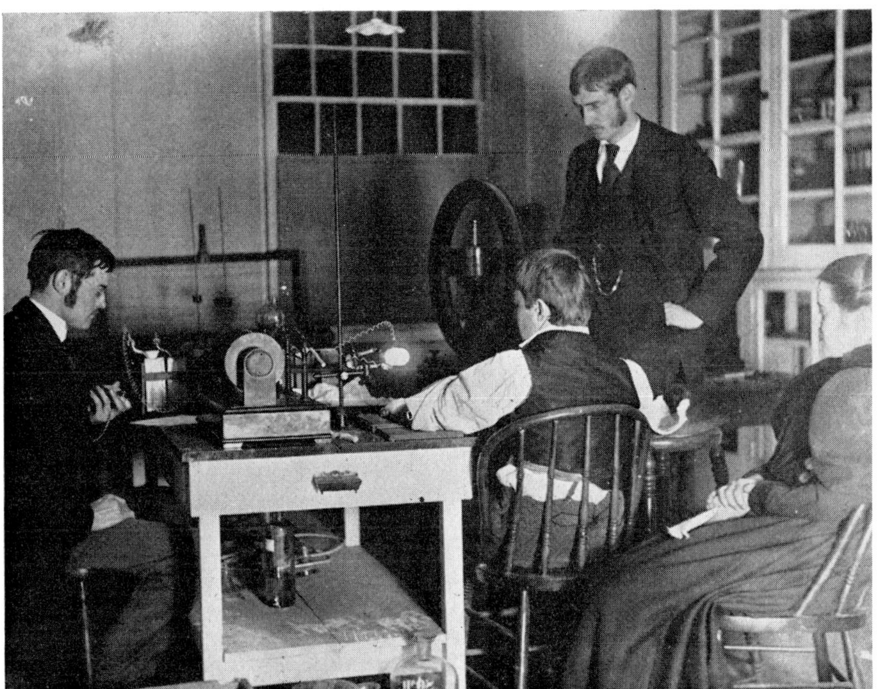

PLATE III. (Courtesy Trustees of Dartmouth College). Photograph made February 3, 1896, at Dartmouth, showing first diagnostic use of X rays in North America. See page 17.

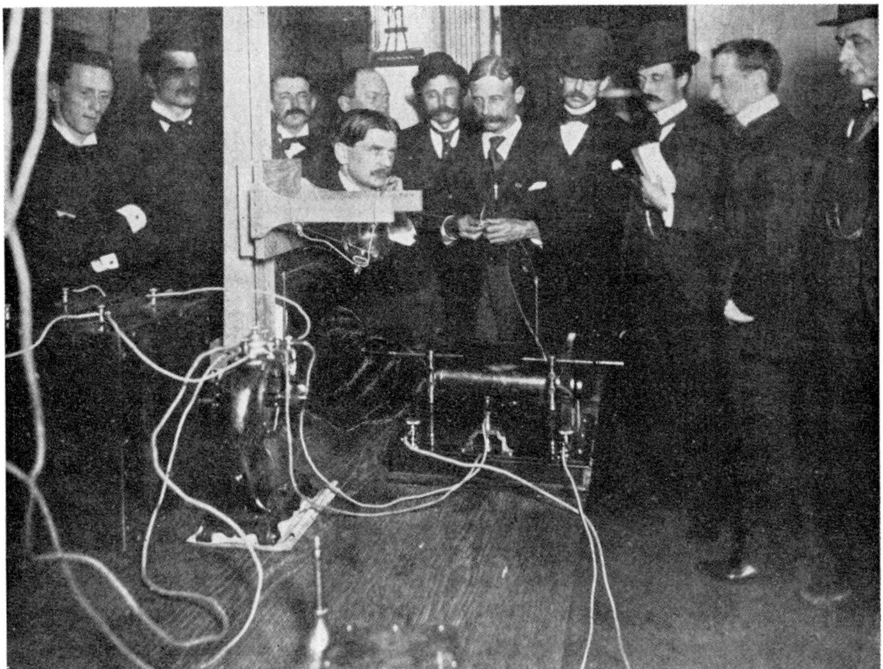

PLATE IV. Photographic experiments in Chicago with Roentgen rays. From *Western Electrician, 18:* February 15, 1896. See page 23.

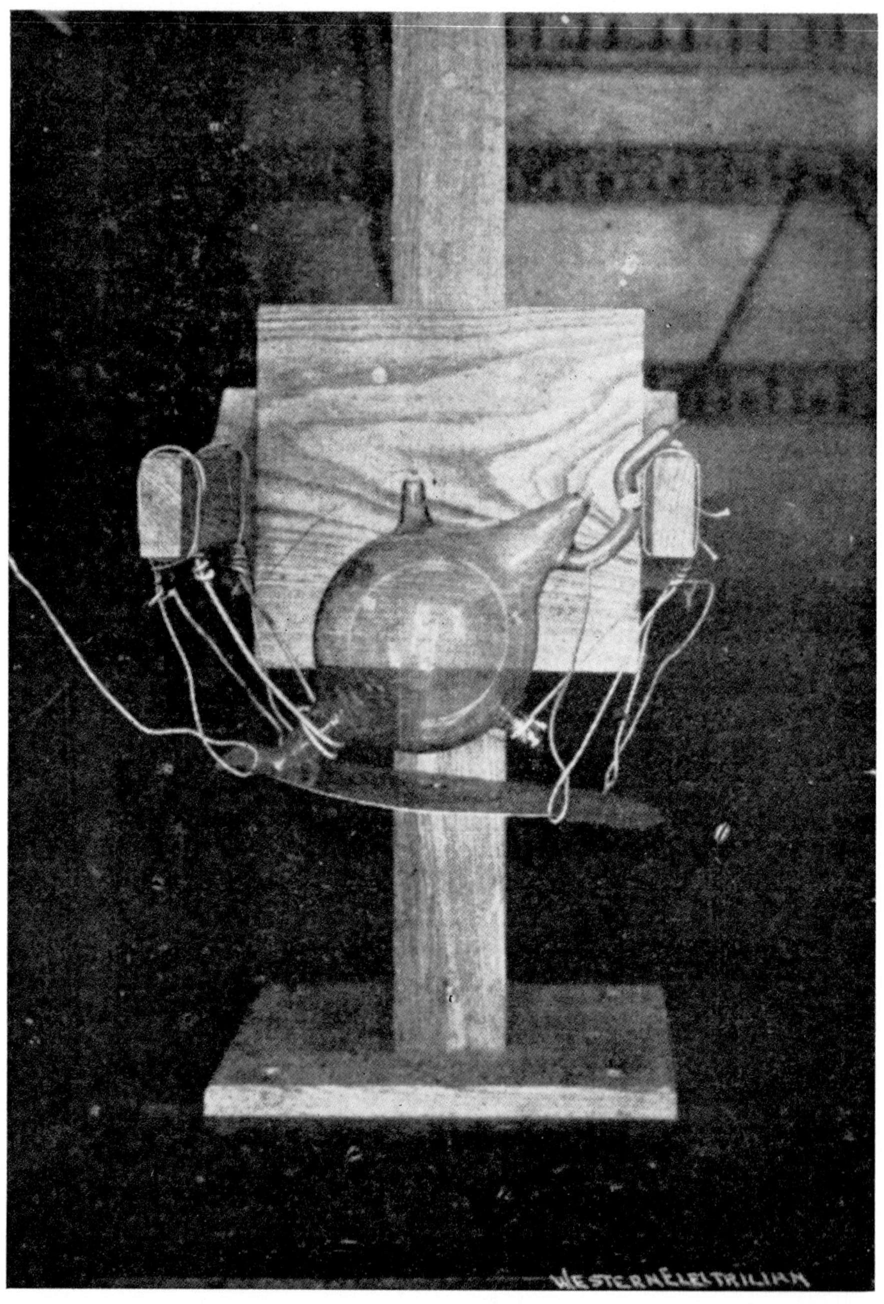

PLATE V. Photographic experiments in Chicago with Roentgen rays—Crookes tube in position over plateholder, lead diaphragm interposed. From *Western Electrician, 18:* February 15, 1896. See page 23.

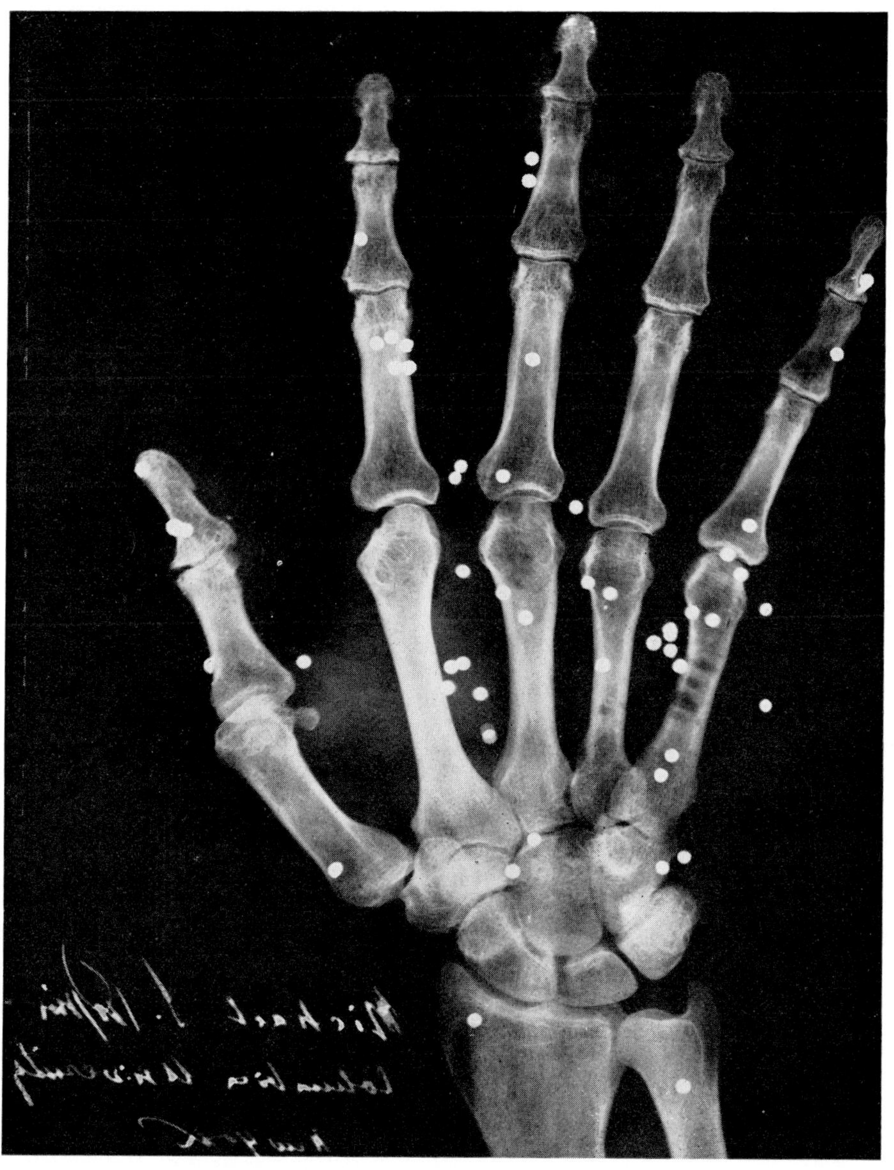

PLATE VI. From American Institute of Radiology. X ray of hand with buckshot made by Professor Michael Pupin in February 1896. See page 56.

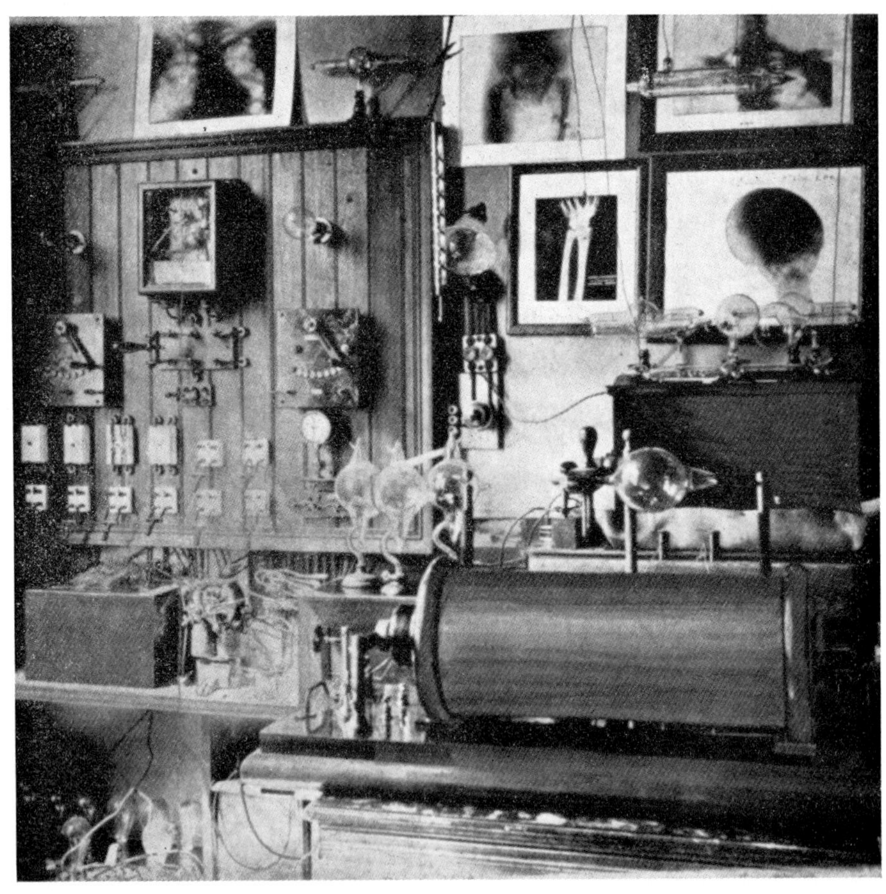

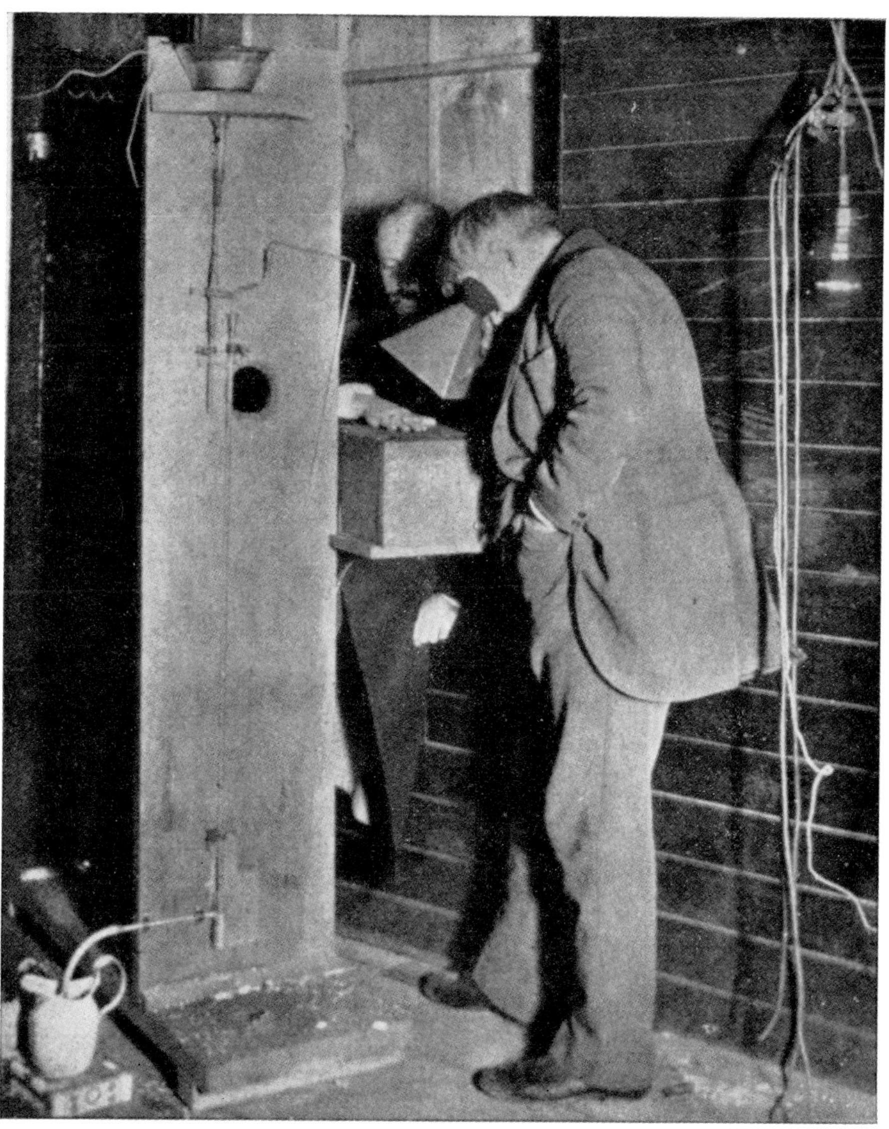

PLATE VIII. From American Institute of Radiology. Thomas A. Edison examining hand through fluoroscope, 1896. The hand may have been that of Clarence Dally, his glassblower. See pages 41, 86, 162.

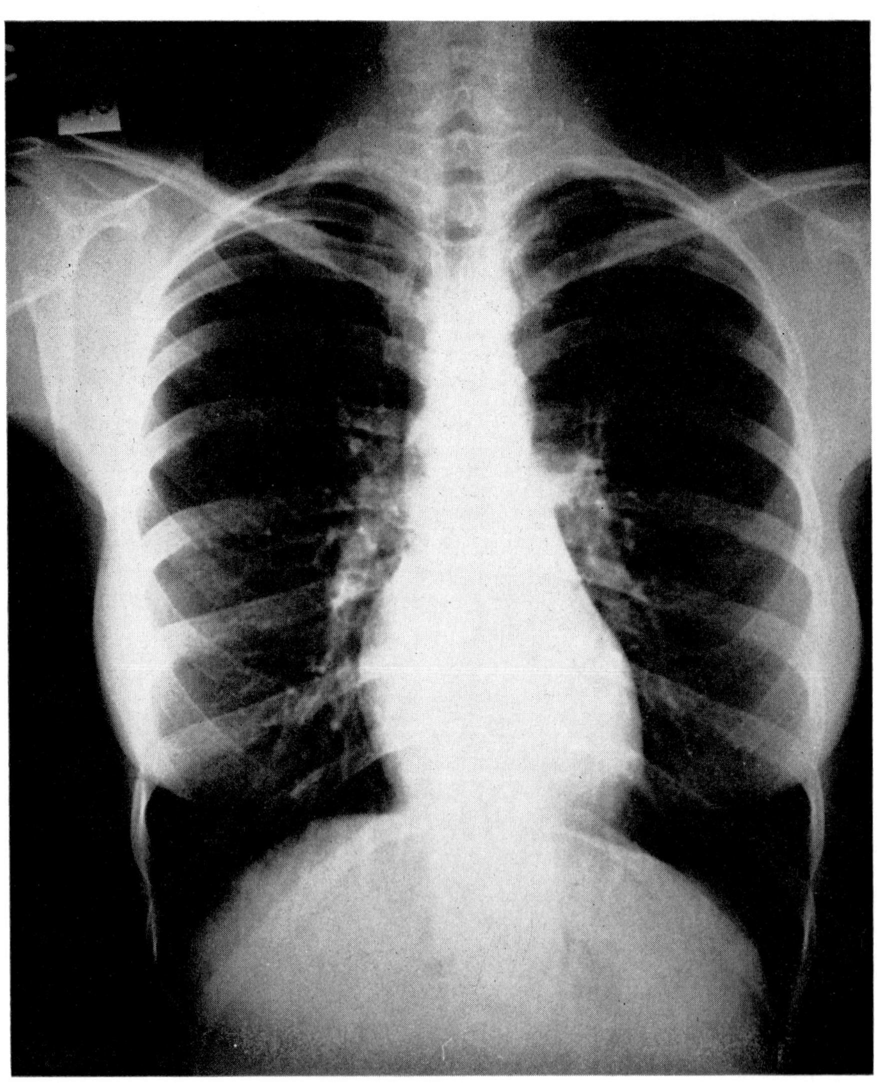

PLATE IX. A modern radiograph of the chest of a normal, healthy young woman.

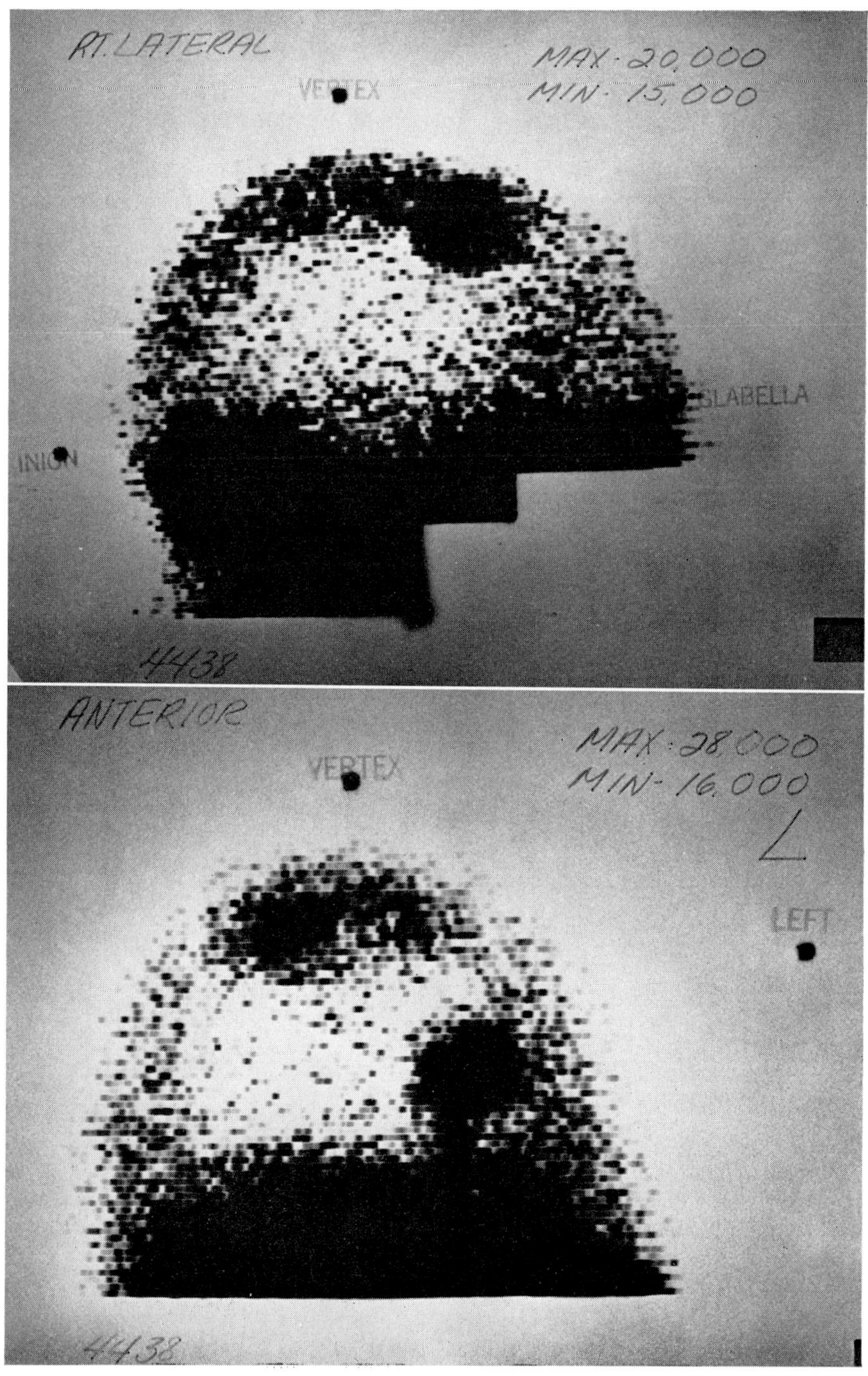

PLATE X. Frontal and lateral isotope scans of the brain. The dark spots provided a tentative diagnosis of tumor. See page 398.

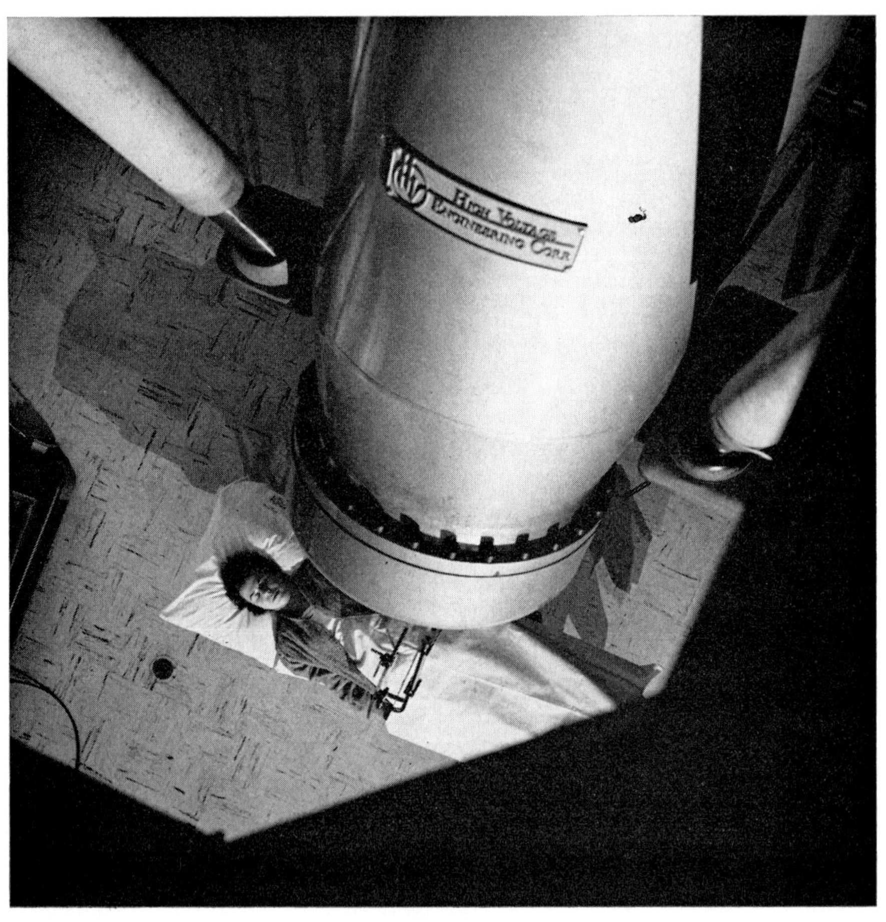

Plate XI. A Van de Graaff-type high-voltage radiation generator used for treating cancer patients (see pages 338–340 and 350–351).

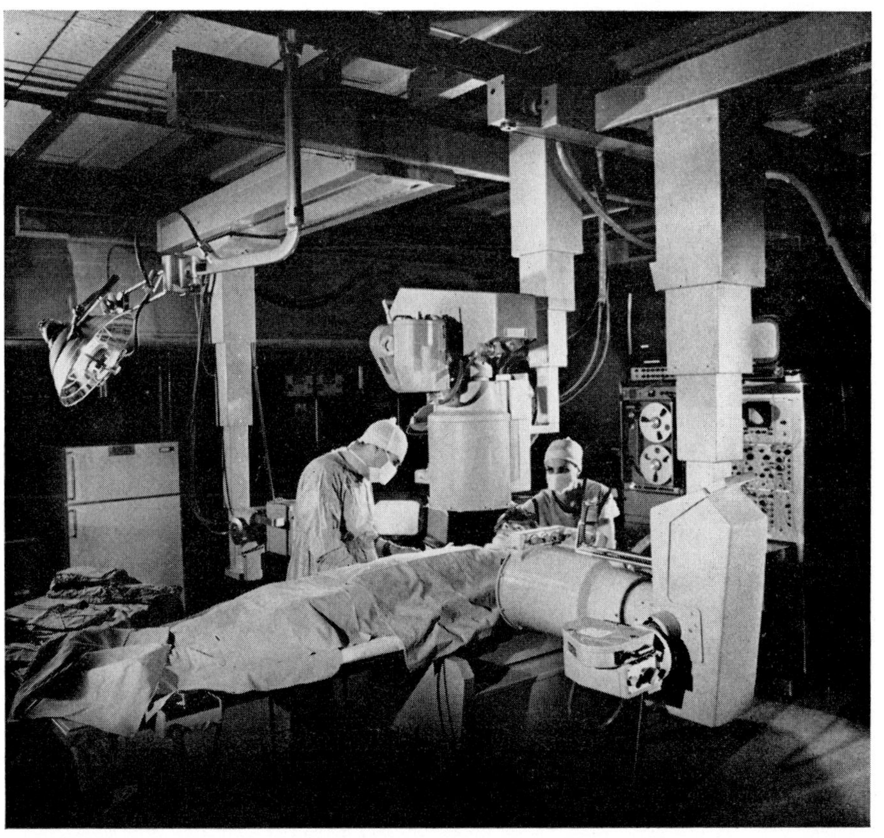

PLATE XII. A modern biplane cineangiographic facility, complete with film and videotape capabilities, such as might be used to diagnose strokes (see pages 443–444).

PLATE XIII

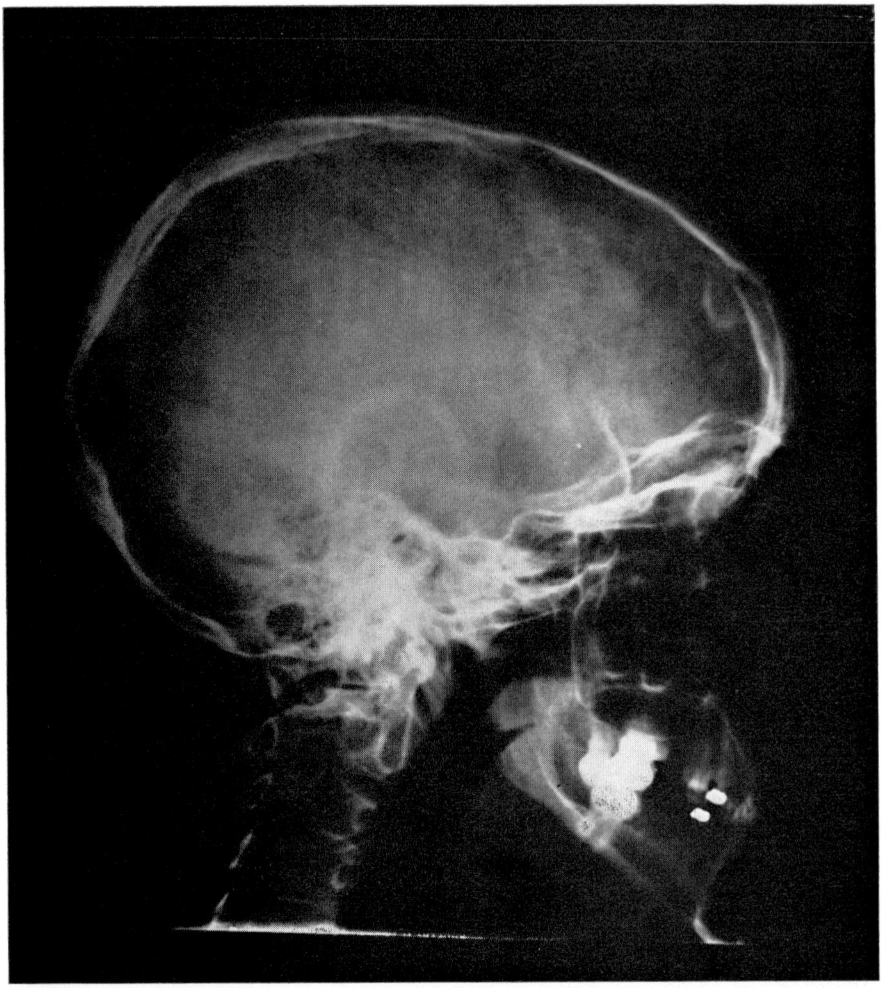

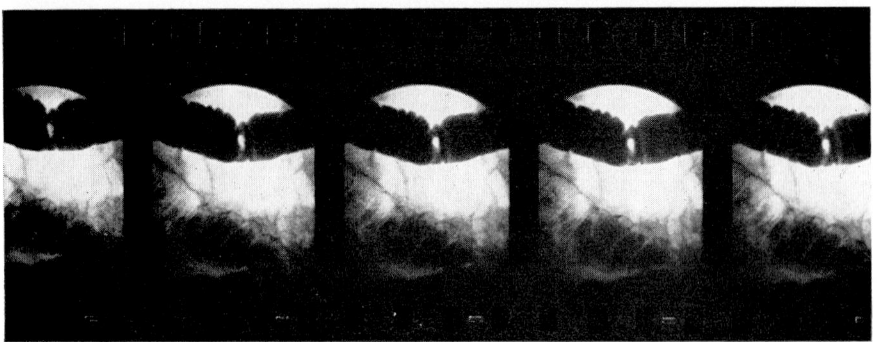

Upper: A lateral view of a normal adult skull.

Lower: A segment of cinefluorography of the small intestine, showing a diseased segment.

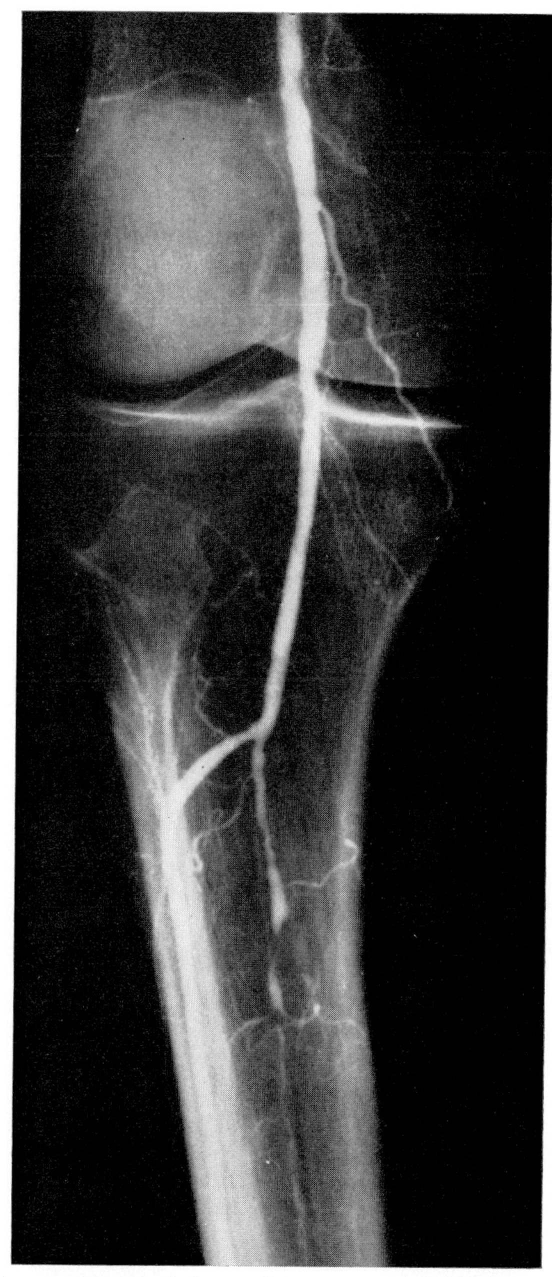

PLATE XIV. An arteriogram of the popliteal artery of the leg, showing partial blockage below the knee caused by arteriosclerosis (see pages 443–444).

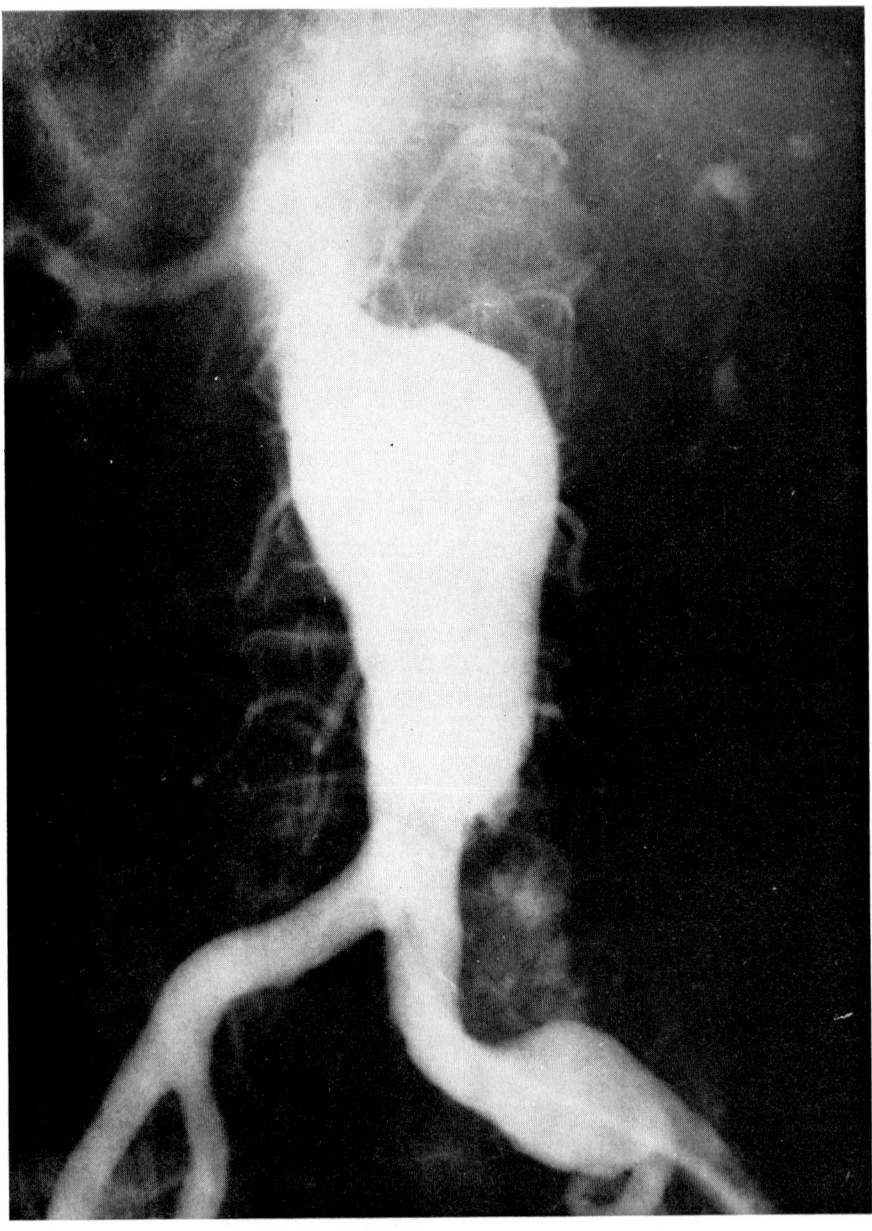

PLATE XV. An abdominal aortogram, or view of the major body artery, showing a large aneurysm (see pages 443–444).

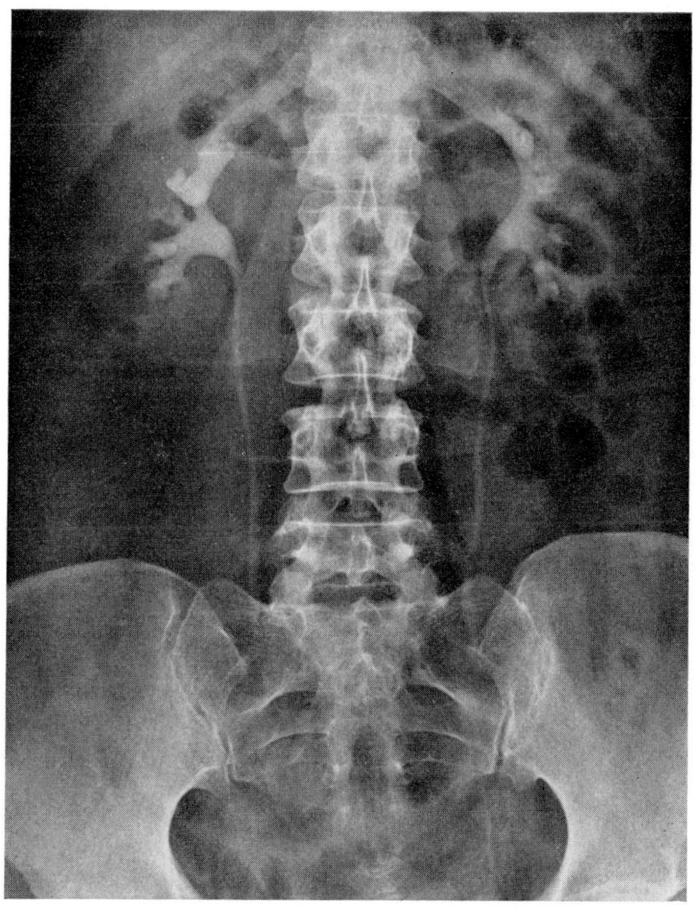

PLATE XVI. A normal pyelogram showing contrast medium in the collecting systems of the kidneys and in the ureters leading from the kidneys to the bladder.

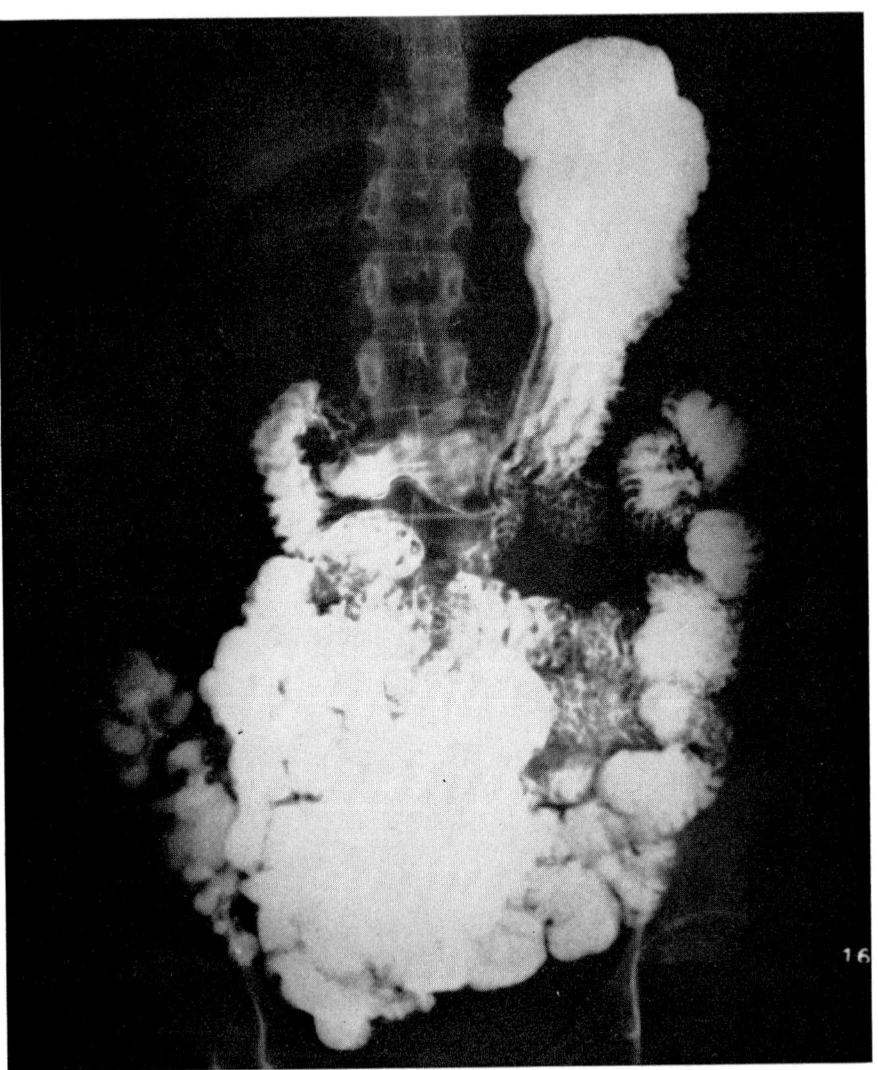

PLATE XVII. A view of the stomach and small intestine after ingestion of a barium mixture (see pages 117–135).

PART I. THE YEAR OF DISCOVERY
(1895–1896)

1 Prelude and Discovery*

On the evening of February 22, 1890, nearly 6 years before the X rays were discovered, two young Philadelphians met in the modest physics laboratory of the University of Pennsylvania.[1] Both were 30 years old, but one had already earned a position of some eminence. He was Arthur Willis Goodspeed (1860–1943), professor of physics at Pennsylvania; his guest was an English-born photographer, William N. Jennings (1860–1945).

Photography was still an experimental art in the early 1890's, and the effects which could be achieved with various types of lighting—such as the light emitted by an electric spark—were of interest to many photographers. Jennings had no doubt read of experiments with spark photography, and wished to try some himself. Professor Goodspeed was willing to cooperate, and Jennings accordingly brought to Goodspeed's laboratory that evening his camera and a stack of photographic plates wrapped in black paper.

The equipment needed for Jennings' spark photographs was quite simple: a spark gap and an induction coil—that is, a "voltage multiplier" capable of transforming a low-voltage into a high-voltage current. Professor Goodspeed connected his induction coil to his spark gap and, with the light from the sparks thus generated, Jennings made a series of plates of coins and other small objects.

The evening was still young when he finished, and so the talk of the two men naturally drifted to other scientific matters. The induction coil that Professor Goodspeed had used to generate the sparks was the one ordinarily used to demonstrate the properties of "Crookes tubes." These devices—named for Sir William Crookes (1832–1919), who had performed many experiments with them during the 1870's[2]—consisted essentially of two or more electrodes sealed into a glass bulb from which most of the air was evacuated. When the negative terminal of a high-voltage supply such as an induction coil was attached to one electrode (the cathode) and the positive terminal to another (the anode), a beam of "cathode rays," identified years later as electrons, streamed out of the

---

* The references are found at the end of each chapter (see page 10). Quotations whose source is stated in the text are not cited. When successive quotations come from the same source, only the first is cited.

cathode and caused the glass of the tube to fluoresce. Even small physics laboratories maintained a supply of such tubes. After completion of the spark-photography experiments on the evening of February 22, Professor Goodspeed proceeded to demonstrate the characteristics of a number of his own Crookes tubes for the "pleasure and amusement" of his guest.[3]

In one type of tube commonly available in 1890, a windmill or "raymill" was lodged between the cathode and anode; when the electric potential was applied, the cathode rays caused the mill to revolve, suggesting that the rays were not waves but rather were composed of particles having a finite mass (Fig. 1).

In another form of the tube, a metal cross was placed in the path of the rays; its shadow could then be seen sharply silhouetted on the fluorescing glass of the tube, indicating that the rays traveled in a straight line (Fig. 2).

When a magnet was held near the tube, this shadow was displaced toward its positive pole, which suggested that the cathode rays were composed of negatively charged particles of some kind (Fig. 3).

In general, the cathode rays seemed to leave the cathode at right

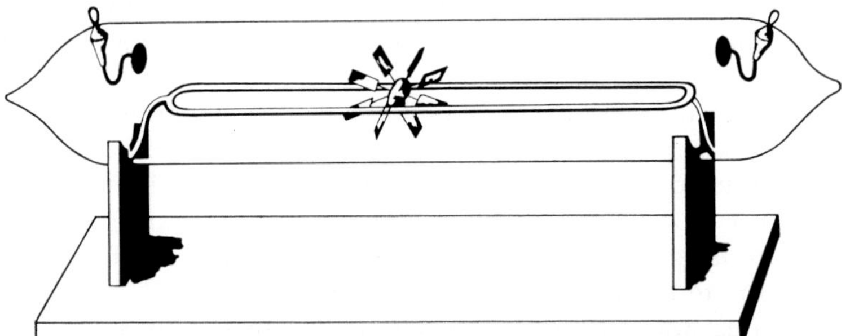

Fig. 1. From *Electrical Engineer (New York)*, *21:* 237, March 4, 1896.

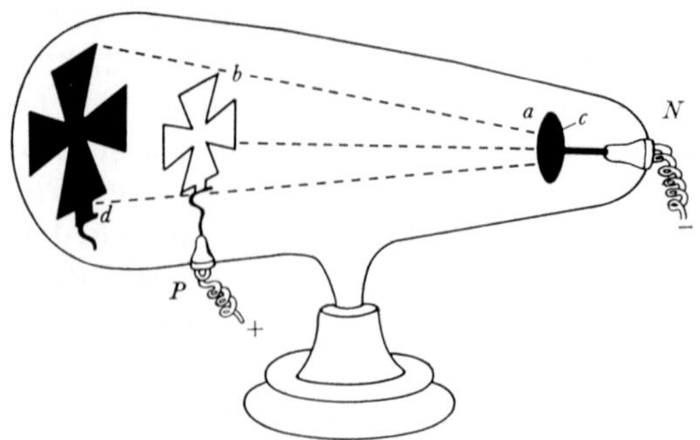

Fig. 2. From *Electrical Engineer (New York)*, *21·* 236, March 4, 1896.

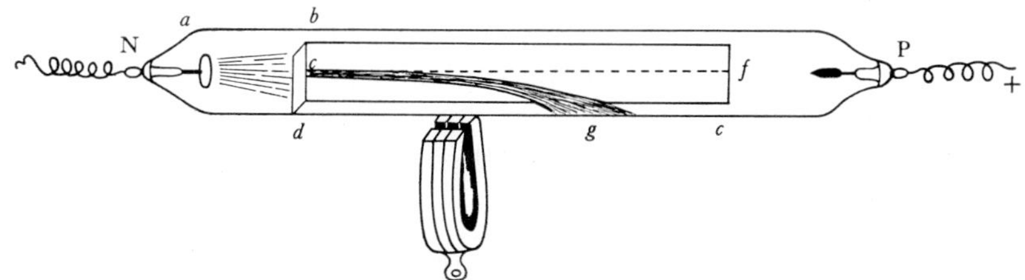

FIG. 3. From *Electrical Engineer (New York)*, 21: 259, March 4, 1896.

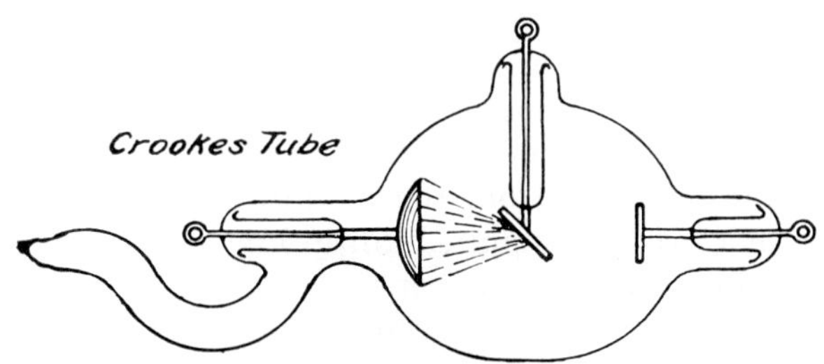

FIG. 4. From Fuchs collection, Eastman Kodak Company.

angles to its surface. Thus, if the cathode was cup-shaped and if the anode was a flat piece of metal placed at a proper distance from it, the cathode rays converged on a single spot on the anode as if they were focused on it (Fig. 4).

While Professor Goodspeed was demonstrating his array of Crookes tubes to Jennings, a stack of unexposed plates left over from the photographic experiments stood near by, and two coins which Jennings had used as photographic objects rested on top of them. At the conclusion of the Crookes-tube demonstration, Jennings departed for home, taking with him both his exposed and his unexposed plates.

A few days later, Jennings reported to Professor Goodspeed a very curious circumstance. Some of the presumably unexposed plates, although still tightly wrapped in their lightproof black paper, had somehow or other become fogged, and on one of them images of two "very mysterious discs" [4] appeared when it was developed.

"No explanation was found at the time to account for the phenomenon," Goodspeed later reported, "and the matter was forgotten" for nearly 6 years.[4] Jennings was sufficiently impressed by the mysterious disk-shaped images on the unexposed plate, however, to file it safely away.

No doubt through the decades prior to November 8, 1895, when the X rays were actually discovered, many similar incidents occurred in laboratories where Crookes tubes were in use. Sir William Crookes himself is said to have complained to the Ilford Company, English makers of photographic materials, that the plates they sent him were often fogged and useless.[5] The Philadelphia X-ray plate of February 22, 1890, was unique, however, in one respect: it was preserved, and is reproduced as Plate I—the oldest North American X-ray plate of which a record survives.

WÜRZBURG, 1895

During the years between 1890 and 1895, European physicists made a number of additional discoveries about the cathode rays generated in Crookes tubes. The German physicist Heinrich Hertz (1857–1894), the discoverer of Hertzian waves (now known as radio waves), reported that the rays would pass through a thin foil of aluminum within the tube. This suggested that cathode rays were waves rather than particles, in contrast to the evidence from the raymill and magnet experiments, and it led one of Hertz's assistants, Philipp Lenard (1862–1947), to carry the research an important step further.[6]

All previous experimenters had been handicapped by the fact that the cathode rays could not travel through glass and could therefore be studied only within the tube in which they were generated. Lenard constructed a tube with a thin aluminum-foil window and discovered that the rays emerged through the window and could be detected several inches away. In some Lenard experiments, the rays were detected by means of their effect on photographic plates held in their path just beyond the aluminum window; in others, the detector was a screen made of paper or cardboard covered with a thin layer of crystals which fluoresced when the cathode rays struck them.

Lenard's 1894 and 1895 reports on these phenomena drew renewed attention to the cathode rays. Among the physicists who resolved to study the matter further was Wilhelm Conrad Roentgen (1845–1923; spelled Röntgen and pronounced "Rentgen" in German), professor of physics and director of the Physical Institute at the University of Würzburg. In 1894 or 1895, Roentgen added to his laboratory's supply of Crookes tubes a Lenard tube with a thin aluminum window and a fluorescing barium platinocyanide screen with which to detect the presence of cathode rays outside the tubes.

Late on a Friday afternoon, November 8, 1895, Roentgen prepared to perform an experiment very much like those that Professor Goodspeed had demonstrated to Jennings in 1890. An ordinary Crookes tube, lacking an aluminum window, was connected to an induction coil. In only three respects was Roentgen's experiment different: the room was completely darkened; the Crookes tube was encased in a lightproof cardboard jacket; and Roentgen's barium platinocyanide screen happened to be lying on a bench a few feet from the tube.

Roentgen's foremost biographer, Dr. Otto Glasser, has explained what was on Roentgen's mind that afternoon.[7] Earlier experiments with Crookes tubes had been performed with the glass uncovered in order to permit inspection of the phenomena inside the tube. Lenard had darkened the room and covered the tube glass with lightproof paper or cardboard so that light coming directly from the tube would not obscure the faint luminescence caused by the rays emerging through the aluminum window. Perhaps, Roentgen suspected, the aluminum window in the Lenard tube was quite unnecessary. Perhaps the cathode rays emerged through the glass itself. Earlier experimenters would have missed this effect because they lacked the means to detect the presence of the rays outside the tube or because the light coming directly from the tube blinded them to the fainter phenomena visible outside the tube. Roentgen's November 8 experiment was admirably designed to test this possibility.

He was quickly distracted from his original intention, however, by a quite unexpected phenomenon which made its appearance when he activated the lightproofed tube in the pitch-black room. Professor Glasser has poignantly described the next moments.

> Suddenly, about a yard from the tube, [Roentgen] saw a weak light that shimmered on a little bench he knew was located nearby. It was as though a ray of light or a faint spark from the induction coil had been reflected by a mirror. Not believing this possible, he passed another series of discharges through the tube, and again the same fluorescence appeared, this time looking like faint green clouds.... Highly excited, Roentgen lit a match and to his great surprise discovered that the source of the mysterious light was the little barium platinocyanide screen lying on the bench. He repeated the experiment again and again, each time moving the little screen farther away from the tube and each time getting the same result.[9]

The screen had lit up even though there was no aluminum window through which the cathode rays could escape from the tube!

The cause of the fluorescence could not be cathode rays, for the screen lit up at a distance of 6 or 7 feet from the tube, and Lenard had shown that cathode rays would not penetrate that far, even through an aluminum window. Only one inference was possible, and Roentgen boldly drew it. Some new kind of radiation—neither visible light nor cathode rays—must be emanating from the tube and causing the barium platinocyanide screen to fluoresce.

"I have discovered something interesting," Roentgen remarked casually to a friend, Theodore Boveri, shortly afterward, "but I do not know whether or not my observations are correct." [9]

During the weeks of intensive day-and-night experimentation which followed, Roentgen's doubt was erased, and he went on to explore in greater and greater detail the behavior of this "new kind of light," which he tentatively dubbed "X rays" ("X Strahlen") to indicate that they were rays of an unknown kind. He noted, for example, that, unlike cathode rays, the X rays were not emitted by the cathode, but seemed to come from the glass bulb which was being bombarded by the cathode rays; unlike the cathode rays, they did not emerge at right angles from the surface but, like visible light, they streamed out in all directions; also, the X rays, unlike the cathode rays, could not be deflected by a magnet, and they traveled much further through air than cathode rays.

Roentgen's very first observation had established the fact that his X rays would pass through lightproof black cardboard. A series of further experiments elaborated this observation. Substances varied greatly, he learned, in their transparency or opacity to the new rays. Clear glass, for example, is almost perfectly transparent to ordinary light, yet it seemed more opaque to X rays than an equal thickness of aluminum. Lead cast a denser shadow than copper. Of the utmost interest to Roentgen, and to the whole civilized world ever since, was the fact that human bones cast a denser shadow than soft tissues. Hence, when a hand was placed between the Crookes tube and the fluorescent screen in one of his experiments, he was amazed to see the bones inside the skin and flesh clearly outlined on the screen.

Could Roentgen believe his own eyes? He did not have to. To check his vision, he placed a photographic plate in the path of the rays, and was delighted to learn that it captured a permanent record of the event for all to see.

One such shadowgram—or "skiagram," as it soon came to be called —is reproduced as Plate II. It was made by Roentgen himself on December 22, 1895, presumably of his wife's hand, and it shows much more than the mere outline of the bones. Because the density of the shadow cast varies not only with the substance of the objects in the path of the rays but also with their thickness, the photographic plate records the varying thickness of the bones, and gives an indication of the modeling of the bony contours. The potential significance of the X rays for medical and surgical diagnosis all but leapt from the surface of the plate.

Roentgen delivered the manuscript of his preliminary report on these and other findings, entitled "On a New Kind of Rays," to the secretary of the Physical-Medical Society of Würzburg on December 28, 1895, for publication in the *Proceedings* of that society. He received back reprints, Dr. Glasser reports, within a few days and mailed copies, along with some sample X-ray prints, to a number of eminent physicists on New Year's Day, 1896.[9]

THE NEWS SPREADS

The news of Roentgen's discovery reached the United States by a roundabout route. One of the reprints which Roentgen had mailed to a physicist in Vienna was passed on to the editor of the Vienna *Presse*, who broke the story with much fanfare on the front page of the *Presse* for Sunday, January 5, 1896. The Viennese correspondent of the London *Daily Chronicle* telegraphed a summary to London; this was promptly relayed to New York. The New York *Sun* announced on January 6, 1896:

> The noise of war's alarms should not distract attention from the marvellous triumph of science which is reported from Vienna. It is announced that Professor Routgen [*sic*], of the Würzburg University, has discovered a light which, for the purposes of photography, will penetrate wood, flesh, and most other organic substances. The professor has succeeded in photographing metal weights which were in a closed wooden case; also a man's hand, which shows only the bones, the flesh being invisible.
>
> The *Chronicle* correspondent says the discovery is simple. The professor takes a so-called Crookes pipe, *viz.*, a vacuum glass pipe with an induction current going through it, and, by means of rays which the pipe emits, photographs on ordinary photographic plates.
>
> In contrast with the ordinary rays of light, these rays penetrate organic matter and other opaque substances just as ordinary rays penetrate glass.
>
> He has also succeeded in photographing hidden metals with a cloth thrown over the camera. The rays penetrated not only the wooden case containing the metals, but the fabric in front of the negative.
>
> The professor is already using his discovery to photograph broken limbs and bullets in human bodies.

Other American newspapers picked up the story. The *Sun's* January 6 cable was reprinted, for example, in the St. Louis *Post-Dispatch* for January 7, including the misspelling of Professor Roentgen's name. The newspaper accounts also erred in stating that Roentgen was already putting his discovery to medical use. The *New York Times* had a paragraph on January 12:

> Scientists are greatly interested in the report of the experiments at Würzburg, repeated at Buda-Pesth, by which a positive picture is

obtained by the agency of the Crookes tube through barriers of wood, cloth, and flesh. . . .

On January 16, the *Times* was still misspelling Roentgen's name:

> Men of science in this city are awaiting with the utmost impatience the arrival of European technical journals which will give them the full particulars of Professor Routgen's great discovery. . . .

But until the end of January, these and other similar stories were for the most part restrained and tucked away on inside pages. Not until American experimenters repeated and confirmed Roentgen's findings, and American reporters were thus able to see for themselves the amazing phenomena, did the X rays become front-page news.

During the subsequent decades, Roentgen's discovery was to help revolutionize the science of physics, open new paths in medicine and surgery, and arouse an unprecedented enthusiasm among scientists and laymen alike. The effects on medicine and surgery within the United States and Canada are the central theme of this volume.

REFERENCES

1. *Proc. Amer. Phil. Soc., 35:* 17–24, 1896.
2. Crookes, W., Lecture delivered before the British Association for the Advancement of Science Aug. 22, 1879; reprinted in *Electrical Engineer (New York), 21:* 189–190; 211–212; 236–237; 258–259; 283–284.
3. *Proc. Amer. Phil. Soc., 35:* 23, 1896.
4. *Science (n.s.), 3:* 394–396, 1896.
5. Glasser, O.: *William Conrad Roentgen and the Early History of the Roentgen Rays,* pp. 223–224. Charles C Thomas, Publisher, Baltimore, 1934.
6. *Wiedemann's Annalen der Physik, 56:* 255, 1895.
7. Glasser, *op. cit.,* pp. 1–51.
8. Glasser, O., *Dr. W. C. Roentgen,* Ed. 2, p. 36. Charles C Thomas, Publisher, Springfield, Ill., 1958.
9. *Ibid.,* p. 39.

2 The North American Pioneers

THE RAYS IN NEW HAVEN AND CAMBRIDGE—JANUARY 1896

European physicists had available Roentgen's original paper, or reprints of it, during the first weeks of January 1896, and were thus able to repeat and confirm Roentgen's findings promptly. Americans, however, had to wait for more detailed news to cross the Atlantic; the early cables supplied little or no information on how the rays were generated. Not until the last week of January did any American announce that he had successfully captured images of hidden objects by means of Roentgen's rays. Then, in rapid succession, parallel announcements came from Yale and Harvard.

Arthur Williams Wright

The Yale investigator was Arthur Williams Wright (1836–1915), professor of experimental physics and director of Yale's Sloane Physical Laboratory. Wright was known on the campus as "Buffalo" Wright because of a bushy black beard which distinguished him from his Yale colleague "Baldy" Wright. In 1861 he had received his Ph.D. in physics from Yale—the first American to be awarded a Ph.D. in a scientific subject by any American university.[1] In 1877, when the interest in Crookes tubes was at its height, he had published a paper on the deposition of thin metallic films on the walls of Crookes tubes whose cathodes were made of gold or other readily volatilized metals.[2] Subsequently, his attention had turned to other branches of physics, but he continued to maintain a supply of Crookes tubes in his laboratory. He was thus one of the many "men of science" awaiting "with the utmost impatience" further news of Roentgen's discovery after the first cable came.

On the afternoon of January 27, 1896, Professor Wright connected a Crookes tube to an induction coil in the usual way, and powered the coil by a battery of five cells. Under the tube he placed a photographic plateholder, as shown in a sketch which Wright himself drew up at the time or shortly thereafter (Fig. 5).

In the plateholder, which lay about 5 inches below the tube, he placed a sheet of light-sensitive bromide photographic paper, wrapped in thick black paper to keep out ordinary light. Between the tube

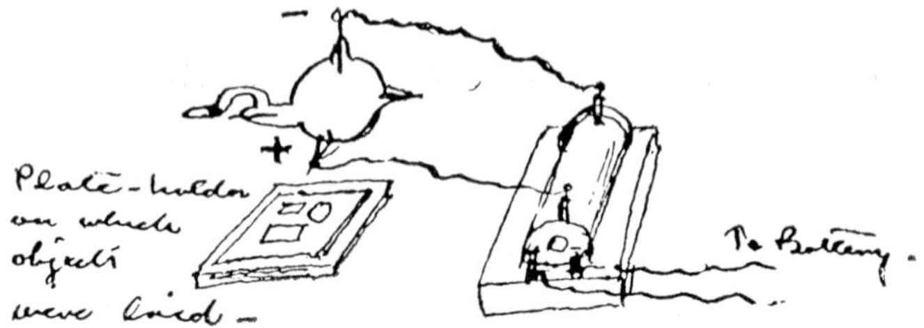

Fig. 5. From *Electrical Engineer, 21:* 134, 1896.

and the plate he placed several small objects: a lead pencil, a pair of scissors, and a 25-cent piece. Then he turned on the current and kept it on for 15 minutes.

When the photographic paper was developed, it revealed "very clear representations of the objects employed." [3] Wright returned to his laboratory that evening and performed additional experiments, using glass photographic plates instead of bromide paper. He interposed a hand as well as other objects between the tube and the plates, and, to make the test harder, he also placed in the path of the rays a whitewood board $5/16$ inch thick so that the rays would have to pass through the board as well as the hand or small objects. To compensate for this, he lengthened the time of exposure to 1 hour. Again "a strong picture" resulted.

In later years, a number of Americans were to claim that they had successfully exposed X-ray plates prior to January 27, 1896, but these claims lack contemporary verification. Wright's success was reported in the *Engineering and Mining Journal* for February 1, 1896, just 4 days after the event; in the New York *Journal* for February 2; and in the *Electrical Engineer* for February 5. He himself published a full account of his experiments, dated February 22, in the *American Journal of Science* for March 1896. He preserved, moreover, his contemporary notes on his January 27 and 28 X-ray trials; these remained with his family and came to light again among the Wright family papers in December 1966 (Fig. 6).[4] Although Wright himself never claimed to be the first in North America, Yale University made that claim posthumously in his behalf in October 1966, and named in his honor its newly erected Arthur Williams Wright Nuclear Structure Laboratory.

"For the production of the cathode rays," Wright wrote on February 22, "a Crookes tube, nearly spherical in shape, was used." [3] This tube had four electrodes. One of them, as was not uncommon in Crookes tubes, was "a slightly concave disk or cup about two centimeters in diameter." This was fortunate, for, as Wright pointed out, such a disk, when used as a cathode, "concentrates the cathode rays, issuing normally

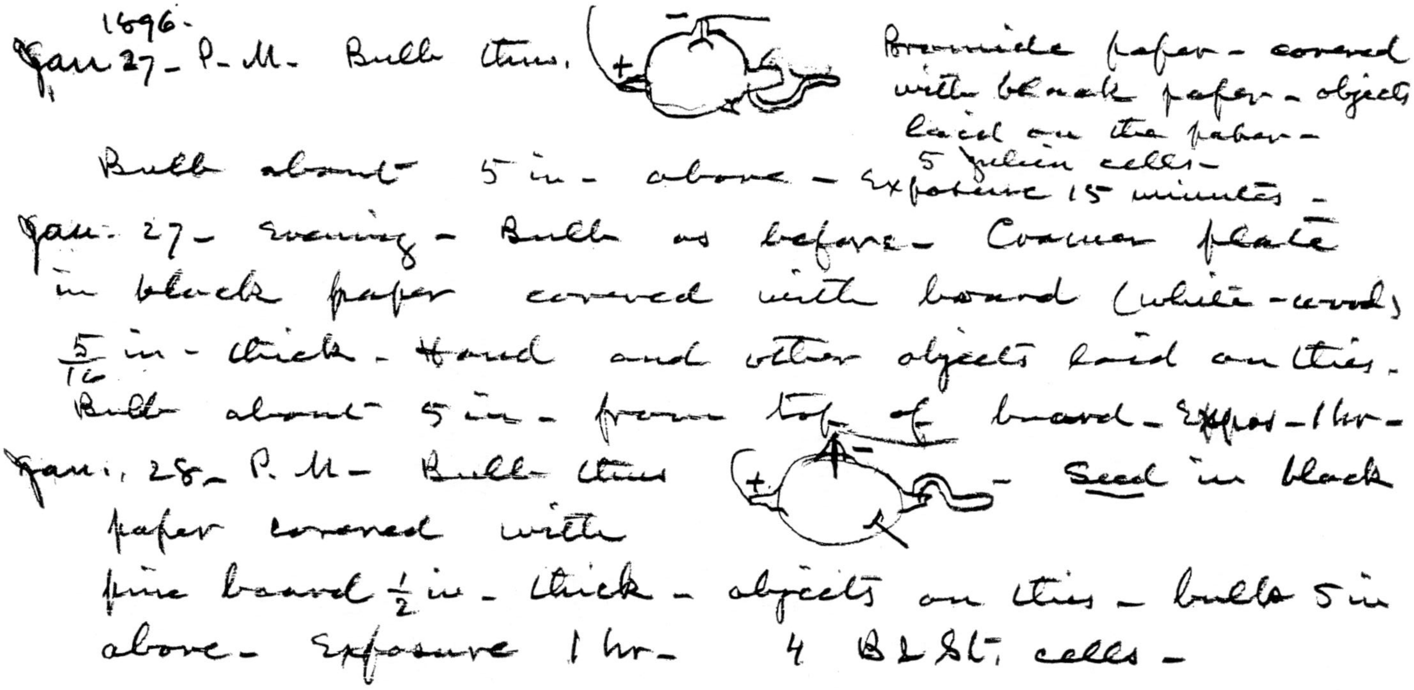
1896.
Jan 27 - P.M. - Bulb thus. Bromide paper - covered with black paper - objects laid on the paper - 5 Julien cells -
Bulb about 5 in. - above - Exposure 15 minutes -
Jan. 27 - evening - Bulb as before - Common plate in black paper covered with board (white-wood) 5/16 in. - thick - Hand and other objects laid on this. Bulb about 5 in. - from top of board - Expos - 1 hr -
Jan. 28 - P.M. - Bulb thus - Seed in black paper covered with fine board 1/2 in - thick - objects on this - bulb 5 in above - Exposure 1 hr - 4 BLSt. cells -

FIG. 6. A. W. Wright's notes on what was undoubtedly the first successful North American X-ray experiment. From Wright family papers, New Haven, Connecticut.

[at right angles] from its surface, at a point near the opposite surface of the tube, sending them through a small area of the glass wall, which becomes strongly heated. The photographic plates show this concentration of the rays plainly." The tube was activated by an induction coil that gave a spark of about $2\frac{1}{2}$ inches, indicating a current of about 35,000 volts.

Much the same conditions were required for a sharp Roentgen photograph, Wright concluded, as for a sharp picture taken with light, "especially the greater distance of the radiating source, and nearness of the object to the surface upon which it is to be projected . . . Increasing the distance of the vacuum tube improved the pictures in the matter of sharpness, fullness of detail, and accuracy of form and dimensions, but the time of exposure was correspondingly increased."

"Other experiments were made," Wright continued, "upon the bodies of animals and the human hand. A rabbit, purchased in one of the markets of the city, after an exposure of one hour to the rays, left upon the plate a complete representation of the bony skeleton, the bones of the legs being very sharply and perfectly represented. The region of the lungs was more transparent than the rest of the body, and the heart still more so, being somewhat definitely outlined. The cartilages at the base of the ears left a distinct trace, the ears themselves scarcely any. Particularly interesting in this photograph were several small round spots which appeared dark in the positive print. These were at once surmised to be shot, and from the indication of their location in the print were readily found and extracted. The mode of death of the animal was not previously known."

Some commentators, reading the early European dispatches, had supposed that X rays could give mere "shadow pictures," and were capable only of silhouetting bones in their path. Wright strongly dissented.

"The photograph of the hand," he pointed out, "shows the bones and their articulations very clearly and well defined. On the side of each finger the plexus of nerves and blood-vessels is distinctly shown as it divides into several branches for distribution to the ball of the finger. When the negative is held to the light the hand appears as if modelled in a translucent, luminous material, with the full appearance of roundness and solidity. It is as if it had become nearly transparent, so that the structure of the interior could be seen, not only in respect to the particulars already mentioned, but also with respect to the distribution, or relative abundance, of the blood in its different parts. . . . The pictures are not merely flat shadows, but the partial opacity, varying with the thickness, gives a corresponding depth of shade in the picture, thus producing an effect of perspective, which in the negative, or a negative transparency projected upon a screen, has a striking effect of relief, and a luminous solidity often of great beauty." Few radiologists since have written a more perceptive description of what can be seen on an X-ray negative. In the process of examining such a negative, as a New York experimenter, Dr. William J. Morton, remarked a little later, "the mind walks in among the tissues themselves." [5]

John Trowbridge

At about the same time that Wright began his X-ray experiments, but almost certainly a few days later, John Trowbridge (1843–1923), Rumford Professor of Science at Harvard and director of Harvard's Jefferson Physical Laboratory, undertook similar work. Professor Trowbridge had previously published in a number of fields of physics, and had also written two popular scientific novels for boys: *The Electrical Boy, or the Career of Greatman and Greatthings* (1891), and *Three Boys in an Electrical Boat* (1894).[6] No doubt the amazing news from Würzburg appealed to Professor Trowbridge's science-fiction as well as purely scientific interests.

The Boston correspondent of the *Western Electrician* stated that the "first thoroughly successful experiment" at Harvard was made "about the last of January." [7] Professor Trowbridge himself never announced the precise date, but he published a signed report on his initial experiments, dated January 31, 1896, in the New York *Journal* for February 2. It was accompanied by a woodcut made from an X-ray plate of a human hand, signed by Trowbridge and marked in his handwriting, "Taken in Jefferson Physical Laboratory Cambridge, Jan. 31, 1896." Because his February 2 report in the New York *Journal* has never been reprinted, it is quoted here and later at some length.

> Interested to discover how true the reports of Roentgen's success were, I arranged a "Crookes tube" in such a manner that the rays from the cathode, after passing outside the Crookes tube, should fall upon a sensitive [photographic] plate tightly enclosed in a wooden box. The thickness of the wood was not far from one inch, that is, the rays had to pass through an inch of ordinary board before they reached the sensitive film. There is no difficulty, I find, in obtaining photographs of a peculiar pattern in this manner through solid wood. The pattern was made out of strips of glass a few inches apart. There were therefore spaces free from glass, so that the rays of a portion of the pattern would have to pass through the glass, and other rays through the portions not covered by the glass. All the rays had to pass through a thickness of wood. On developing the plate it was found that a thickness of glass of about an eighth of an inch cut off the cathode rays, or, we might say, stopped them. But these rays had easily passed through the wood not protected by the

> glass, and through the solid wood had made their appearance on the sensitive plate. In other words, a thickness of glass of an eighth of an inch was sufficient to stop the cathode rays, although it was perfectly transparent to ordinary light rays, and the cathode rays passed through the wood, which is opaque to ordinary light. You will readily see the strange difference between the cathode rays and those of ordinary light, which pass with utmost ease through ordinary glass but are stopped by most other substances.

Trowbridge's amazement can be sensed across the years.

Professor Trowbridge then described an effort to refract the strange rays (see below, page 29), which he mistakenly thought were cathode rays, and continued:

> The next experiment that I tried was an endeavor to obtain a photograph of the bones of the human hand. I placed a sensitive plate in a wooden box, and, having brought the box near a Crookes tube, opposite the cathode, I placed my hand between the cathode and the wooden box, so that the rays should pass through my hand before they reached the sensitive films in the wooden box. I exposed the plate to the rays for a minute and a half, and on development perceived an image of the hand with the principal lines of the bones, the knuckles and the phalanges. A clear and distinct representation of the bones was obtained down to the middle of the palm. Careful inspection of the negative showed considerable detail, although the entire picture was somewhat of the nature of a shadow picture. A longer exposure would doubtless have given more detail; but I was afraid the Crookes tube would not stand the powerful current which I was obliged to use. These have been my principal experiments.

After a further description of his equipment (see below, page 52), Trowbridge discussed "the important bearing of this subject on surgery" and added, "I propose before long to pass the rays through the entire body. To do this . . . will require much longer exposure and more powerful currents."

Like Professor Wright, Professor Trowbridge scrupulously refrained from making any priority claim at the time or thereafter.

THE "X-RAY RUSH"—FEBRUARY 1896

The Wright and Trowbridge reports were followed in the next few weeks by literally scores of announcements of other successful X-ray experiments.

Edwin Brant Frost

Professor Edwin Brant Frost (1866–1935) is of particular importance as the first American to apply the new rays in clinical medicine. Frost, at the age of 30, was professor of astronomy at Dartmouth in 1896, but during the years from 1887 to 1889 he had served as assistant to C. F. Emerson, Dartmouth's professor of physics, and had become familiar with physical apparatus. "When the cable hints were received about Roentgen's success," Frost later wrote, "it immediately seemed worthwhile to test the numerous vacuum tubes in our laboratory for their capacity to produce the mysterious rays." [8] The first tests were made on a "Saturday evening, either January 24, or February 1, 1896, probably the latter," by Professors Frost and Emerson; Frost wrote on February 4 a report of the two men's work which appeared in *Science* for February 14, 1896. "Experiments with Roentgen's newly detected X rays have been carried on during the past few days," this report noted, thus fixing the date as almost certainly February 1.

Four Crookes tubes were tried, but only one "emitted rays which (with the exposure given) made a visual impression upon a photographic plate protected from the ordinary luminous rays." The tubes were usually excited by an induction coil, as in other early experiments, but Frost noted that a static machine (see below, page 52) "has served about equally well."

The first successful Frost-Emerson experiment produced an image of a knife and pair of scissors hung on the side of a whitewood box 1 centimeter thick, after an exposure of 12 minutes. Subsequently "a coin concealed between two boards of total thickness, 24 mm., were shown after an exposure of 11 minutes, the tube being 15 cm. above the plate. The power of transmitting the X rays has been tested for a number of substances. Silver and gold seem to be the most opaque of the metals yet tried.... Glass is more opaque.... Cork transmits better than any other substance examined.... With the tube 9 cm. above the plate an exposure of 15 minutes clearly brought out the bones of a hand laid upon the plate holder, and subsequent plates have revealed the bones of the hand and arm with startling distinctness." One of these plates was reproduced with Professor Frost's communication in the February 14 issue of *Science*.

After these preliminaries, Professor Frost put his Crookes tubes to practical use. A Hanover boy, Eddie McCarthy, had broken his forearm a couple of weeks earlier and was under treatment by Professor Frost's brother, Dr. G. D. Frost. On February 3, 1896, Dr. Frost brought Eddie to the Dartmouth physical laboratory for diagnostic examination; also present were Dr. Frost's wife and a Hanover photographer, H. H. Langill, "who was always glad to assist in scientific experiments." [8] Eddie's hand was placed on a photographic plate enclosed in a light-proof plateholder, and the Crookes tube was suspended above it; the photographer recorded the event for posterity (Plate III). "No one could ever forget the interest felt in watching the development of those first plates," Professor Frost later recalled.[8] The image secured was "satisfactory" after a 20-minute exposure, and showed "the fracture in the ulna very distinctly." This was, so far as the surviving record reveals, the first diagnostic X-ray made in North America. "Comment on the numerous applications of the new method in the sciences and arts would be superfluous," Professor Frost concluded his February 4 report.

John Cox

John Cox (1851–1923), professor of physics at the Macdonald Physical Laboratory of McGill University in Montreal, made his first X-ray plate on February 3, 1896, and was no doubt the first in North America to use the X rays successfully as an adjunct to surgery, on the morning of February 7, 1896. A reporter was present for the occasion, and the New York *Journal* recounted the event at length the next day:

"On Christmas Day last," the *Journal* noted, "Tolson Cunning, a young man, was shot in the leg during a scrimmage." Cunning was taken to the Montreal General Hospital, and an attempt was made, without success, to locate the bullet by probing. The wound healed, but early in February it again began to bother young Cunning. Accordingly, his surgeon, Dr. Robert C. Kirkpatrick of McGill, brought him to Professor Cox for X-ray diagnosis. The *Journal* continued:

> The experiment was made this morning in one of the laboratories of McGill's physics building. A table was procured, a chair placed upon it, the left leg of the young man was stripped, and when he had taken his seat, a camera holder containing a sensitized Stanley plate was placed against a heavy block of wood at one side of the leg, the latter being held in a steady position by means of bandages and towels.
>
> When all was in readiness the electric current was turned on. The light immediately began to flare and flicker, but after a short interval became quite steady. At the end of forty-five minutes the current was cut off, the bandages loosened, and the plates taken to the dark room for developing.
>
> After the lapse of fifteen minutes Professor Cox reappeared. One could detect at once, from the beaming countenance, the success of the experiment.

Professor Cox was naturally gratified. "The bones in the calf of the leg," he was quoted as saying, "are plainly discernible in the plate, and in addition there is a solid substance there which I am convinced is the bullet."

The news soon spread through the city, and Professor Cox was asked to describe his work at the monthly meeting of the Montreal Medico-Chirurgical Society that same night.[9] "The meeting was fully attended," the Montreal *Daily Witness* reported on February 8, "the rooms not being able to accommodate the crowd." Cox first explained Roentgen's discovery, and then went on to describe his own work during the past few days.

With the splendid Macdonald collection of apparatus at hand, he declared, he "found no difficulty" in reproducing Roentgen's results on February 3. "Wasting no time over photographs of coins or other small objects, we have obtained the pictures of hands"—pictures which he then proceeded to pass around. An induction coil capable of generating a 10-inch spark (about 110,000 volts) was used as power supply.

On February 5, 2 days after his initial success, a Montreal physician had sent Professor Cox a patient with a hip injury, "but I am sorry to say," Cox declared, "that after one hour's exposure we obtained not a trace upon the plate (22 in. × 18 in.)."

Tolson Cunning, the young man with the bullet in his leg, was present in person at the meeting, and Professor Cox next proceeded to discuss his case. "As this was probably one of the earliest cases of the successful application of Roentgen's rays, especially in penetrating such a thickness of flesh," he said, "the negative, which clearly shows the flattened bullet lying between the tibia and fibula, will be seen with interest. The plate was a Stanley . . . and the exposure 45 minutes. It was clearly underexposed, and should have had at least an hour and a half. Near the top of the plate may be observed a copper wire tied around the leg, three centimeters above the entrance to the wound, from which to measure distances . . . The bullet was six centimeters below the wire, where indeed it had been suspected to lie. It may be said that in this case the new process converted a surmise into a certainty."

The bullet was removed. Dr. Robert C. Kirkpatrick of McGill, surgeon in the case, later reported, "The patient recovered rapidly and left the hospital ten days after the operation."

But the story did not end there. The patient, Mr. Cunning, later brought suit against the man who had shot him, and Cox's X-ray plate was relevant to his suit. The *Canadian Medical Review* for March 4, 1896, reported:

ROENTGEN RAYS IN COURT

The Court of Queen's Bench in the City of Montreal will be the first court on record where Professor Roentgen's new photographic discovery will be used in evidence. A photograph of the leg of Tolson Cunning, who was shot on New Year's Eve, will be filed, showing the location of the bullet. The photograph was taken by Prof. Cox, of McGill University. The case is now before the grand jury. . . .

Arthur W. Goodspeed

Meanwhile, at the University of Pennsylvania, Professor Arthur W. Goodspeed had not been idle. On January 22, 1896, he began his efforts to secure deliberately X-ray images of the kind that he and his photographer friend Mr. Jennings had secured accidentally 6 years before (see above, page 3); but he was not successful in capturing an image on a photographic plate until February 5.[10] He reported his early results in a paper dated February 8, which appeared in *Science* for February 14; he gave a further report at a meeting in Philadelphia of the American Philosophical Society on February 21[11]; and he published a second paper in *Science* for March 13.

For his first plate on February 5, Goodspeed reported, "a small slip of glass and a piece of sheet lead, together with a wedge of wood, were held in place upon a sensitive photographic plate by elastic bands, and the whole enclosed light tight in an ordinary plate holder. This was placed horizontally upon a table, eight or ten centimeters below the large end of the Crookes tube." [11] The tube itself he described as "a beautiful, large pear-shaped one . . . about 27 centimeters long and 11 centimeters in diameter at the largest end." [10] The current was turned on, and "an exposure of twenty minutes produced, upon development, a sharp impression of the objects. . . . The sight was startling at first, as every experimenter who gets the result for the first time can testify." [11]

"Impressions of several surgical cases, including deformed fingers, fractures, etc., have been successfully produced," Goodspeed wrote on February 8. "The results seem to be best where the tube is about five inches from the sensitive plate, with its longer axis vertical and the cathode at the top." [10]

Goodspeed exhibited several of his recent plates at the February 21, 1896, meeting of the American Philosophical Society, but the sensation of the meeting was the plate that he and Jennings had made 6 years earlier, on February 22, 1890.

When he secured, in the course of his recent work, the image of some coins inside a purse, Goodspeed recounted, he was reminded immediately of the two "very mysterious discs" recorded on Jennings' plate years before. He accordingly asked Jennings if he could find the old plate, and Jennings produced it from his files. Its resemblance to an X-ray plate was unmistakable.

To clinch the matter, Goodspeed and Jennings re-enacted in mid-February 1896 the events of February 22, 1890. "On repeating the experiment by operating a Crookes tube for ten minutes in the vicinity of an enclosed photographic plate having two coins on the outside of the box, it is found that the coin shadows are strikingly similar to the mysterious discs upon the old plate," Goodspeed reported.

No doubt Professor Goodspeed thus deserves a place in the history of radiology, along with Crookes, Hertz, Lenard, and many others, as one of the men who *might* have discovered X rays before Roentgen, but who did not. Indeed, Goodspeed came even closer than the others, for he actually recorded an X-ray image. But he failed to recognize its value, and failed to pursue the matter further. "The writer and his associate [Jennings]," he stated, "wish to claim no credit for the interesting accident, but the fact remains that without a doubt the *first* Roentgen picture was produced on February 22, 1890, in the physical lecture room of the University of Pennsylvania."

William Francis Magie

William Francis Magie (1858–1943), professor of physics at Princeton, made his first X-ray negative prior to February 6, 1896. On that day, the *New York Times* reported on February 7, "he exhibited a specimen photograph of his own hand, which had been photographed through a wooden board." On February 8, he wrote a report on his research which was published in *Medical News* (New York) for February 15. This report was concerned with a new diagnostic device which Magie named the "skiascope" but which soon became known as the fluoroscope:

> The instrument here proposed for examination with the Röntgen rays I have not seen described elsewhere, and therefore present a brief account of it in the hope that it will be of use to investigators in this interesting subject.
>
> A sheet of black paper, coated on one face with platinum-bari cyanide, is placed with the coated side inward across the end of a tube or box, into which the observer looks, and which is so fitted to the face or shielded by cloths that the phosphorescent substance and the eyes are protected from all extraneous light. If this tube be then directed toward the excited Crookes' tube, which is giving the Röntgen rays, the phosphorescent paper in the tube glows, and the shadows of objects interposed between it and the Crookes' tube appear upon it. The advantage of this arrangement consists in its avoiding the experimental inconvenience of working in a dark room, and likewise the delays involved in the plan used by Röntgen. By this instrument the phenomena of the Röntgen rays can be most conveniently investigated. Its obvious applicability in diagnosis has led to my giving an account of it here.

Magie published a fuller account of his device in the March 1896 *American Journal of the Medical Sciences,* but by then he had learned that he had been anticipated by an Italian scientist. "In describing this instrument as my own," Magie modestly pointed out in his second paper, "I do not wish to be considered as asserting priority over Professor [Enrico] Salvioni, of Perugia, who has described an instrument essentially similar, but only independence in the invention." [12]

Professor Salvioni had indeed described such a device at a meeting of the Perugia Medico-Chirurgical Society on February 5 or 6, 1896[13]; he also was preceded by two other Italians, Angelo Batteli and Antonio Garbasso, who described a fluoroscope in a January 1896 issue of *Il Nuovo Cimento*, published in Pisa.[14]

James Burry

Wright, Trowbridge, Frost, Cox, and Magie were all physicists; the first American physician to announce an X-ray success was Dr. James Burry (1853–1919), a Chicago surgeon who made his first X-ray plate on February 6, 1896. Dr. Burry's work was mentioned in the Chicago *Tribune* for February 9, and he published a fuller account in the *Journal of the American Medical Association*.

When he read the early announcements of Roentgen's discovery, Dr. Burry explained, "the surgical importance . . . appealed to me strongly." [15] His first effort to produce an X-ray plate was made on February 4, when, no doubt misled by newspaper reports circulating at the time, he used an ordinary incandescent bulb instead of a Crookes tube and an induction coil which gave only a ½-inch spark. Naturally, no results were obtained. Dr. Burry accordingly wired the country's best-known inventor, Thomas Alva Edison, who was then, according to newspaper accounts, just launching his own X-ray experiments (see below, pages 32–43).[16]

February 4, 1896

From: CHICAGO, ILLINOIS
To: THOMAS A. EDISON
    ORANGE, N.J.
    IT IS NECESSARY FOR ME TO PROCURE ROENTGEN PHOTOGRAPHS FOR HOSPITAL PURPOSES AT ONCE IF POSSIBLE. PLEASE ADVISE BY WIRE AT MY EXPENSE. DO YOU USE BATTERY OR DYNAMIC CURRENT. DOES YOUR EXPERIENCE INDICATE POSSIBILITY OF OBTAINING PHOTOGRAPHS OF BONY OUTLINE THROUGH LIVING SUBJECTS. WHAT SIZE INDUCTION COIL IS ADVISABLE. DO YOU USE CROOKES TUBES IF SO WHAT SIZE OR SHAPES DO YOU SUGGEST. NO CROOKES TUBES IN CHICAGO. WHERE CAN WE GET THEM. HAVE WRITTEN.

DR. JAMES BURRY
ROOKERY BUILDING
CHIC.

Edison's reply was not helpful[16]:

February 4, 1896
THING IS TOO NEW TO GIVE DEFINITE DIRECTIONS, IT WILL REQUIRE TWO OR THREE MORE DAYS EXPERIMENTING BEFORE PROPER DIRECTIONS CAN BE GIVEN I USE TEN INCH SPARK COIL PRIMARY WORKED BY ALTERNATING DYNAMO—HAVE TROUBLE WITH TUBES, AM MAKING THEM MYSELF, HAVING BROKEN THOSE OF CROOKES MAKE.

EDISON

But Dr. Burry did not desist. He telegraphed fruitlessly for a genuine Crookes tube to New York and Boston, and then located two for sale in Philadelphia. They arrived in Chicago on February 6, and Dr. Burry took them forthwith to the laboratory of the Western Electric Company, where Charles E. Scribner and F. R. McBerty of Western Electric helped him hook them up to a suitable source of current.

The first exposures, Burry wrote, were made for $\frac{1}{2}$ hour. Shadowgraphs of a hand were secured; however, "they gave but dim and indistinct outlines of the bones." [15] So, like countless other experimenters before and since, Dr. Burry and his associates began systematically to vary the conditions—time of exposure, distance from the tube to photographic plate, voltage of the current—in order to get a better image. The equipment is shown in Plate IV. Soon "a perfect shadowgraph of the bones in the hand, wrist, and a part of the forearm was obtained."

Five days later, on February 11, Dr. Burry as a surgeon was enabled to put his new Crookes tube to practical use. "A small buckshot was located in the hand of a painter," he wrote, "between the fourth and fifth metacarpal bones near their carpal ends by means of the shadowgraph; and this shot I removed at Mercy Hospital. This is the first instance in America, so far as I can learn, of the removal of a foreign body following its location by such means, and where it could not be located by any other means." News of Burry's experiment appeared in the *New York Times* for February 13, 1896.

THE RAYS MAKE NEWS

These and other experiments performed in the United States and Canada during the last days of January and early February 1896 converted the X rays from a distant miracle reported only by cable into a close-to-home marvel; no prior scientific discovery in history, it seems likely, aroused such interest and enthusiasm among American newspapers and their readers.

"Photographing the Unseen" was the headline in the New York *Daily Tribune* for February 2. Three days later the *New York Times* reported:

SOME STARTLING RESULTS AT YALE

Professor Bumstead Secures Some Very Interesting Pictures

The Toronto *Globe* ran a two-column story on February 10:

TRIED IN TORONTO

Marvelous Feats of the New Photography

SUCCESSFUL EXPERIMENTS

Pictures of Objects Taken Through Opaque Bodies

Toronto University Professor Makes Use of the Cathode
Light—Possibilities of the Discovery

The Chicago *Tribune* ran an editorial on February 2, and 10 stories between February 7 and 23; on February 9 the story was on the front page. The Hartford *Courant* ran a series of daily stories beginning on February 11:

THE ROENTGEN RAYS

Successful Experiments at Trinity College

THE WONDERFUL X RAYS

KEYS INSIDE A PURSE CLEARLY PHOTOGRAPHED

The *Nevada State Chronicle* ran stories on February 12 and 13, as did many other papers across the continent during the weeks that followed. An exceptionally well-written local account appeared in the Galveston (Texas) *Daily News* for February 22:

FIND HIDDEN THINGS

A Succinct Statement of What Is Accomplished by the
Roentgen Rays

A BOON TO ANATOMY

Bones of Frogs and Fish Photographed Through the Flesh—
Facts About Prof. Roentgen

Some of the reports tried to make fun of the X rays; there were cartoons and satiric poems. The *Electrical Engineer* for February 26, 1896, reported that a legislator had introduced a bill in the New Jersey House of Representatives "prohibiting the use of X rays in opera glasses in theaters." But with few exceptions, the reporting was serious and competent.

The scientific and technical journals also covered the discovery creditably. The American scientific news weekly, *Science,* printed in its issue for January 31, 1896, a remarkably precise and useful account of the new rays and how they could be generated, written on January 15 by the Harvard philosopher and psychologist Hugo Münsterberg, who happened to be in Germany at the time.[17] *Science* also reprinted in its issue of February 14 a translation into English of Roentgen's original paper; this translation originally appeared in the English weekly, *Nature,* and was reprinted during early February in *Electricity* (New York), *Electrical Engineer* (New York), *Western Electrician* (Chicago), *Electrical World* (New York), and perhaps other American periodicals. Thus, by mid-February, the basic facts about the X rays were widely known among both scientists and laymen throughout North America, and the flood of publicity was accompanied by a flood of experimentation.

On February 5, 1896, the *Electrical Engineer* reported, "The demand for Crookes tubes has, we understand, created a 'corner' in that commodity," and, on February 12, "It is safe to say that there is probably no one possessed of a vacuum tube and an induction coil, who has not undertaken to repeat Professor Roentgen's experiments." *Electrical World* announced on February 22, "All the Crookes tubes in Philadelphia for sale have been purchased, which certainly illustrates the universal interest in these new and important phenomena." Four days later the *Electrical Engineer* reported, "Messrs. Baker & Company, the platinum refiners of Newark, New Jersey, inform us that they have sold more of the particular salt recommended by Roentgen as most suitable for X-ray experiments, namely, barium platinocyanide, than ever before in the history of their business, and that in consequence of the undiminished demand for this salt they have been obliged to increase their laboratory force." Also on February 26, the *Electrical Review* estimated that "hundreds of American physicists and electricians have been repeating and verifying the experiments of Professor Roentgen." By early March Professor D. W. Hering of the University of the City of New York was describing "hosts of inquirers and imitators," all experimenting with X rays and all engaged in "a scientific scramble, the like of which has probably never before been seen. It has been like a rush to the gold fields, and might perhaps recall to a forty-niner some of the incidents of that eventful period of discovery." [18] Professor A. E. Dolbear of Tufts College noted similarly, "The physical laboratories of the world appear to have well-nigh dropped everything else in order to duplicate that work and ring the changes on it, and the experimenters are daily besieged by the multitude of reporters from the daily press, anxious to be the first to describe whatever is done." [19]

By mid-February, experimentation had even spread to some high schools. The New York *Daily Tribune* for February 14 reported, "Dr. S. Oscar Myers, of Mount Vernon, has succeeded with one or two experiments with the cathodograph method which he has made this week. In making the experiments he had the use of the vacuum tube and other apparatus of the laboratory at the High School, in connection with the regular apparatus of a photographer. The most successful experiment was begun on Tuesday, that of taking a picture of a gall-stone inside of an artificial gall-bladder made of tripe.... Dr. Myers ... thinks that in the matter of the gall-stone the practical value of the Roentgen discovery has been demonstrated."

To follow in detail these hundreds of February experiments would serve no useful purpose. The tabulation below, although no doubt incomplete, records the names of more than 50 physicists, physicians, photographers, teachers, students, and others who, according to the voluminous contemporary record, successfully experimented with the new rays prior to March 1, 1896.

During the years after 1896, many other people recalled, or thought they recalled, that they or their friends had recorded X-ray images prior to March 1, 1896; some even claimed to have anticipated Wright's first plate made on January 27. Some unrecorded experiments, of course, may in fact have occurred. Public enthusiasm was high, however, and newspaper reporters were enterprising in ferreting out X-ray experiments. Hence, the likelihood that others preceded Wright, or worked with the X rays in early February, without leaving a contemporary trace, is relatively slight. The man whose priority claims have been most often accepted at face value in the radiological literature was Dr. Emil H. Grubbé of Chicago; for the details of his story, see Chapter 8.

Some North American X-Ray Experimenters during February 1896

Name	Place	Source
Dr. Wellington Adams and Prof. Nipher	Washington University, St. Louis	*Nature*, March 5, 1896

Henry A. Bumstead	Yale University	*New York Times*, Feb. 5, 1896
James Burry, Charles E. Scribner, and F. R. McBerty	Western Electric Laboratory, Chicago	See above, page 22
Henry W. Cattell	University of Pennsylvania	Chicago *Tribune*, Feb. 14, 1896
Clark and Webster	Clark University	*Western Electrician*, Feb. 29, 1896
John Cox	McGill University, Montreal	See above, page 18
J. Grosvenor Cross	Rochester, Minn.	Rochester *Post*, Feb. 21, 1896
John Daniel	Vanderbilt University	See below, page 81
Edward P. Davis	Jefferson Medical College, Philadelphia	*American Journal of the Medical Sciences*, March 1896
Amos E. Dolbear	Tufts College	*Western Electrician*, March 7, 1896
Thomas A. Duncan and A. B. Crowe	Fort Wayne, Ind.	*Western Electrician*, March 7, 1896
Thomas A. Edison	Edison Laboratory, Orange, N. J.	See below, pages 32–43
Edwin B. Frost and C. F. Emerson	Dartmouth College	See above, page 16
Arthur W. Goodspeed	University of Pennsylvania	See above, page 20
Goodwin	Massachusetts Institute of Technology	*Western Electrician*, March 7, 1896
Griffiths	New Paltz (N.Y.) Normal School	New York *Daily Tribune*, Feb. 16, 1896
Eugene Hannel and W. H. Jakway	Syracuse University	*New York Times*, Feb. 11, 1896
D. W. Hering	University of the City of York	New York *Daily Tribune*, Feb. 13, 1896
E. J. Houston and A. E. Kennelly	Houston-Kennelly Laboratory	*Journal of the Franklin Institute*, April 1896
W. W. Keen	Jefferson Medical College, Philadelphia	*American Journal of the Medical Sciences*, March 1896
Ralph R. Lawrence	Massachusetts Institute of Technology	*Nature*, March 12, 1896
Lawrence	University of Rochester	New York *Daily Tribune*, Feb. 29, 1896
William F. Magie	Princeton University	See above, page 21
John S. McKay	Packer Institute, Brooklyn	*New York Times*, Feb. 25, 1896
J. C. McLennan and H. C. Wright	University College, Toronto	Toronto *Globe*, Feb. 10, 1896
McRae	University of Texas, Austin	Galveston *Daily News*, March 2, 1896
Father Meiner and others	St. Ignatius College, Chicago	*Western Electrician*, March 7, 1896

Dayton C. Miller	Case School of Applied Science, Cleveland	*Electrical World*, March 21, 1896
W. L. Miller and C. A. Chant	University of Toronto	Toronto *Globe*, Feb. 12, 1896
William James Morton	New York City	Toronto *Globe*, Feb. 12, 1896, citing New York World
S. Oscar Myers	Mt. Vernon (N.Y.) High School	New York *Daily Tribune*, Feb. 14, 1896
William C. Peckham	Adelphi Academy, Brooklyn	*New York Times*, Feb. 18, 1896
Michael I. Pupin	Columbia University	See below, pages 55–57
J. O. Reed	University of Michigan	*Western Electrician*, March 7, 1896
William L. Robb and Arthur J. Wolff	Trinity College, Hartford	Hartford *Courant*, Feb. 11, 1896
Ogden N. Rood and Henry S. Curtis	Columbia University	*Harper's Weekly*, Feb. 22, 1896
Henry A. Rowland	Johns Hopkins University	New York *Daily Tribune*, Feb. 10, 1896
Charles R. Sanger and A. S. Cushman	Washington University, St. Louis	St. Louis *Post-Dispatch*, Feb. 21, 1896
Samuel Sheldon	Brooklyn Polytechnical Institute	New York *Herald*, Feb. 18, 1896
Henry L. Smith	Davidson College, N.C.	Charlotte (N.C.) *Observer*, Feb. 27, 1896
W. M. Stine	Armour Institute of Technology, Chicago	Chicago *Tribune*, Feb. 19, 1896
Nikola Tesla	New York City	New York *Journal*, Feb. 9, 1896
Elihu Thomson	General Electric Company, Lynn, Mass.	*Electrical Engineer*, Feb. 12, 1896
Tilman	U.S. Military Academy, West Point	*New York Times*, Feb. 11, 1896
John Trowbridge	Harvard University	See above, page 15
F. L. Woodward	Harvard University	*New York Times*, March 2, 1896
Arthur W. Wright	Yale University	See above, page 11

What Are These Mysterious Rays?

In addition to generating X rays, American scientists during 1896 speculated freely concerning the true nature of the rays. Attention was centered on four rival theories: (1) The X rays were composed of waves like light waves, but with a *longer* wavelength. (2) They were composed of waves like light waves, but with a *shorter* wavelength. (3) They were composed of *longitudinal* waves in the ether. (4) X rays were not wavelike at all, but composed of particles.

Roentgen himself had concluded that his new rays were waves because they cast shadows as light did, and emerged from the source in all directions, like light. He cautiously suggested, however, that unlike the transverse light waves the X rays might be longitudinal waves—that is, waves whose peaks and valleys were in the same plane as the forward motion of the ray rather than at right angles to it. From the very beginning, American experimenters were concerned with these issues and sought to solve the mystery.

Professor Wright at Yale, for example, was one of many who reasoned that if Roentgen's rays were light waves they should be reflected from a surface, should be refracted when they passed through a prism, should be diffracted when passed through narrow slits, and should be doubly refracted when passed through certain crystals such as those of Iceland spar. He tried all of these experiments, and reported in the *American Journal of Science* that he found little or no reflection, refraction, diffraction, or double refraction.[4]

Professor Trowbridge at Harvard was similarly concerned from the beginning with the inherent nature of the rays. One of his experiments, he reported in his New York *Journal* paper on Feb. 2, 1896, was "to determine whether the cathode rays were refracted like ordinary light waves." By "cathode rays," Professor Trowbridge meant X rays; he was as yet unconvinced that Roentgen's rays differed from those studied earlier by Crookes, Lenard, and many others. To test for refraction, Trowbridge used two prisms, one of wood and one of vulcanite; he could not use ordinary glass prisms, since the rays did not pass through glass. He arranged the prisms and two strips of glass in such a way that some of the rays from the Crookes tube were blocked by the two glass strips, some of them passed through an air gap between the strips to strike the photographic film, and some after passing through the air gap had to pass also through the prisms.

If the rays were being refracted, Professor Trowbridge explained, the image of the edges of the glass would not have been perfectly straight; they would have been bent like the image of a stick which is partly in air and partly submerged in water. "On developing the image, however, the image of the two portions of the air gap was not broken but perfectly straight. This appeared to show that the prisms of wood and vulcanite did not refract the rays."

Professor Cox of McGill was concerned with the speed of the rays. Did they proceed relatively slowly, like cathode rays, or move at the speed of light? He and an associate used quite subtle techniques to measure the speed of the X rays, and he concluded in his May 1896 paper that it must exceed 200 kilometers per second.[20]

The wavelength of the rays—if, indeed, they were waves and had a length—was also a source of much bewilderment in 1896. All the evidence initially available suggested that the shorter the waves, the greater difficulty they had in passing through matter. The longest waves known, Hertzian waves, passed readily through almost everything. The infrared waves, next in order, passed through sheets of matter impervious to visible light. Visible light itself passed only through glass and a few other transparent materials. Ultraviolet rays were blocked even by glass, and the shorter the ultraviolet waves, the more completely were they blocked. Extrapolating from these data, theoreticians in 1896 found it hard to believe that waves even shorter than ultraviolet waves could pass through matter as readily as the X rays did.

Yet early tests seemed to show that the waves must be very short. In general, long waves are readily diffracted, and the longer the wave, the greater the diffraction. The X rays, in contrast, seemed not to be diffracted at all—and remarkably sensitive methods were used to look for this effect. Professor Henry A. Rowland and his associates at the Johns Hopkins, for example, performed X-ray tests in April 1896 which would have revealed the presence of diffraction if the waves were even 0.000007 centimeter long—one-seventh the wavelength of yellow light. They found none, indicating that the X rays could not be waves longer than that.

Roentgen's own suggestion, that the X rays might differ from light waves in being longitudinal rather than transverse waves, was accordingly a welcome solution to the many theoretical dilemmas surrounding the new rays. But how could this hypothesis be tested? No longitudinal waves had ever been detected, and no one knew how they would behave if they did exist; hence, no experiments could be devised to determine whether the X rays behaved in the ways required by the hypothesis.

The physicist Nikola Tesla (1856–1943) and some others held in 1896 that the X rays were not wavelike at all but, like the cathode rays, were composed of particles. If so, of course, the particles must be very small indeed to pass through solid matter. Particles small enough to pass through bone, tissue, and even aluminum placed quite a strain on the scientific imagination of 1896.

In addition to these "respectable" theories, many implausible guesses were hazarded. Some men continued to insist, for example, that the X rays were really just Crookes's cathode rays, despite all the evidence to the contrary, such as proof that the X rays could not be deflected by a magnet. Edison at one time announced that X rays were very high-pitched sound waves in the air. Elihu Thomson promptly showed that this was nonsense. Roentgen rays, he pointed out, pass through a glass bulb from which almost all of the air has been exhausted, whereas sound waves cannot travel through a vacuum. Professor A. A. Michelson suggested in April 1896 that the X rays were electromagnetic whirlpools or *vortices* swirling through the ether. This was another theory which could neither be proved nor disproved.

Many years were to elapse before these and related issues were settled. Then it was determined that the X rays are indeed composed of waves, like radio or light waves, but exceedingly short ones. The failure of the 1896 pioneers to demonstrate refraction, diffraction, and other phenomena of wave behavior was due to the shortness of the waves; with the subtler techniques later available, the wavelike nature of the X rays was readily demonstrated. Still later it was found that the energy of the X rays is present in packets or *quanta*, as is the case with light and radio waves; thus, in some respects the X rays are particle-like as well as wavelike.

That the early X-ray workers accomplished as much as they did, despite their ignorance of the basic nature of the rays with which they were dealing, is one of the striking features of early X-ray research.

REFERENCES

1. PIERSON, G. W., *Yale College, An Educational History*. Yale University Press, New Haven, 1952.
2. *Amer. J. Sci. Arts*, ser. 3, *13*: 49–55, 1877.
3. *Amer. J. Sci.*, Ser. 4, *1*: 235–244, 1896.
4. Unpublished papers in the possession of Mrs. Norman Pearson, Hamden, Connecticut.
5. MORTON, W. J., *The X-Ray*. American Technical Book Company, New York, 1896.
6. For biographical information on John Trowbridge, see the *Dictionary of American Biography*.
7. *Western Electrician, 18:* 104, 1896.
8. *Dartmouth Alumni Magazine*, pp. 383–384, April 1930.
9. *Montreal Med. J., 24:* 661–665, 1896.
10. *Science (n.s.), 3:* 236–237 and 394–396, 1896.
11. *Proc. Amer. Phil. Soc., 35:* 17–24, 1896.
12. *Amer. J. Med. Sci., 111:* 251–255, 1896.
13. *Nature (London), 53:* 399, 1896 (quoting the Rome correspondent of *Brit. Med. J.*).
14. *Proc. Acad. Med.-Chir. (Perugia), 8:* nos. 1 and 2, 1896 (quoted in *Nature (London), 53:* 424–425, 1896).
15. *J.A.M.A, 26:* 402–404, 1896.
16. Quoted by Arthur W. Fuchs, in BRUWER, A. J., *Classic Descriptions in Diagnostic Roentgenology*, p. 120. Charles C Thomas, Publisher, Springfield, Illinois, 1964.
17. *Science (n.s.), 3:* 161–163, 1896.
18. *Electrical World, 27:* 255, 1896.
19. *J. Franklin Inst., 141:* 241–278, 1896.
20. *Trans. Roy. Soc. Canad.*, Ser. 2, *2:* sect. III, 171–191, 1896.

3 The Dual Role of Thomas Alva Edison

Most of the Americans who experimented with the X rays in January and February 1896 were essentially followers of Roentgen, using his methods to confirm and where possible to expand and apply his findings. Thomas Alva Edison (1847–1931) played a different and much more complex role—indeed, a double role—both as organizer of legitimate X-ray research and as a sort of county-fair barker, publicizing the activities of his laboratory and spouting off-the-cuff dicta about Roentgen's "new kind of ray."

Edison was 49 in 1896, and renowned as "America's foremost inventor" for his work on the electric light and power system, the phonograph, the moving picture, and other "miracles of modern science." During the years after 1890, however, his attention had turned in considerable part from invention to a grandiose scheme for mining iron ore on a large scale in western New Jersey, and for separating the iron from the ore by means of a magnetic process that he had developed. This project was to prove a failure, and it was already in difficulty early in 1896 when the news of Roentgen's discovery reached Edison. To return from the headaches of mining iron ore to his beloved West Orange, New Jersey, laboratory must therefore have been a relief.

Edison appears to have begun his speculations concerning Roentgen's rays quite early. He was quoted in the Washington *Post* for January 18, 1896, as saying, "The cardinal factor of the whole matter is this radiant heat, but I am satisfied that the Würzburg inventor had special rays thereof and special chemical plates." There was no indication on that date, however, that he had done any experimenting himself. On January 27, he wired a former associate, Professor A. E. Kennelly: HOW WOULD YOU LIKE TO COME OVER AND EXPERIMENT ON ROENTGEN'S NEW RADIATIONS.... On February 2, under a headline which read "His Experiments Began Last Week," the New York *World* quoted Edison as explaining:

> One reason for my lack of perfect success thus far has been that I have been using a battery. But I am fixing up a dynamo. When I have a sufficiently powerful engine I am sure that there will be no question of obtaining a good photograph of a man's hand.... I ex-

pect to have my dynamo in operation by Tuesday [February 4] at the latest.

On February 5, William Randolph Hearst, then publisher of the New York *Journal,* spurred Edison to further efforts with a telegraphed request:

WILL YOU AS AN ESPECIAL FAVOR TO THE JOURNAL UNDERTAKE TO MAKE CATHODOGRAPH OF HUMAN BRAIN KINDLY TELEGRAPH ANSWER AT OUR EXPENSE

Edison accepted Hearst's challenge. "Tomorrow morning Mr. Edison will attempt further to demonstrate the penetrating powers of the new light by an experiment in photographing a man's brain," a February 7 dispatch to the *New York Times* from Edison's laboratory announced. "... That the best results be obtained, Mr. Edison has made a celluloid vacuum to be especially used in the test. The inventor says he will try to find some practical use for the X rays." Edison was also quoted as claiming to have improved on the basic Crookes tube by making one out of an ordinary incandescent light bulb with glass only $\frac{1}{64}$ inch thick. The cost was only a trifle, Edison told a reporter, "yet the bulb gave better satisfaction than the expensive one, no doubt because the thin glass offered less resistance to the rays." Such premature claims were to issue repeatedly from the Edison laboratory during subsequent weeks.

The announcement that Edison was about to use X rays to "photograph the living human brain" attracted hordes of reporters and onlookers to West Orange (Fig. 7). "For three weeks," Edison's assistant William H. Meadowcraft later recalled, "more than twenty newspaper reporters were stationed at the Laboratory, the work going on nights, days, and Sundays." The pace was feverish. "Edison is a man who knows nothing of the passing of day and night," said the *Electrical Review.* "... He had 'the boys,' as he calls his assistants, working most of the time. When Saturday night came, Edison had been working steadily for the better part of 70 hours, so he went home to rest on Sunday. Bright and early Monday morning he appeared at the laboratory as chipper as a lark...." [1] The *Electrical World* reported similarly, "Edison himself has been having a severe attack of the Roentgen mania. The newspapers having reporters in attendance at his laboratory did not suffer for copy, as the yards of sensational matter printed emanating from that source attest, and we learn that last week Mr. Edison and his staff worked through 70 hours without any intermission, a hand-organ being employed during the latter hours to assist in keeping the force awake." [2]

Despite all the hullabuloo, however, the photographing of a man's

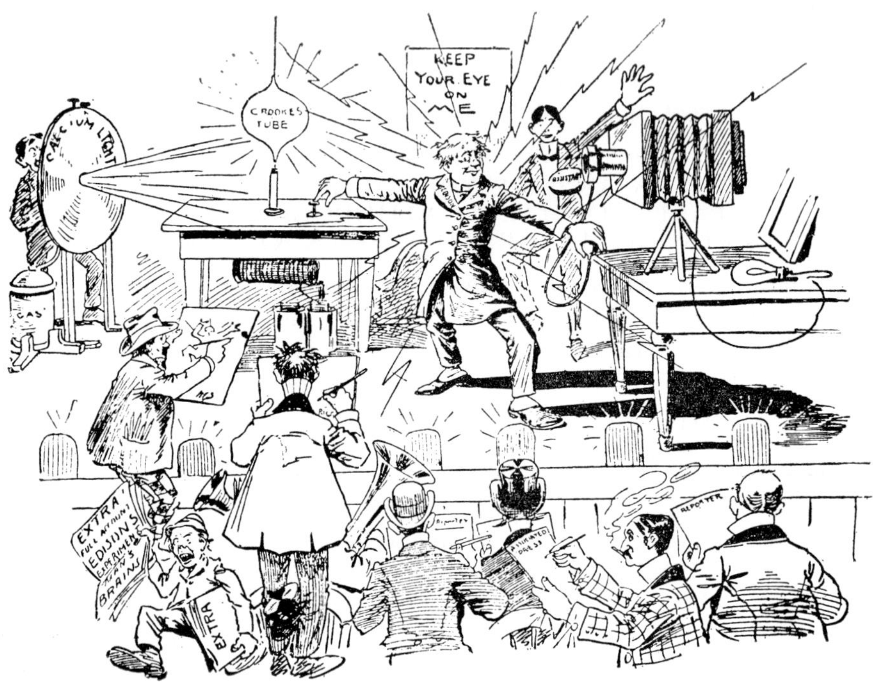

Fig. 7. Cartoon from the New York *World,* reprinted in the *Western Electrician* for February 22, 1896, p. 87.

brain, scheduled for February 8, did not take place. A *Times* reporter questioned Edison and quoted him as explaining, "Yes, we are making some special long tubes which will give a five-inch distance between the poles in the vacuum. Some day next week one of our boys will lay his head down on the table, and we shall suspend a battery of five of these large tubes over his head so as to get a profile and side-face combination."

Yet along with pseudo-scientific flummery, Edison also talked sense to the *Times* reporter. "Whether Roentgen's discovery has a commercial value or not," he was quoted as saying in the *Times* for February 9, 1896, "is something which has not yet been determined. He is a pure scientist, and cares nothing about that aspect of the question. He needs others, like myself, whose chief aim is to turn the great discoveries of science into practical use and adapt them, so that the world will receive the benefit from them."

By February 11, the fact that Edison had *not* taken a photograph of a man's brain the previous day was deemed important news. "The tubes which are being prepared for that purpose," the *Times* of that date explained, "were not ready. He spent a busy day, however, in making experiments designed to bring out the properties of the X rays."

Now the whole country was looking over Edison's shoulder. The *Nevada State Chronicle* for February 12 carried a typical dispatch of this period:

> *Orange, N.J., Feb. 11*—Thomas Edison was hard at work all day in his laboratory in West Orange preparing for his experiment of photographing the human body and brain with the aid of the newly discovered ray.... Surrounded by a score or more of reporters and other visitors, Edison sat for hours watching progress of the work and he displayed a wonderful amount of patience, when after repeated trials the desired result was not obtained.... Mr. Edison explained to the reporters that he was trying to see whether the rays were longitudinal etheric vibrations going straight out into space or local magnetic waves circulating from one electrode to the other....

There was much more verbiage of this kind, but Edison's true purpose of the moment was also succinctly stated: "He was desirous of finding the degree of vacuum in the tube which would give the best effects...."

By now the reporters camped in West Orange were getting a little impatient for that promised picture of a human brain, but it was not forthcoming. In one experiment watched by the reporters February 12, the photographic plate was exposed for 1 full hour; when it was developed, nothing could be seen but a murkiness plus a curved line which Edison could not explain. Edison's apology was quoted in the *New York Times* for February 13: "A man making experiments may count himself lucky if he has successful results in ten out of every hundred experiments which he makes. At the same time, each negative result obtained under proper conditions closes up some avenue along which no further experiments are needed."

On February 14 the *New York Times* reported, "Thomas A. Edison made a huge stride forward yesterday in his experiments with the Roentgen rays . . . and he is now confident of his ability to pierce through the densest substances...." But the long-awaited plate of the human brain still was not forthcoming. Indeed, according to the New York *Daily Tribune* of February 14, "With regard to his . . . brain experiments, [Edison] said that he was extremely skeptical as to reaching any results that would be of value. He thought that the opacity of the bony structure of the cranium would offer insuperable obstacles...." Yet there remained a ray of hope. "It would perhaps be possible to succeed by taking a test through the brain down into a plateholder held in the mouth of the subject. In this way only one thickness of bone would have to be penetrated by the rays." So far, however, Edison's X rays would penetrate only 2 inches of wood, and he declared that he would not attempt the brain experiment "until he had so far perfected his tubes that he could pass the X rays through a solid block of wood three inches thick."

Some of the reporters went home, but hope continued to emanate from West Orange like X rays from a Crookes tube. On February 19 the Spokane (Washington) *Review* announced that Edison would soon X-ray a human brain, and on February 20 the New York *Daily Tribune* gave details:

> Thomas A. Edison said yesterday that he believed he could get a fairly good shadowgraph of the brain, or of a portion of the skull, with his present appliances, and that he would in all probability make the experiment on Friday or Saturday night.... Edison said that he had got his tubes perfected.

Bad luck, it seems, intervened. "I have had every kind of accident during the past week," Edison was quoted as saying in the *Times* for February 23. "My tubes have burst, I have not been able to get as high a vacuum as desired, and I have had to substitute two Leyden jars for the condensers which I have used heretofore.... I tried [a] German glass [tube]... and at first got good results.... Afterward it failed to act altogether." Still, he could now get the rays to pierce 5 inches of wood, so that "I may try to get a photograph of the living skull any day now."

Week after week the extravaganza at West Orange continued, although it was playing to a diminishing audience. "Mr. Edison is steadily continuing his experiments," *Electrical Engineer* reported on March 25, "and last week succeeded in making visible... the bones of the hand through a block of wood eight inches thick." So far as is known, however, Edison never did succeed in producing that promised X-ray plate of a human brain or skull, nor did many of his other promises, predictions, theories, or miscellaneous pronouncements bear fruit.

Yet Edison should not be dismissed as a mere charlatan or entertainer, for, while he was performing out front for the visiting reporters, solid work of some importance was in fact going on in his laboratory.

RESEARCH IN THE LABORATORY

Edison's greatest invention, as his most perceptive biographer, Matthew Josephson, has pointed out, was neither the electric light not the phonograph but *the concept of an industrial research laboratory*.[3] Flush with profits from his inventions and corporate operations, Edison had built his great laboratory on Main Street in West Orange back in 1890, on what was for that day a Gargantuan scale. It was, says Josephson, "the largest and most complete private research laboratory in the world," about 250 feet long, three stories high, with 60,000 feet of floor space, machine shops, an engine room, glass-blowing and pumping rooms, chemical and photographic departments, rooms for electrical testing, a comprehensive library, and "eight thousand kinds of chemicals"—the ideal site, in short, for intensive research on the new rays. At times it was staffed with as many as 60 employees, some of them eminent scientists in their own right. Many professors of physics in those days, and for years thereafter, thought themselves lucky to have two basement cubicles and one assistant.

To back up his X-ray research in 1896, Edison brought to this laboratory experts of many kinds: the chemical consultant J. W. Aylsworth, for example; the physicist Dr. Arthur E. Kennelly, later co-discoverer of the Kennelly-Heaviside layer; and even Professor Edwin J. Houston, an old enemy of Edison's, co-founder of the Thomson-Houston Company which had "jumped" his electric light patents a few years before and which became the General Electric Company. When photographic consultation was needed, Edison summoned the eminent Walter E. Woodbury, editor of the *Photographic Times*. Merely by bringing many such men as these together under one capacious roof, Edison established the conditions in which new ideas were likely to be sparked and significant progress made. The other great industrial research laboratories of the period—General Electric's in Schenectady, for example, Westinghouse's near Pittsburgh, and the Thomson-Houston laboratory in Lynn, Massachusetts—were all patterned after West Orange.[3]

Edison's laboratory during this period also maintained close liaison with researchers at other centers. The Chicago *Tribune* noted on February 9, for example, that Burry and others at work in the Western Electric laboratory there "have been in telegraphic communication with Thomas A. Edison and Prof. Trowbridge of Harvard University, who are seeking like results. As fast as one establishes a fact he gives the others the benefit of it." One such communication has been preserved in the Edison archives, a wire to Dr. Burry on February 7:

> WE ARE MAKING OUR OWN TUBES AND OBTAINING VERY FINE RESULTS. STATE OF EXHAUSTION OF TUBE IS IMPORTANT FACTOR. DISK ELECTRODES BEST. EDISON.[4]

Each industrial laboratory, like each individual scientist, develops through the years a characteristic pattern of attack on scientific problems. The characteristic approach of the Edison laboratory had been established years before, when many thousands of substances had been tested as filaments for incandescent light bulbs and a highly practical filament had thus been developed. One important X-ray endeavor of Edison's West Orange laboratory was patterned directly on this earlier filament project.

Edison had read Roentgen's original paper and noted that Roentgen had used only barium platinocyanide and a few other fluorescent materials to detect the presence of X rays. Was it not possible, he asked, that other chemicals might be found to fluoresce even more brightly when excited by the new rays?

Years later, Edison's chemical consultant J. W. Aylsworth recalled how the search for such substances was launched. Edison took him to the chemical storeroom and told him, "Aylsworth, start up there at the top and work down. If there is a suitable fluorescent salt or combination of salts that will fluoresce, we will get it. Stick at this and let me know with what substances you get results." [5]

During the weeks which followed, laboratory assistants under Aylsworth's supervision tested scores and then hundreds of substances, systematically exposing them to X rays and watching for fluorescence. Quite early the discovery was made that a cheaper and more readily available compound, calcium tungstate, fluoresced even more brightly than barium platinocyanide—6 times as brightly, according to Edison's estimate.[6] He jubilantly cabled the news to England (Fig. 8):

PLEASE INFORM LORD KELVIN THAT HAVE JUST FOUND CALCIUM TUNGSTATE PROPERLY CRYSTALLIZED GIVES SPLENDID FLUORESCENCE WITH ROENTGEN RAY FAR EXCEEDING PLATINOCYANIDE RENDERING PHOTOGRAPHS UNNECESSARY. EDISON. MARCH 17, 1896.[7]

Edison preserved Lord Kelvin's cordial reply (Fig. 9):

THANKS FOR INTERESTING DISCOVERY HAVE INFORMED ELECTRICIAN NATURE ELECTRICAL REVIEW[4]

But this discovery did not end the search. By late March Edison could report: "After trying over 1,800 different salts, I have found 72 that fluoresce. The best of these is tungstate of calcium; but as I am still continuing my work in this direction, I may find something even better." [8]

When his "boys" had exhausted the supply of relatively simple chemical compounds—lithium bromide, barium chloride, cadmium sulfate, and so on—Edison cracked the whip and turned them loose on more complicated compounds: potassium benzene disulfonate, calcium fluosili-

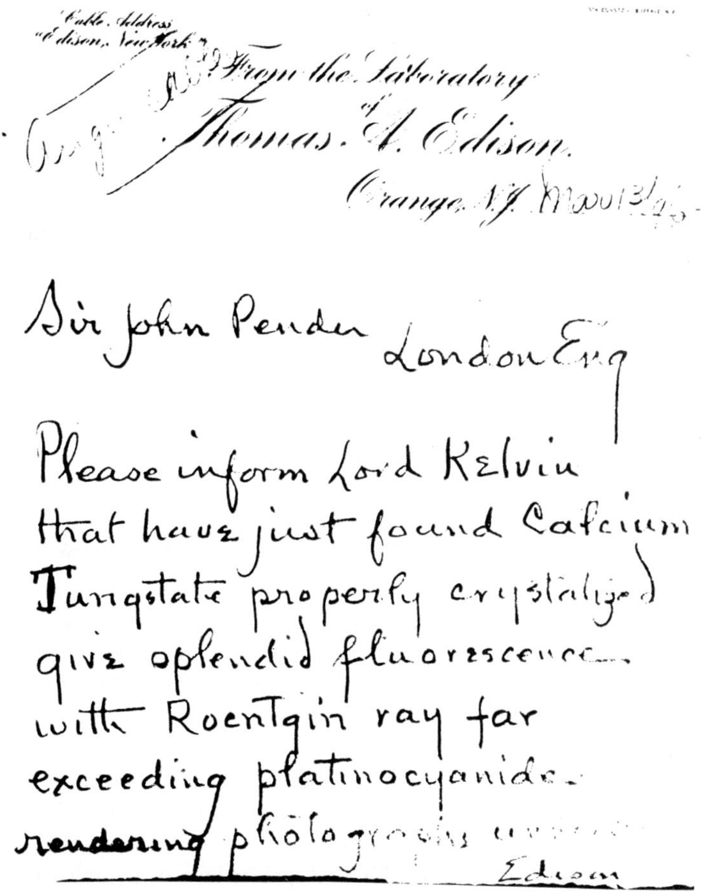

FIG. 8. Edison's cable to Sir John Pender (Edison Archives).

cate, potassium chromium salicylate. By November 1896, some 8000 substances had been tested, according to Edison's count, and 63 more had
been found to fluoresce, but none so brightly as calcium tungstate,
which remains today the compound of choice for several radiological
applications.[9]

The search for fluorescing substances also broadened in other dimensions. After Roentgen's first announcement, the newspapers had carried
a rash of stories about new kinds of rays emanating from sources other
than Crookes tubes—rays from arc lights, from sparks, and even from
the sun, all capable (it was alleged) of penetrating opaque matter.
Edison could have refuted such claims by exposing calcium tungstate
to the alleged rays and showing that it did not fluoresce, but he was

THE DIRECT UNITED STATES CABLE COMPANY, (LTD.)

Head Office, 50 Old Broad Street, London, England.

No.______

PRINCIPAL OFFICES:

NEW YORK, 40 Broadway and 51 New Street.
"   444 Broome Street.
"   21½ Spruce Street.
BOSTON,   Old State House.
"   General Post Office Building.
HALIFAX,   Queen Buildings, Hollis Street.
LONDON,   39 Mark Lane.
LIVERPOOL, D 6 Exchange Buildings.
GLASGOW,   4 Waterloo Street.
BRISTOL,   Back Hall Chambers.

RECEIVED
MAR 17 1896
ANSWERED
MAR 17 1896

The following **CABLEGRAM RECEIVED "Via Direct Cable."**

GLASGOW 15

EDISON NY,

THANKS FOR INTERESTING DISCOVERY HAVE INFORMED .

ELECTRICIAN NATURE ELECTRICAL REVIEW,

KELVIN

FIG. 9. Cable from Lord Kelvin to Edison (Edison Archives).

not satisfied with so easy a refutation. Soon his "boys" were hard at work exposing *other* substances, enclosed in lightproof containers, to arc lights, sparks, and the direct rays of the sun from 11 a.m. to 2 p.m. In all, it was reported, 1200 substances were thus tested, with uniformly negative results.[10]

Other massive inquiries were also undertaken. Edison knew, of course, as Crookes had also known, that if a tube were too highly evacuated no cathode rays would be generated, and no X rays would emerge— at least, no X rays detectable by barium platinocyanide or calcium tungstate. But Edison was not content with testing only two substances. Might it not be that some other compound would fluoresce in the presence of a tube too highly evacuated to produce rays detectable in the usual ways? So those 1200 substances were tested once again, this time in the presence of a highly evacuated tube. Again all results were negative. An individual researcher, working alone in a laboratory like Roentgen's, might well have spent a lifetime exploring even part of the ground which Edison's well-organized team covered in 1896.

Improving the Crookes tube, as has been noted, was one of Edison's main goals. By early March 1896, his "boys" had completed experiments with 150 tube designs, testing each tube at varying degrees of vacuum with varying voltages. It was easy to show that the thinner the glass (all other factors being constant) the more X rays emerged.[11]

But what kind of glass was best, when tube envelopes of equal thickness were compared? Day after day Edison's glassblower, Clarence Dally, blew tubes of various kinds of glass for him. One tube was even blown of a rare kind of "Scotch glass" ordinarily used for the water gauges on boilers. The results were necessarily inconclusive, since there were no ways to measure the X-ray output accurately or to maintain optimal conditions in each tube during the test, but Edison could report in March that "German glass appears to give better results than lead glass." [12]

As the work progressed, a goal gradually evolved in Edison's thinking. Some day soon he would market a complete X-ray "outfit."

To what degree of vacuum should the tube in such an installation be exhausted? To find out, Edison tested each tube while it was still connected to the vacuum pump, and pumped out air until the X-ray output reached a maximum. Then he sealed off the tube.[6] Unfortunately, he soon encountered a whole series of puzzling and troublesome phenomena which were to plague radiologists throughout the next 16 years.

First of all, the vacuum promptly deteriorated. If a tube were tested even 3 or 4 hours after being sealed up with the ideal vacuum, it was found to be already too "soft," and to emit only weak X rays or none at all.

If a high-voltage current were run through such a tube, Edison learned, the vacuum would gradually improve again, but this phenomenon was variable, almost capricious. If a bulb were left cold for 24 hours, for example, the vacuum might deteriorate so greatly that $4\frac{1}{2}$ hours of current were needed to bring it back to a condition in which X rays could be generated. (Many of the prolonged exposures to X rays reported during the first weeks of experimentation—exposures of several hours, for example—were no doubt the result of this phenomenon. Although the tubes were kept on for many hours, actual X rays were in all probability being generated during only a fraction of the presumed period of exposure. The rest of the time was wasted because of too low or too high a vacuum.)

Since tube vacuums deteriorated after the tube was sealed off, an obvious gambit was to overexhaust the tube initially, but this did not work very well, either. True, such a tube began to emit X rays more promptly when first turned on; then, as the current was continued, the vacuum continued to increase until the tube went dark, no cathode rays were generated, and no X rays emerged.[6]

Many other aspects of tube design—the size of the tube, for example, and the composition of the cathode and anode—were systematically explored in the Edison laboratory in a similar manner. The sensitivity of various types of photographic plates was also explored, for Edison correctly perceived that the plate most sensitive to light might not necessarily be the one most sensitive to X rays. In addition, countless man-hours were devoted to repeating the experiments and refuting the findings reported from other laboratories.

In February, for example, an experimenter named Piltchikoff had reported in a French scientific journal that the X-ray output of Crookes tubes could be raised, and hence the time needed for producing an X-ray negative could be shortened, by placing a fluorescent material inside the tube. If true, this announcement might prove of major importance. To test it, Edison had a tube blown with an internal coating of calcium tungstate. Only feeble X rays were emitted, much more feeble than those from an identical tube without the calcium tungstate. Such negative findings win no Nobel Prizes, nor do they earn large sums for the industrial laboratories which repeat the experiments, yet they play an important role in the workaday progress of science. Somebody

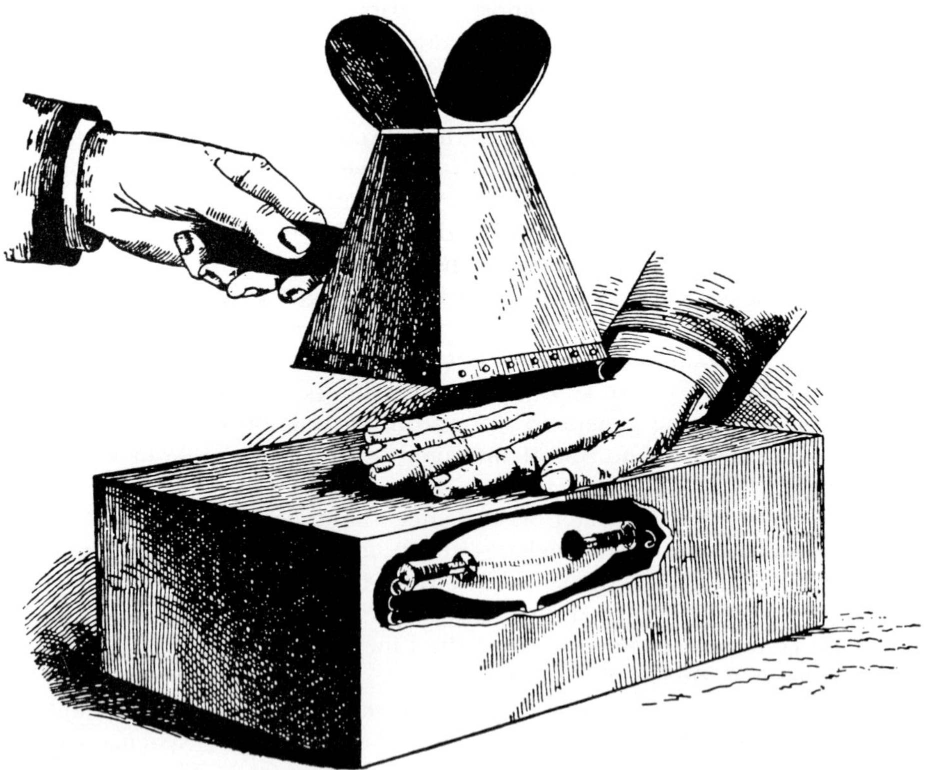

Fig. 10. Edison's fluoroscope.

has to do the weary work, and the modern industrial laboratory patterned after West Orange is ideally suited to the role. Other scientists and other laboratories both in the United States and abroad were engaged in similar projects. Some of them no doubt made findings similar to or identical with Edison's a few days or a few weeks earlier than he did. But this hardly detracts from the credit due to the Edison laboratory.

Out of all this research, Edison emerged in the popular mind as the inventor of the fluoroscope. As noted above (page 22), Batteli, Garbasso, and Salvioni in Italy, Magie at Princeton, and no doubt others as well had preceded him. His fluoroscope was, in principle, Magie's "skiascope." Although he did not invent the fluoroscope, his contributions to its development deserve recognition and clearly illustrate why science needs its Edisons as well as its Roentgens.

First, Edison's fluoroscope was shaped like the familiar stereoscope, so that both eyes could be comfortably focused on the image simultaneously—an exceedingly simple change, but an important one. Second, Edison coated the fluorescent screen of his fluoroscope with calcium tungstate instead of barium platinocyanide, thus enhancing its sensitivity. Finally, and most important, Edison turned his fluoroscope over to an associated company, Aylsworth & Jackson, to manufacture and sell at a low price. Thus, by March 25, 1896, the fluoroscope was no longer merely a device to be read about in scientific publications, but an article which could be purchased on the open market (Fig. 10).[13]

Only a little later, Edison reached his primary goal. A complete set of X-ray apparatus, which could be bought as a unit, "designed under the personal supervision of Thomas A. Edison," was being advertised in the scientific journals.

REFERENCES

1. *Electrical Rev., 28:* 87, 1896.
2. *Electrical World, 27:* 170, 1896.
3. JOSEPHSON, M., *Edison, A Biography.* McGraw-Hill Book Company, New York, 1959.
4. Edison Archives, West Orange, New Jersey.
5. *Amer. J. Roentgen., 57:* 145–156, 1948.
6. *Electrical Engineer, 21:* 305, 1896.
7. GLASSER, O., *William Conrad Roentgen and the Early History of the Roentgen Rays,* p. 236. Charles C Thomas, Publisher, Baltimore, 1934.
8. *Electrical Rev., 28:* 166, 1896.
9. *Electrical Engineer, 22:* 520, 1896.
10. *Electrical Engineer, 21:* 378, 1896.
11. *Electrical World, 27:* 308, 1896.
12. *Electrical Engineer, 21:* 163, 1896.
13. *Ibid.,* p. 327.

4   Early Equipment

The Crookes tube used to generate X rays in 1896 was far from a standardized device; Sir William Crookes himself used multitudinous forms of the tube during the 1870's. With so many different forms of Crookes tube, it was natural that disputes arose concerning the way the tubes functioned. Some experimenters were convinced that the X rays were emitted, like the cathode rays, by the cathode. Others thought that they were emitted by the anode or by the glass bulb of the tube. Roentgen had reported in his preliminary communication that the rays were emitted by the glass. Gradually this confusion was cleared up.

X rays are generated, it was established, whenever cathode rays strike a *target* or *anti-cathode* of any kind. In Roentgen's initial experiments, the rays bombarded the glass bulb directly; hence, he was right in saying that the glass was the source of the rays. But in a Crookes tube which had a metal target or anti-cathode placed in the path of the cathode-ray beam, the X rays were generated in and emerged in all directions from this target. Generally the same metal surface which served as target was also connected to the positive terminal of the power supply and thus functioned also as the anode. All parties to the initial dispute were partially right, except those who insisted that the X rays came from the cathode.

In the *British Medical Journal* for March 7, 1896, what was said to be a major improvement in X-ray tube design was announced, and a similarly "improved" tube was also described in the *Electrical Review* (London) for March 13, 1896. These tubes featured a concave or cup-shaped cathode. Since, as noted above, cathode rays emerge at right angles from the surface, the effect was to bring the cathode rays together at a point or very nearly a point. In the "new" type of tube (Fig. 11) a flat target or anode of platinum was placed in the path of the converging cathode rays, so that the point where the cathode rays came together lay on or close to its surface, and the surface of the anode was tilted so that the X rays generated when the cathode rays struck it could emerge from the tube without being blocked by the cathode.

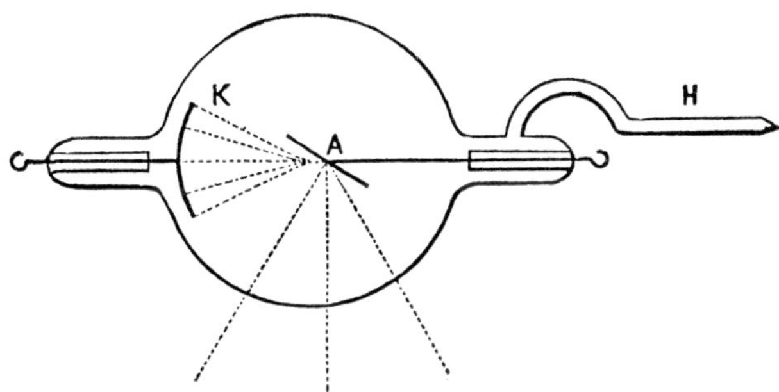

FIG. 11. From *Electrical World, 27: 377*, April 4, 1896.

Two important results followed. Because most of the X rays emerged from a very small region on the surface of the anode, they cast a much sharper shadow, with less blurring. Also, because the heat generated by cathode-ray bombardment was concentrated in the platinum target rather than in the glass bulb, the glass was less likely to melt or crack; a longer tube life resulted.

The *Boston Medical and Surgical Journal* for March 26, 1896, the *Electrical Engineer* for April 1, and the *Electrical World* for April 4 all brought news of this "new" tube design to American readers. High praise accompanied the description. It was claimed to be "a very great improvement over anything that has previously been produced," and a London publication was quoted as having called it "the greatest advance in X-ray photography that has been made since the announcement of Roentgen's discovery." [1] Most of the X-ray tubes used today for medical diagnosis and for some other purposes are, in principle, focus tubes, not unlike the one announced in England on March 7 and 13, 1896.

But who had really invented the focus tube? The first American announcement said that it "was recently designed by one of the professors at King's College, London." Professor Sidney Rowland and also Reginald Jackson, both in England, were sometimes named. Another English focus tube based on much the same principles was attributed to A. A. Campbell Swinton and was said to give "a sharpness of definition not otherwise obtainable."

These English claims to priority did not go unchallenged, however. Herbert B. Schallenberger, working in the Westinghouse laboratory in Rochester, Pennsylvania, insisted that he had used a very similar tube as early as February 15, 1896. Indeed, a picture of his tube had appeared in the *Electrical World*, March 7, 1896. "The only difference between my tube and the focus tube of Professor Rowland," Schallenberger wrote in April, "is that he placed the platinum disc [combination target

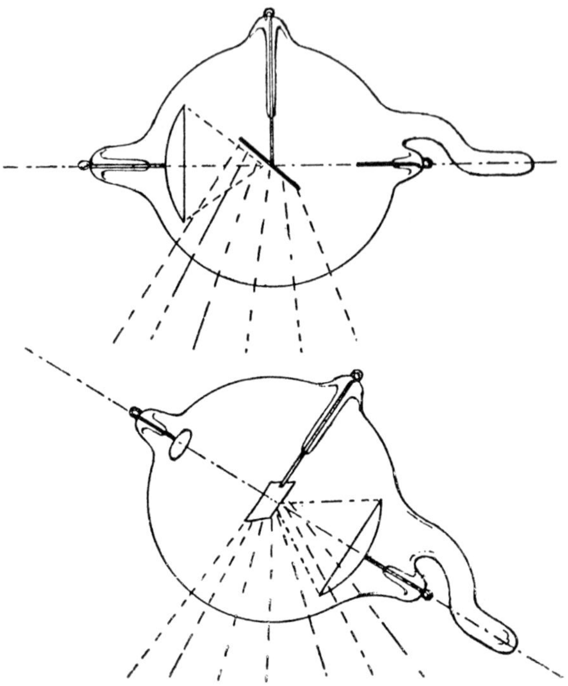

Fig. 12. From *Electrical World, 27:* 433, April 18, 1896.

and anode] at an angle, while I tilt my entire tube—but in both cases
to secure the same results—the proper relation of the photograph
plate to the point of radiation of the rays." [2] To illustrate this negligible
difference, Schallenberger offered a drawing (Fig. 12). Other claimants
were also heard from, both in the United States and in other countries.

While these claims and counterclaims were still resounding, Sir
Oliver Lodge cleared up the mystery in the *Electrician* (London),
April 10, 1896. The focus tube had been designed, Sir Oliver pointed
out, by Crookes himself, many years before Roentgen. It was just another
of the countless forms of Crookes tubes, developed for special purposes, collecting dust through the years in the racks of physics laboratories. "I first saw it at work in Professor Carey Foster's laboratory
at University College, London, last January," Sir Oliver testified, "and
that particular tube still gives about the best defined results possible."
Professor Wright at Yale, it will be recalled, also used a focus tube
for some of his January 1896 experiments (see above, pages 13–14).

Although they were often called "vacuum tubes" in the 1890's, an
inherent characteristic of Crookes tubes was their need to have a
little air or other gas left inside; hence, they later came to be called

"gas tubes." If the vacuum was either too low or too high, the tube would not emit X rays; as the tube heated up, as noted above (page 40), more and more gas particles were deposited on the interior surfaces, until the tube became too "hard" and X-ray emission ceased.

A much-touted "improvement" designed to minimize this problem was introduced early in 1896. An elongated protuberance was added to the glass bulb of the tube, and a chemical such as potassium carbonate, which emits a gas when heated, was placed in the protuberance. Then, if the vacuum rose too high, heat was applied to the chemical in the "regulator," whereupon the gas from the chemical lowered the vacuum and the tube began to function again. But this, too, turned out to be a mistaken 1896 priority claim; Crookes and others had used tubes with regulators of this kind at least as early as the 1870's.

Late in 1896 or early in 1897, however, a young Philadelphian did introduce a related improvement of substantial value. He was Henry Lyman Sayen (1875–1918), and he had begun work on the design of scientific equipment in 1893, when he was 17 years old, in the shop of Queen & Co., manufacturer of induction coils and related devices.[3] Sayen devised a tube in which, whenever the vacuum rose too high, the current produced sparks between a second pair of electrodes. This *automatically* heated the potassium carbonate or other chemical lodged in the path of the sparks, released a little gas, and thus started the tube up again. Known as the Queen self-regulating tube (Fig. 13), Sayen's tube became quite popular, and a later advertisement for it quoted praise from eminent authorities:

> "Especially ingenious."—Prof. W. C. Roentgen
> "Most satisfactory."—Lord Kelvin
> "The best I have yet seen."—Dr. A. W. Goodspeed
> "It can take care of itself."—Dr. H. P. Bowditch, Harvard College

Countless other variations on the Crookes design were introduced in 1896 (Fig. 14). Professor Woodward at Harvard developed an all-metal tube[4] and Professor Trowbridge designed an oil-immersed tube to keep the glass cool and to eliminate the sparking which sometimes cracked or melted the glass of ordinary tubes.[5] Elihu Thomson of General Electric applied for a patent on a "new" tube on August 21, 1896; it was essentially a focus tube with two cup-shaped cathodes instead of one and with a built-in vacuum regulator. His patent was granted January 26, 1897—no doubt the first to be issued to an American for an X-ray device. Yet little or nothing new was revealed in the Thomson patent application; even the dual-cathode arrangement had been used by Crookes himself decades before, and was described in a paper by Roentgen dated March 9, 1896.[6]

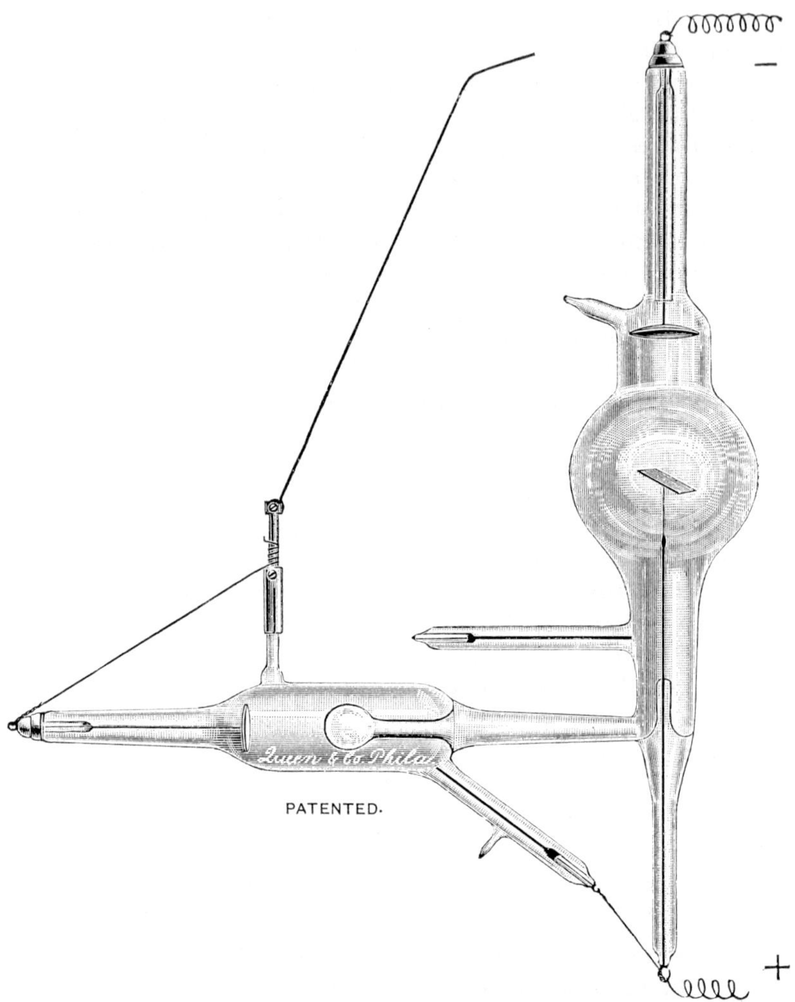

Fig. 13. From Queen & Co. catalogue.

The best tubes at the end of the year were basically similar to the Crookes tubes available at the beginning. What was accomplished during the year was a better understanding of the way in which the tubes generated X rays, greater skill in handling them, and a selection from among the countless features available in earlier tubes of those specific features best suited for X-ray uses.

FILTERS AND DIAPHRAGMS

Two important auxiliary devices familiar to modern radiologists are the *filter*, usually made of aluminum, which when placed in the path

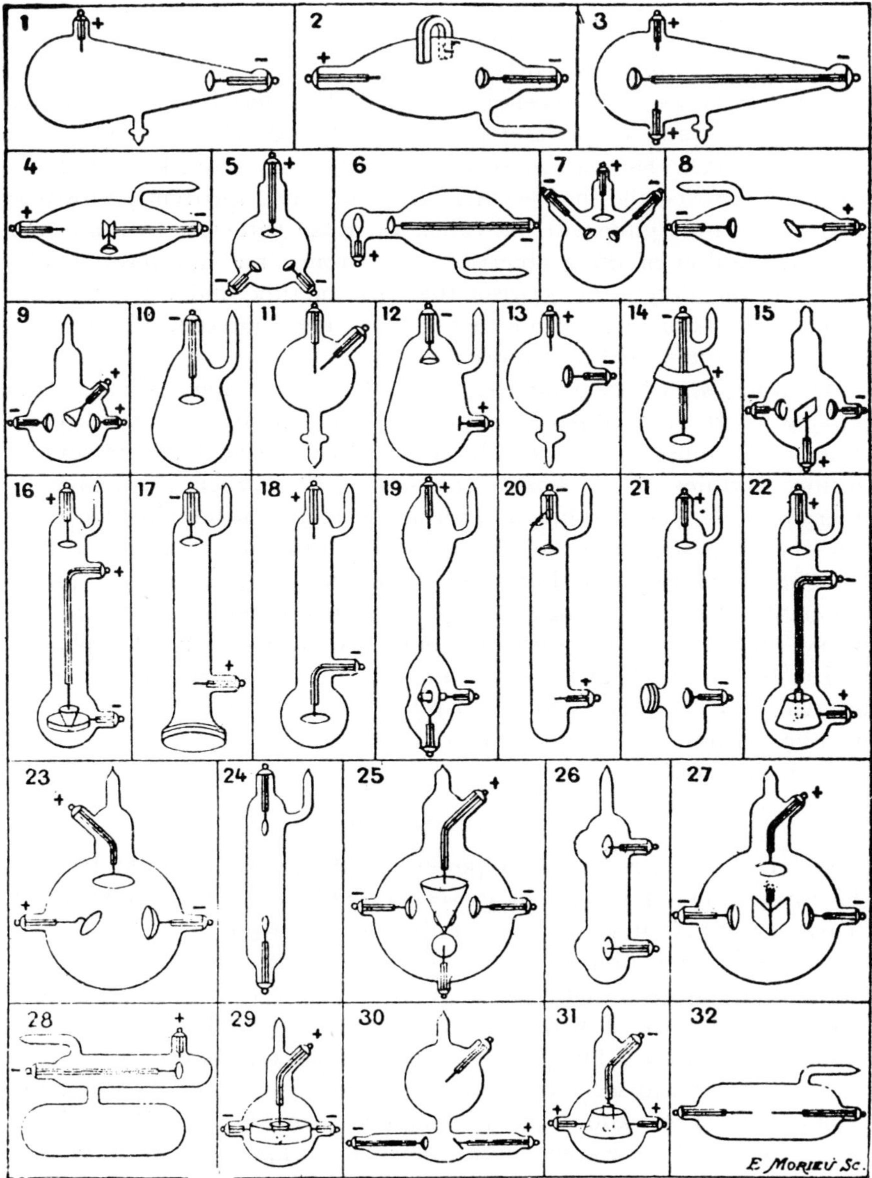

Fig. 14. From *Electrical Engineer, 22:* 668.

of the X rays filters out the softer ones and thus tends to sharpen the shadows cast, and the *diaphragm,* a sheet of lead or other metal opaque to the X rays, with a hole in the middle of it. By cutting off "stray rays," the diaphragm also sharpens the image, much as does the iris diaphragm in an ordinary camera. Both of these devices, interestingly enough, were discovered by American experimenters in February 1896, and perhaps by European workers as well.

Professor Magie of Princeton described the effectiveness of the aluminum filter quite simply and precisely in his March 1896 paper cited above (page 21). He was amazed to note that an obstacle to the rays actually improved the shadows that they cast, and, apparently unwilling to trust his own judgment, he called in other witnesses to confirm it. "In the opinion of three observers," he wrote, "the interposition of a thin plate of aluminum between the vacuum tube and the fluorescent paper of the skiascope did not merely leave the fluorescence undimmed, but actually intensified it considerably."

Dr. Burry in Chicago (above, page 22) was familiar with the "diaphragm effect" in ordinary photography. When his first X-ray plates made of a human hand on February 6, 1896, "gave but dim and indistinct outlines of the bones," he sought to sharpen the images by interposing "a lead diaphragm with an aperture one-half inch in diameter" between the Crookes tube and the photographic plate (see Plate V). The results promptly improved, although a ½-inch aperture proved too small. "By . . . increasing the aperture in the lead diaphragm," Dr. Burry continued, "and with the bulb six inches from the plate, a perfect shadowgraph of the bones in the hand, wrist, and a part of the forearm was obtained." No record has survived, however, of anyone in 1896 using both a diaphragm and a filter—common practice in modern radiology.

Power Supplies

No major improvements in power supplies were reported in 1896; the three common sources of power available previously continued to be used by the X-ray workers with only minor changes.

Like Roentgen himself, Professor Wright and most of the other American pioneers usually used an *induction coil*. It consisted essentially of two coils of wire, a primary and a secondary, both wound around an iron core. The primary winding was composed of a few turns of heavy wire; the secondary contained many turns of fine wire. One popular model was known as the Ruhmkorff coil (Fig. 15). These induction coils acted as voltage multipliers and amperage reducers; when current of low voltage and high amperage was fed into the primary, current of high voltage but low amperage emerged from the secondary.

But the induction coil had several drawbacks. It would not work on steady direct current, only on an alternating current, or on a pulsating current turned on and off many times a second by an "interrupter." Each

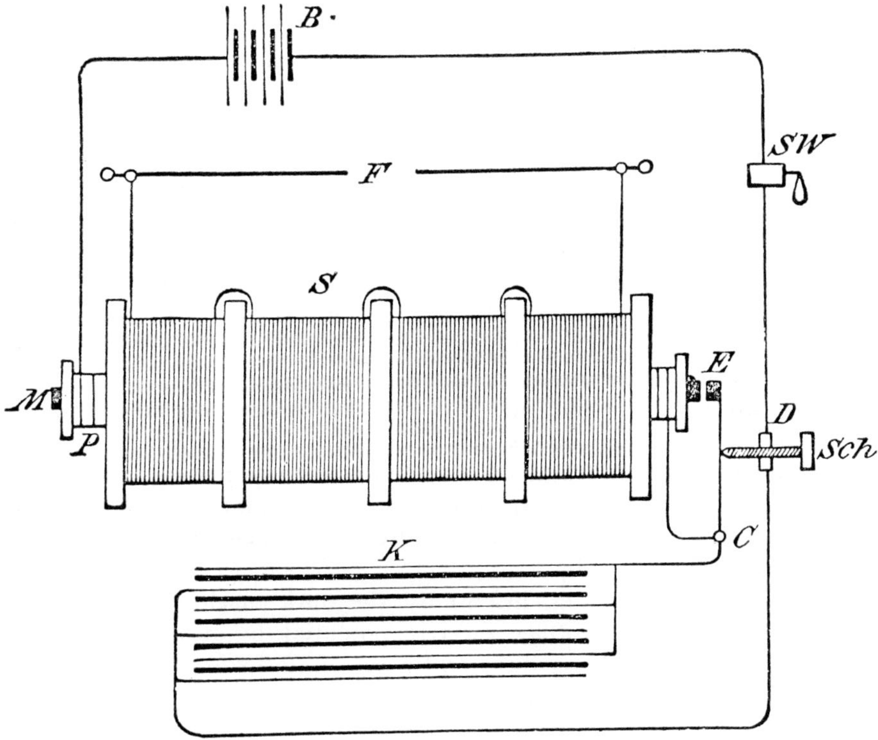

FIG. 15. From FREUND, LEOPOLD, *Elements of General Radio-therapy*, p. 57. Redman Co., New York, 1904.

time that the primary current was turned on, a surge of current moved in one direction through the secondary; each time that it was turned off, a surge in the opposite direction resulted. Thus, the induction coil yielded alternating current even when direct current was fed into it. Crookes tubes, however, worked best when fed with a steady direct current. In an effort to match the induction coil to the Crookes tube, several devices invented earlier were sometimes used.

In some laboratories, for example, direct current from storage batteries, from a generator, or from a d.c. city power system was fed into the primary of an induction coil through an interrupter which turned the current on and off at very brief intervals. A second interrupter, supposedly synchronized with the first, was then introduced into the secondary circuit; it fed half of each power cycle into the tube, so that all the current reaching the tube flowed in one direction. The difficulty was that the tube was actuated less than half the time.

A more sophisticated type of equipment was designed to feed the current into the tube in one direction during the first half of each cycle and in the reverse direction during the second half.

The interrupters available in 1896, however, were mostly rotating wheels, the rims of which were edged with alternating strips of metal and of insulating material. A metal brush rubbed against the rim, making electrical contact as each metal strip reached it and breaking contact when an insulating strip followed. The noise of the X-ray apparatus, referred to in early reports, was noise from the interrupter. Keeping one such device in good working order was difficult; keeping two of them operating synchronously was far harder. Not until 1908, when the Snook "interrupterless transformer" became available (see below, p. 202), was the power supply problem adequately solved.

As an alternative to the induction coil, Professor Frost at Dartmouth and some other X-ray workers in 1896 used a *static machine*—a type of electrical generator in common use before 1896 for the treatment of various diseases (electrotherapeutics) and for laboratory demonstration of electrical phenomena. Several hundred static machines, it was said, were also being used by lightning-rod salesmen to demonstrate the effectiveness of their wares. Essentially, the static machine was a device for producing a high-voltage electric potential by means of friction between a set of revolving disks and a set of stationary disks (Fig. 16). The disks were made of glass, hard rubber, or mica. The current generated was direct rather than alternating, and continuous rather than interrupted; it was thus excellently suited to X-ray work.

Static machines capable of delivering very high voltages were readily available in 1896; the difficulty was that they delivered very little amperage. To increase the amperage, larger and larger static machines were built in later years. They, too, were noisy, and many of them worked poorly on humid days. Thus, the 1896 radiologist's choice between induction coil and static machine was a Hobson's choice at best; he could anticipate difficulties no matter which he used.

Professor Trowbridge at Harvard used in some of his earliest experiments a *Tesla apparatus,* named for Nikola Tesla, who had developed it a few years before (Fig. 17). This was essentially a series of coils designed to step up the voltage to very high potentials, and simultaneously to increase the frequency of current alternation to millions of cycles per second by passing the current through condensers and spark gaps. It was with the help of the Tesla apparatus that Professor Trowbridge was able to capture an X-ray image in $1\frac{1}{2}$ minutes late in January 1896—as contrasted with the 15 minutes, $\frac{1}{2}$ hour, or even longer required initially by the other pioneers. But the Tesla apparatus was far from ideal for X-ray purposes; it delivered alternating instead

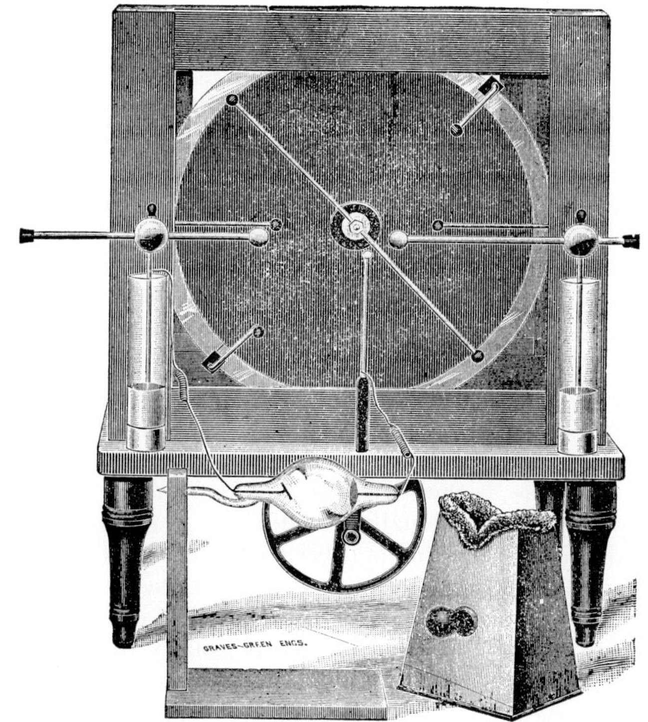

Fig. 16. Advertisement. Lent by Dr. Traian Leucutia.

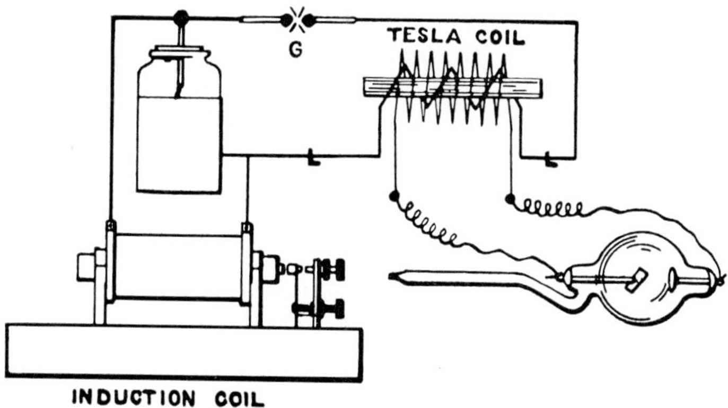

Fig. 17. From *Journal of the Franklin Institute, 143:* 212, March 1897.

of direct current, and it frequently blew out tubes. Hence, few of the pioneers preferred it to the available alternatives.

With induction coils, static machines, and the Tesla apparatus alike, moreover, three related problems plagued the early experimenters.

First, no precise measurement of the outputs of these various kinds of power supply was possible in 1896. Voltage could only be measured by a rough rule of thumb. The current was fed to a spark gap and the widest gap across which the spark would jump was measured. The number of inches of spark, multiplied by 10,000, plus 10,000, gave a rough estimate of the voltage; thus, a potential which produced a spark across a 3-inch gap was deemed to be 40,000 volts. Amperage was judged on the basis of the "fatness" of the spark; the fatter it was, the higher the presumed amperage. With such primitive measuring techniques, it was obviously difficult to know just what current was being fed into a tube, or to duplicate in one laboratory the findings reported by another.

Second, the degree of vacuum, as has been noted, varied from tube to tube and even from minute to minute within a single tube. To generate X rays in abundance, the voltage fed into the tube had to be matched to the vacuum; the higher the vacuum, the higher the voltage required. Experimenters gradually learned to gauge the characteristics and power requirements of their tubes by the tint and brightness of the fluorescence observed, and they could thus raise or lower the input voltage to keep the tube fluorescing. But again, it was difficult to repeat an experiment precisely, and impossible to convey the conditions of an experiment in repeatable form to experimenters operating different tubes in other laboratories.

The *third* vagary which plagued 1896 researchers was so subtle that most of them were unaware of its existence. X rays were later found to be nonhomogeneous. They cover a considerable band in the spectrum, varying in wavelength much as light varies in color. When a Crookes tube is activated, it emits a beam composed of X rays having varying degrees of penetrance. Some rays in the beam are "soft," barely able to pass through skin, while others may be so "hard" that they pass with ease through the thickest bones. In general, the higher the voltage fed into the tube, the "harder" the X rays emitted, but some soft rays accompany the hard rays even at maximum voltages.

At least one 1896 experimenter realized that X-ray penetration varied with input voltage. Professor Fred S. Jones of the University of Minnesota reported in the *Western Electrician* for March 21 that very high voltages produced rays which passed through bone while very low voltage produced rays to which even connective tissue was opaque. "These and other experiments," he concluded, "justify the theory that the Roentgen rays vary greatly in penetrating power, and that potential applied to the vacuum tube plays much the same role in exciting these different rays as temperature does in producing light rays, new wave lengths being excited as the temperature rises."

But Jones's report in the *Western Electrician* was either not read, or not believed, or forgotten, or simply lumped with many other reports as interesting if true. Most experimenters through the remainder of 1896 were at the mercy of whatever rays might emerge from their tubes at the voltage they happened to be using. They were thus in much the same position as photographers using a light which varied in color from minute to minute—but able neither to see the light nor to determine its color in other ways.

The story of how these and other vagaries of power supply were overcome is told in later chapters. Perhaps enough has been said here, however, to enhance our respect for the 1896 pioneers. They were like mariners with few stars and no compass, yet they explored many distant shores.

Photographic Plates

Three alternative methods of recording the X-ray image were available in 1896. Wright at Yale used bromide-coated photographic paper in his very first experiment, and for a few experiments he used Celluloid film. But he, and almost everyone else, used glass plates coated with a photographic emulsion most of the time. Hour-long "sittings" to secure an image were often needed as a result of the combined shortcomings of the tubes, the power supplies, and the photographic plates. One of the major steps taken in 1896 to shorten the time of exposure was the introduction of a fluorescent substance to supplement the direct effect of the X-rays on the photographic emulsion.

In contemporary radiology, this is accomplished by sandwiching a photographic film, coated with a light-sensitive emulsion on both sides, in between two fluorescing screens held in a filmholder or *cassette*. When the X rays reach the film, they directly affect the two emulsions. In addition, they cause the two screens to fluoresce, and the light from the screens is recorded by the emulsions along with the direct action of the X rays. Indeed, some 98 per cent of the total effect on the film is said to be contributed by the fluorescence rather than by the direct impact of the rays.

One of the pioneers who discovered this important principle was Professor Michael Pupin (1858–1935) of Columbia University. "Among the experiments made by Professor Pupin," the *Electrical World* reported on February 15, 1896, "was one to test the effect of treating the film of the negative with a fluorescent substance, which treatment appeared to increase the effect, though not so markedly as to permit any definite conclusions to be drawn." A pupil of Professor Pupin's, Max Osterberg, gave a fuller account in the *Photographic Times* for March 1896.

"It occurred to Professor Pupin," Osterberg wrote, "to paint the back of the plate shutter [cassette] with luminous paint, or to dip the sensitized plate in a luminous substance. His idea was, and the first preliminary experiments seem to be promising, that the energy from the Roentgen rays would undergo a re-transformation behind the plate shutter and, by becoming luminous, mark a greater contrast between light and shadow."

In later years, Professor Pupin's account of his discovery grew by accretion. Thus, he wrote in his 1930 autobiography, *From Immigrant to Inventor:*

> The late Dr. Bull of New York sent me a patient, a Mr. Prescott Hall Butler, with nearly a hundred small shot in his left hand. He was in agony; he and I had mutual friends who begged me to make an X-ray photograph of his hand and thus enable Dr. Bull to locate the numerous shot and extract them. The first attempts were unsuccessful, because the patient was too weak and too nervous to stand a photographic exposure of nearly an hour. My good friend, Thomas Edison, had sent me several most excellent fluorescent screens, and by their fluorescence I could see the numerous little shot, and so could my patient. The combination of the screen and the eyes was evidently much more sensitive than the photographic plate. I decided to try a combination of Edison's fluorescent screen and the photographic plate. The fluorescent screen was placed on the photographic plate and the patient's hand was placed upon the screen. The X rays acted upon the screen first and the screen by its fluorescent light acted upon the plate. The combination succeeded, even better than I had expected. A beautiful photograph was obtained with the exposure of a few seconds. The photographic plate showed the numerous shot as if they had been drawn with pen and ink.

Pupin mistakenly added, "That was the first X-ray picture obtained by that process during the first part of February 1896, and it was also the first surgical operation performed in America under the guidance of an X-ray picture."

Pupin's memory erred in several respects. The New York *Daily Tribune* reported February 16, 1896, that Dr. Bull's patient had come to Professor Pupin only the day before, "with about 20 small shot lodged in his hand and wrist." He wanted an X-ray taken, but Professor Pupin could not oblige because his tubes were not ready. The patient returned 2 days later, and this time, the *Daily Tribune* reported, "Professor Pupin subjected the hand to an hour's exposure"—not an "exposure of a few seconds"—with a fluorescent screen. The image secured by Professor Pupin revealed about 50 shots in the hand; it is reproduced as Plate VI. Edison's fluoroscope had nothing to do with the matter; indeed, Pupin conceived the idea of intensifying the photographic effect with the help of a fluorescing substance before Edison conceived of the fluoroscope.

In Philadelphia at about the same time, a well-known manufacturer of photographic plates, John Carbutt (1832–1905), was also experimenting with techniques for producing X-ray plates with shorter exposure times.

"Naturally," Carbutt explained, "the announcement of Professor Roentgen's discovery of photographing the invisible, with what he terms X rays, attracted my attention, the more so as I saw that a new field had been opened up for the use of dry plates. The length of exposure required particularly interested me, and I therefore commenced experiments to produce, if possible, a plate that should be more sensitive to these X rays than the ordinary rapid plate." [7] He was promptly successful. Using Professor Goodspeed's equipment at the University of Pennsylvania, he was able to produce with a 20-minute exposure negatives superior to those taken with ordinary plates during 1-hour exposure.

Carbutt reported his success, and exhibited two of his plates, at a meeting of the Franklin Institute in Philadelphia on February 19, but he pointedly did not reveal what he had done to speed up the plates.

Professor Goodspeed let Carbutt's secret slip at a meeting of the American Philosophical Society in Philadelphia 2 nights later. He displayed there slides of negatives which had been successfully exposed for a mere 1 to 5 minutes. "These slides," he explained, "were . . . prepared to demonstrate the efficiency of a plate especially sensitized by Mr. John Carbutt of this city for this work. He conceived the idea that the photographic plate might be rendered more sensitive to this energy, *if the film were treated with some fluorescent substance.* Mr. Carbutt very kindly placed in our hands some of the special plates."* Goodspeed compared them with very rapid untreated photographic plates and reported that the Carbutt plate after fluorescent treament "seems to have been considerably more sensitive than the other." [8] Carbutt may or may not have picked up the idea by reading the *Electrical World*'s account of Professor Pupin's experiment, published a few days before.

In Montreal, much the same plan as Pupin's and Carbutt's was emerging also in the mind of John Cox of McGill at about the same time. In a letter dated February 18, 1896, Cox described two "main ideas I have found time to try—increasing the sensitiveness of the

---

* Italics added.

plate by (1) placing a fluorescing screen inside the holder in contact with it; (2) soaking the plate in the fluorescing substances." [9]

However, Cox did not claim priority. On the contrary, he pointed out in his letter of February 18 that the same experiments "have been successfully carried out by Heinrich Geissler, of Bonn [Germany]; so that I have nothing new...." Others, of course, may have preceded Geissler.

Although the principle of using fluorescence to buttress the direct effect of the X rays on photographic emulsions was thus repeatedly discovered in February 1896, the practical application of the principle was not perfected for many years. The images produced with the help of fluorescence tended to be "grainy," matching the grain of the fluorescing substance, and it was often difficult to determine whether variations seen on the plate were due to variations in the object being X-rayed or to variations in the fluorescing screen. In this as in a number of other respects, the ingenuity of the 1896 pioneers tended to exceed the capacity of the materials and equipment available to them. That they accomplished as much as they did in the face of the obstacles they encountered was the most remarkable feature of the first year of radiology.

REFERENCES

1. *Electrical World, 27:* 377, 1896.
2. *Ibid.,* p. 484.
3. Unpublished biographical data made available by Miss Ann Sayen.
4. *Electrical World, 27:* 219, 1896.
5. *Amer. J. Sci.,* 4th series, *1:* 245–246, 1896.
6. GLASSER, O., *Dr. W. C. Roentgen,* Ed. 2, pp. 73–74. Charles C Thomas, Springfield, Ill., 1958.
7. *J. Franklin Inst., 141:* 261–265, 1896.
8. *Proc. Amer. Phil. Soc., 35:* 22, 1896.
9. *Ibid.,* pp. 34–35.

5   Putting the X Rays to Work

Armed only with unreliable Crookes tubes, inadequate power supplies, and relatively insensitive photographic plates, the 1896 X-ray workers proceeded industriously to explore the potential usefulness of the new rays in many branches of medicine and in other fields as well.

At McGill University in Montreal, Professor Cox (above, page 18) and his associate, Professor Hugh L. Calendar, reported in May 1896 on a series of patients brought to them by physicians for X-ray examination. The following half-dozen they described as "the more difficult cases which we have attempted":

Bullet in brain of child, aged 12. The bullet and the hole by which it entered are clearly shown in a photograph with an exposure of nine minutes. The bullet was faintly visible on another plate with an exposure of three minutes. It was found to have settled down nearly in the centre of the brain.

Broken hip joint. An exposure of fifteen minutes was allowed for this case, as the subject was a man of solid build. The head of the thigh bone was found to have been broken off and twisted round. The foramina and other details of the pelvis are clearly shown. The negative is so dense that it takes more than half an hour to print in bright sunshine.

Drainage tube in lung. This was a case of a small drainage tube of ebonite, No. 9 catheter, which was lost in the lung eleven years ago. Owing to its thinness and to the comparative transparency of ebonite, the tube was a somewhat faint object, but was quite unmistakeably visible in the negative.

Fracture of the skull. The subject had been gored by a bull two years previously, and had lost one eye and part of the bone of the orbit. He had lately become subject to fits. The negative showed a vague white shadow in the neighborhood of the gap in the skull, which may have been due to a piece of displaced bone, or to some bony growth. The indications are too indefinite, however, to be of much use in diagnosis.

Pus cavity in lung. In this case the diagnosis from the ordinary methods was very uncertain. A cavity, however, was very clearly indicated as a dark shadow in the negative. If the cavity had been full of pus at the time, it would have been indicated by a lighter patch, the transparency of liquid being less than that of lung tissue when distended with air.

Stone in kidney. Some of the typical symptoms were absent in this case. The X-ray negative showed a faint white patch in the region of the kidney.

In addition to the above, which include the more difficult medical cases, a very large number of simpler cases of fractures, etc., of the extremities were taken, as well as photographs of various parts of the healthy body including the skull and trunk.[1]

A number of the 1896 X-ray workers were concerned with medical research as well as practice. Among the first was Dr. Edward Parker Davis (1856–1937), professor of obstetrics at Jefferson Medical College, who performed his first X-ray trials in February 1896 and reported on them in the March issue of the *American Journal of the Medical Sciences*.

Dr. Davis's goal was to secure the image of an unborn fetus inside the maternal uterus. Assisted by electricians and photographers, his first step was to X-ray a fetal skull inside a female pelvis taken from a cadaver. The results indicated at least the possibility that a living fetus *in utero* might be successfully portrayed on an X-ray plate. X rays were accordingly next taken of a living 3-day-old baby, and the baby was examined with one of Magie's "skiascopes." Only after these preliminary trials were successful did Dr. Davis venture to try his equipment on a pregnant woman.

The patient was "a girl, aged eighteen years, pregnant eight and a half months, her fetus occupying the usual position in the womb." She was stretched out comfortably on a clinical table, and a photographic plate was placed against her abdomen. "It was interesting to observe . . . ," Dr. Davis declared, "that the proximity of the electrical apparatus seemed to have no disturbing effect on the patient. She was informed that an effort would be made to ascertain the position of the child by the use of the electric light; she readily consented to the attempt, and, aside from the slight fatigue from remaining quiet in one position, she seemed to be soothed by the constant sound of the apparatus, her pulse not varying through the entire time."

The first exposure of this patient lasted 1 hour and failed. The second lasted 1¼ hours. ". . . The faint outline of the trunk of her fetus could be recognized," Dr. Davis stated, "the darker shadow of its pelvis occupying the upper right-hand portion of the plate, while projecting downward at about the center were irregular white masses showing the situation of the fetal limbs. The head of the child was so hidden by the mother's pelvis that no indication of its presence was obtained. While this experiment failed to outline distinctly the skeleton of the fetus, it offers information which may be of value in further attempts." Dr. Davis reported in March that he had already examined 10 patients, and he noted that X rays might be of obstetrical use in several ways: to determine the position and attitude of the fetus; to determine the outlines of a contracted pelvis; to diagnose an abnormal condition of the fetus, such as a tumor; to reveal an accumulation of fluid within a cavity of the fetal body, as shown by the abnormal contour of the fetal tissues; to reveal the presence of more than one fetus in the uterus.

"The attempt to obtain information by this method is certainly a justifiable one," Dr. Davis stated, "as it requires no exposure of the patient, no vaginal manipulation, and puts her to no essential discomfort." He concluded, "There has not been the slightest evidence that the passage of the rays through the uterus has affected either mother or child."

The ophthalmologists, too, were soon adapting the new rays to the needs of their specialty. The *Ophthalmic Review* for August 1896 cited two examples. A Dr. Clark of Columbus, Ohio, had a patient with a small fragment of metal buried somewhere in or near his eye. The patient was anesthetized with ether, a tiny photographic plate (probably a strip of film) was introduced into his nostril, and the rays were directed through the eye toward the plate. The metal fragment was found. Dr. Charles H. Williams of Boston reported an even more remarkable case in which a fragment of a copper cartridge case was found deep in the eye during an X-ray exposure in which the rays passed through the entire thickness of the skull (see below, page 72).

Dr. William J. Morton of New York City, one of the most enthusiastic of the pioneers, presented an eloquent account of clinical progress in a paper delivered before the Medical Society of the County of New York on April 27, 1896, published in the *Medical Record* (New York) for July 4.

"Physicians, from time immemorial," Dr. Morton began, "have ever had a keen desire to explore the interior of the animal body. Hence arose dissection, and later on vivisection, and still later on the revelations of the microscope. But none of these methods fully satisfy the wish to know what is actually taking place within the animal organism during life.... No wonder then that the X ray with its marvelous revelations of the hitherto unseen has excited a universal interest."

His audience already knew, of course, how foreign bodies could be located and broken bones precisely set with the aid of the new rays; Dr. Morton pointed out that it was also possible "to detect and to diagnosticate irregularities, deformities, malformations, congenital or otherwise, of bones," and to identify dislocations as well as fractures—"the coexistence of both or the existence of one to the exclusion of the other. Diseases of the bones which vary their density, either by increasing or diminishing it, like exostoses, tuberculosis, and sarcoma, are clearly located. One of the radiographs I have presented ... locates what is presumed to be tuberculous disease, and is certainly some form of disease of bones of the wrist, in a case which has thus far for five years defied diagnosis and treatment. An operation, soon to be made, and not justifiable for mere ordinary exploration, will soon decide upon the nature of this disease."

Another promising field of research, Dr. Morton noted, was "the detection of calcareous infiltrations [calcium deposits] involving, for instance, the arteries, or occurring in the lungs and other tissues." Kidney stones, bladder stones, and stones in the salivary ducts "have already been successfully located."

But Dr. Morton's most sensational announcement went much further. "One of the most unexpected . . . but obviously one of the most useful applications of the X ray," he declared, was in the study of *soft* tissues which do not cast a sharp shadow as bone or calcium deposits do. "In the radiograph of the infant the liver is plainly shown in outline, the heart is shown and mapped out in relation to the usual landmarks. Organs distended with gas, such as the stomach and intestines, allow the X rays to pass freely, and thus the record of their location and size is made." This early recognition of the importance of gas as a "contrast medium" was to be followed by many major radiological advances based both on the natural presence of gas in the body and on its deliberate introduction for X-ray purposes (see below, pp. 219–229). Dr. Morton correctly predicted:

> These findings in relation to the soft tissues upon a radiograph are but the beginnings of a new art of diagnosis. In delineating and demarcating the organs and tissues, we shall soon arrive at refinements of method and of technique in relation to time of exposure, posturing, etc., . . . for an exposure may be so timed as to depict clearly the soft tissues and their interrelations. An overexposure, for instance, effaces every record upon the plate except that of the bones and may even easily efface that, while an underexposure gives a negative which is full of delicate ghost-like and yet clearly defined outlines of skin, muscle, tendon, veins, and arteries. . . .
>
> But stranger still are the revelations of looking through the living fleshly body by aid of the fluoroscope. First are seen the vertebrae, the greater bones, the ribs, and then to the astonished gaze, in dark outline but moving, may be seen the beating of the heart, the rise and fall of the ribs in respiration, and the movements and rhythmic displacement of organs. I have seen these organs plainly outlined and noted changes in their density due to disease.

Stereoscopic X-ray techniques added to the early wonder. Professor Elihu Thomson, in the *Electrical Engineer* for March 11, 1896, was the first to report on this possibility.

"While experimenting with the making of [X-ray] shadow pictures," Thomson wrote, "it occurred to the writer that it would be desirable to secure some indication in space of various imbedded solid objects, or, in other words, to obtain a pair of pictures which, when placed in a stereoscope, would show solidity. This would manifestly be useful in surgical examinations, as the true relations in space of the parts of a bone, or of a foreign body and the bone would become evident."

The technique of making stereoscopic photographs had been well-known for decades; a photographer simply took a picture, moved his camera 1 inch or so, and took a second. When the two pictures were then viewed in a stereoscopic viewer, so that one eye saw only one picture and the other eye only the other, the illusion of depth and solidity was readily achieved, and it was easy to judge the relative position of objects in the foreground, middle ground, and background. Professor Thomson simply followed the same procedure with a Crookes tube instead of a camera, exposing two plates with the tube in slightly different positions. Then paper prints made from the negatives were mounted for use in an ordinary stereoscopic viewer.

"The first trial made by the author was completely successful," he wrote with justifiable pride, "objects appearing in high relief.... The effect is curious. A cork or block of wood having nails or screws driven into it in various directions is clearly shown and the screws or nails in their proper positions. When two heavily insulated wires constitute the object, the metal wires alone are seen, but standing apart in space, one around the other. The bones of two superposed figures are to be seen in their correct positions."

Now that the X rays were readily available, were surgeons justified in continuing to perform operations without first making X-ray studies? This question arose within a few weeks after Wright of Yale and Trowbridge of Harvard made the first North American X-ray plates. An unnamed but "eminent" physician was quoted as remarking at a meeting of the Philadelphia Photographic Society held February 12, 1896, that "even with our present limited knowledge of this new discovery, it would now hardly be admissible to probe for extraneous matter in the human body without the aid of this method." [2] In the March 6 issue of *Science*, Professor Henry W. Cattell of the University of Pennsylvania went considerably further. "The manifold uses to which Roentgen's discovery may be applied in medicine are so obvious," Professor Cattell declared, "that it is even now questionable whether a surgeon would be morally justified in performing a certain class of operations without first having seen pictured by these rays the field of his work—a map, as it were, of the unknown country he is to explore."

Similar remarks are scattered throughout the medical literature of 1896, and many patients consulted X-ray workers seeking evidence on which to base malpractice suits. Before the end of the year, Dr. Maurice H. Richardson, of Harvard and the Massachusetts General Hospital, was stressing this hazard to his fellow surgeons in a lecture on "The Practical Value of the Roentgen-Ray in the Routine Work of Surgical Office Practice." No surgical consulting room, he insisted, "is fully equipped without an apparatus for X-ray investigation." Indeed, he urged that the fluoroscope be used before and the X-ray negative after each operation—the fluoroscope to protect the patient from surgical error, and the negative to protect the surgeon from malpractice charges. Dr. Richardson concluded that an X-ray apparatus of his own "is as essential to the surgeon as the mirror to the laryngologist, or the stethoscope to the general practitioner." [3]

In contrast to Dr. Richardson's suggestion that each surgeon equip his own office with X-ray apparatus, many physicians and surgeons preferred to refer their patients to specialists in the new field. Among the early specialists was Dr. Otto L. Schmidt, professor of medicine at the Chicago Polyclinic and physician at the Alexian Brothers Hospital in Chicago, who opened an X-ray laboratory early in the year. In *Medicine* (Detroit), June 1896, he described a number of cases referred to him by others, and concluded his paper by saying, "Dr. F. C. Harnisch and I, who are associated in this work, desire to extend an invitation to the readers of *Medicine* to inspect the negatives and the apparatus in our laboratory."

Whether or not physicians actually visited the Schmidt-Harnisch laboratory, they sent patients in large numbers; soon Dr. Schmidt and Dr. Harnisch could not handle the crowd and turned the laboratory over to an electrical engineer, the German-born Wolfram C. Fuchs (1865–1908). It became the Fuchs X-Ray Laboratory (Plate VII), and by the end of 1896, it was reported, Fuchs had performed more than 1400 X-ray examinations—striking evidence of the enormous demand for X-ray services.

Photographers, electrical engineers, and laymen of other kinds also made X-ray services available to the public in 1896. "Mr. M. D. Martin has opened an X-ray studio at 110 East 26th Street," the *Electrical Engineer* reported on June 3, "where pictures of the interior human structure, etc., will be taken. The consultation hours are from 1 to 2 and 5 to 6. A lady assistant is in attendance." But none of the others achieved the success or the respect in medical circles earned by the Fuchs Laboratory in Chicago, which continued to play a significant role in the development of X-ray diagnostic techniques until the death of Fuchs from cancer in 1908 (see below, page 165).

Free X-ray service was another 1896 curiosity. In Denver, Colorado, Colonel C. F. Lacombe of the Mountain Electric Company set up an X-ray apparatus for his own interest early in 1896 and offered to make X-ray plates without charge as a public service. His laboratory, Dr. W. Walter Wasson of Denver later recalled, was "besieged by persons who were certain that their physicians were wrong, and wanted X-ray photographs to prove it." [4] Colonel Lacombe thereupon established a rule that no patient would be X-rayed unless his physician was present.

In addition to the X-ray equipment in physical laboratories, doctors' offices, and independent laboratories or "studios," some pioneering hospitals began installing X-ray apparatus early in 1896. The magazine *Electricity* reported on February 12 that the Presbyterian Hospital in New York City and the Surgical Department of Columbia College were securing the necessary equipment. The *University Medical Magazine* noted in September 1896 that the Laboratory of Clinical Medicine at University Hospital in Philadelphia already had a "Roentgen plant," and that "by October 1 another complete plant will be installed in the Department of Clinical Surgery."

Beginnings were also made during 1896 in the exploration of the therapeutic use of the new rays. Attention naturally focused first on its use in killing germs. The *Medical News* reported on February 22:

> It is a well-known fact that sunlight possesses a decidedly germicidal effect, and that if the prismatic rays be passed through a culture-tube containing a fluid medium, the various bacilli therein will exhibit a selective action. And it has occurred to more than one worker along the lines of bacteriological investigation that it was quite within the realm of possibility that the Roentgen ray would be found capable of killing bacteria within the human system.
>
> During the past week, in order to test the influence of the Roentgen rays upon germ life, pure cultures of diphtheria bacilli were obtained from Dr. W. H. Park, of the bacteriological laboratory of the New York Board of Health, and subjected to the direct effect of the rays from a Crookes tube for thirty minutes. Cultures were made both before and after the exposure, which were personally developed in the laboratory by Dr. Park, who reports that no effect whatever was discovered. . . .

Despite these initial negative results, the successful killing of bacteria was later reported from time to time, and many cases of tuberculosis and other infectious diseases were treated with X rays in 1896. Dr. J. William White at the University of Pennsylvania, and perhaps other physicians here and abroad, began cautious experiments in the use of the rays against cancer (see below, page 137).

The remarkable ability of the new rays to suppress inflammation and pain was generally overlooked by physicians—although not by patients. An amusing case was reported in a letter to the editor of the *Boston Medical and Surgical Journal* for September 3, 1896:

A NEW USE FOR THE X-RAYS

BOSTON, August 31, 1896

MR. EDITOR:—About three weeks ago I examined with the Roentgen rays an old fracture near the ankle-joint, in a stout woman of fifty. She had been complaining off and on of the pain in the left ankle. I found a fracture at the lower part of the tibia.... There was slight impairment of the movements of the joint, but the result, on the whole, was good.

After examining with the fluoroscope, I took photographs of the ankle, with an exposure of about five minutes. I have just received the following letter, which suggests a new use for the X-rays:

August 25th.

MY DEAR DR. RICHARDSON:—I feel that I should write and tell you the splendid effect the X-rays had on my foot. It is now three weeks since I was at your office, and I have not had one particle of pain since. The swelling and soreness have disappeared also. My family think it is all imagination, but that is impossible, because all that I expected from the rays was what you might discern....

Yours gratefully,

——— ———

The remarkable improvement in the case reminds me of the occasional cures which are by some patients attributed to the use of the clinical thermometer twice daily.

Yours very truly,
M. H. RICHARDSON, M.D.

In retrospect, it seems quite possible that the patient was right, and that Dr. Richardson was wrong to scoff. Not until many patients had similarly reported benefits did American physicians begin to take seriously the possibility that the X rays might in fact be effective in the relief of inflammation and consequent suppression of pain (see below, page 148).

Among the unusual uses of the X rays in North America was one reported in the *Scientific American* for December 23, 1896. A youth of uncertain age was arrested in Cincinnati for striking and seriously injuring a fellow workman. At the time of his arrest he gave his age as 19, but, upon realizing the seriousness of the criminal charge against him, he and his father insisted that he was only 17 years old and was therefore entitled to the benefits of an Ohio law preventing a prisoner under 18 from being tried in a criminal court. The magazine reported:

Thoroughly convinced that the youth was at least 18 years old, the juvenile court physician decided to have X-ray photographs made of the epiphyseal bones of his hand, elbow, and hip, and also photos of the same bones of a 17-year-old youth. Comparison, it was hoped, would then settle the matter, as it is a known fact in medical circles that when a boy reaches the age of 18 years 'hose bones become hardened.

The photographs developed from the X-ray pictures of the bones of the boys showed that those of the 17-year-old boy had not hardened, but those of the defendant in the case had done so. The physician immediately fixed the age of the prisoner as 18 years or more.

Dental as well as medical uses of the rays were explored quite early. Dr. William J. Morton of New York made what was no doubt the first North American dental X-ray report at a meeting of the New York Odontological Society on April 24, 1896. "The density of the teeth is greater than that of the bone which surrounds them," Dr. Morton explained, "and for that reason pictures of the living teeth may be taken by the X ray, even of each wandering fang or root, however deeply imbedded in its socket. Also, children's teeth may be photographed before they have escaped from the gums, and the extent and area and location of metallic fillings may be sharply delineated, even though concealed from outer view.

"The lost end of a broken drill may be found, and, what is most interesting, even the central cavity of the tooth may be outlined, so that diseases within the tooth may be detected. It is equally obvious that diseases of the bone and other tissues in the neighborhood of the teeth may be observed." [5]

Some dentists promptly took notice. At the meetings of the Southern Dental Association in Ashville, North Carolina, in July 1896, Dr. C. Edmund Kells, Jr., of New Orleans, "exhibited his method of taking skiagraphs of the roots of the teeth *in situ* in living subjects.... A plate, or rather film holder, is made, containing a pocket for holding the film as close to the bone as possible, and having articulated surfaces into which the teeth bite down, thus holding the film absolutely steady during the sitting. [Dr. Kells] presented skiagraphs, taken in from five to fifteen minutes, showing the perfect outlines of the roots of the teeth in the bone...." [6]

A slightly different dental X-ray device was designed by William Rollins of Boston and described in the *Boston Medical and Surgical Journal* for July 23, 1896. It consisted essentially of the familiar dentist's mirror mounted at the end of a rod, but with a small film-holder where the mirror would ordinarily be (Fig. 18). "To use the instrument," Rollins directed, "cut disks from a Kodak film and place six or more [in the holder] with thin disks of aluminum between, enclosing them water and light tight.... Give full exposure to the first film. As each film has less exposure than the one in front of it, the appearances vary and one is sure to give the information sought."

The use of X rays in industry was also pioneered in 1896. Trade papers in February noted that the new rays had been used in an attempt to de-

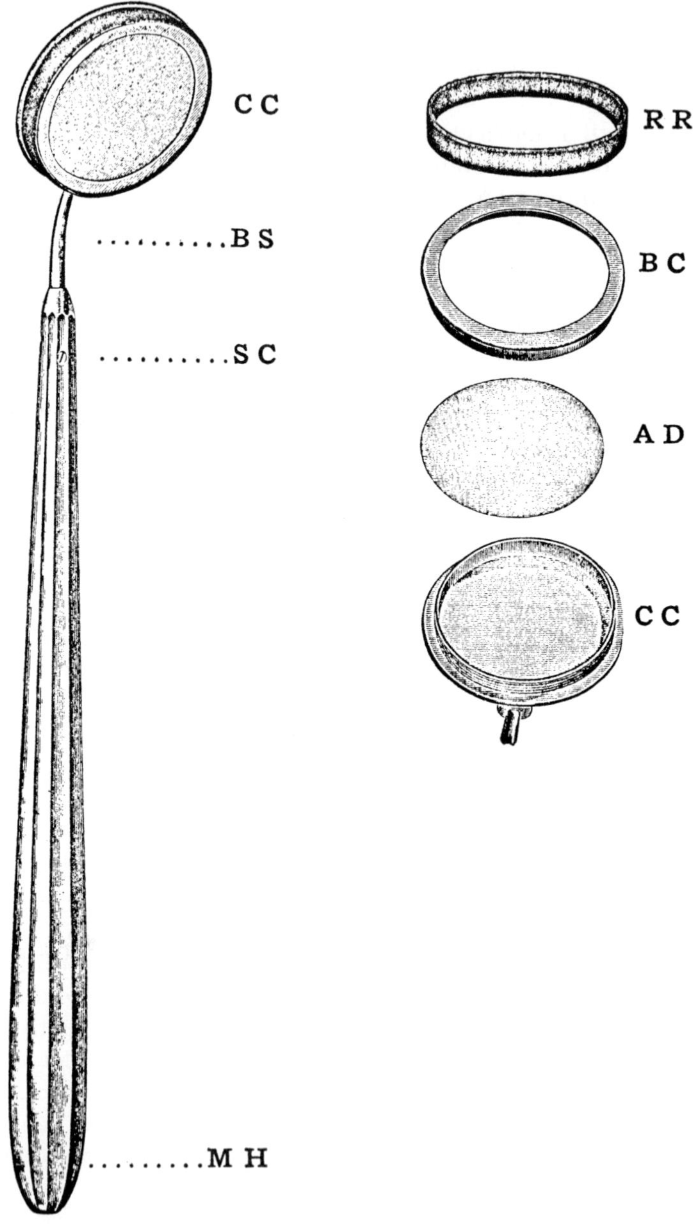

FIG. 18. From ROLLINS, WILLIAMS, *Notes on X-Light*, Plate 2. Privately printed, Boston, 1904.

tect flaws in iron castings at the Carnegie Steel Works. Professor Robb at Trinity College, and no doubt others as well, used X rays in February to distinguished real diamonds (transparent to the rays) from fake diamonds (which were opaque). Also, suggestions were made early that the rays could be used to detect the adulteration of foods, drugs, and other articles of commerce. But the countless subsequent discoveries of nonmedical uses of the rays, here and in Europe, fall outside the scope of this volume.

REFERENCES

1. *Trans. Roy. Soc. Canad.*, Ser. 2, *2:* sect III, 171–191, 1896.
2. *Electrical World, 27:* 201, 1896.
3. *Med. News, 69:* 685–688, 1896.
4. Personal communication.
5. Morton, W. J., *The X-Ray*, p. 150. American Technical Book Company, New York, 1896; see also *Dent. Cosmos, 38:* 478–486, 1896.
6. *Dent. Cosmos, 38:* 1012, 1899.

6 Francis H. Williams: America's First Radiologist

Outstanding among the physicians who turned to the X rays as a specialty during 1896 was Dr. Francis Henry Williams (1852–1936) of Boston, a man admirably suited by training, experience, and temperament to pioneer in the use of Roentgen's rays for medical diagnosis. Dr. Williams had graduated from the Massachusetts Institute of Technology before taking his medical degree; hence, unlike many of his fellow physicians then and now, he could talk to the physicists in their own language. His work with X rays at Boston City Hospital eloquently testifies to the fruitfulness of such close collaboration between the medical and physical sciences.

Collaboration between M.I.T. and City Hospital was first described in the *Boston Medical and Surgical Journal* (now the *New England Journal of Medicine*) for February 20, 1896. "The picture on the opposite page," said an unsigned editorial note in the *Journal,* "exhibits an extremely rare anomaly of the phalangeal bones shown by the Roentgen process. The picture is taken from a patient in the Boston City Hospital, by the kind cooperation of the Department of Physics at the Massachusetts Institute of Technology with gentlemen connected with the hospital. The picture has a twofold attraction: (1) as an excellent example of the new process; (2) as an instance of an interesting and instructive anomaly."

Whether Williams was one of the "gentlemen connected with the hospital" who arranged for this initial cooperative X-ray effort is not known, but 2 months later Williams and his friends at M.I.T.—Messrs. Charles L. Norton and Ralph R. Lawrence—were hard at work together.

"At the meeting of the Suffolk District Medical Society which was held in Walker Hall of the Massachusetts Institute of Technology on April 25th," the same *Journal* reported on April 30, 1896, "Dr. Francis H. Williams gave an extremely interesting demonstration of the work that had been done at the Institute of Technology in developing the application of the X rays, and in particular of the fluoroscope to medical purposes." The usual demonstrations of hand and wrist were shown at the April 25 meeting, but "more wonderful than what was actually shown to the audience," the editor of the *Journal* noted, "was **Dr.** Williams's account of what had been accomplished with the fluoroscope in the diagnosis of diseases of the thorax. Dr. Williams and Messrs. Norton and Lawrence had found the thorax much more transparent to the X rays than the abdomen. The lungs were particularly transparent, the rays passing clearly through them, and the outline of the ribs being plainly seen. The liver was comparatively opaque to the rays, and they were able to mark out accurately the position of the upper border of the liver in extreme inspiration and expiration, and there was found to be a difference of three inches in these levels."

The climax of the April 25 meeting came when Dr. Williams brought in a patient from the City Hospital who had a greatly enlarged heart. The outline of the heart, as determined by percussion, had been drawn on the skin of the man's chest, but this outline could not be seen through the shirt he was wearing. With the shirt still on, Dr. Williams proceeded to draw upon it the outline of the heart as it appeared on the screen of the fluoroscope. When the shirt was removed, the editor of the *Journal* reported, the outline that Williams had drawn on it "everywhere corresponded very closely with the area previously drawn on the skin by percussion." And the editor concluded, "Dr. Williams was warmly applauded at the close of his most interesting and successful demonstration."

No doubt the deeply impressed editor of the *Journal* solicited further details, for the next day Dr. Williams wrote him a letter which also appeared in the April 30 issue. "During the past few weeks, . . . " Williams stated, "I have tested the application of the rays to medical practice in various ways. . . . Our aim has been to make the rays pass through the body; and recently [April 22] this was attained, when Mr. Norton saw in a dark room by means of the fluoroscope the ribs and backbone of an adult. On the same evening I examined Mr. Norton from behind, and saw, besides his ribs and backbone, that the lighter portion of the area of the right lung was limited below by a darker outline at about the height of the fourth rib, and that this outline moved up and down with expiration and inspiration. Evidently this was the upper border of the liver . . ."

Following other preliminaries of this kind, Dr. Williams's letter continued:

> It seemed to me desirable to examine some of my patients by the X rays.
> The first case was that of a man with an enlarged heart (seven inches in transverse diameter). I found that the outline of the heart, as seen from the front of the body through the fluoroscope, corresponded in a general way to the outline drawn on the skin with percussion as a guide. Messrs. Norton and Lawrence confirmed my ob-

servation. It was interesting to note that the heart could be made out through the man's waistcoat and two shirts.

The next case was that of a man with an enlarged spleen who had leukemia. The outline of this spleen could be followed in part; but it was so obvious by palpation that the latter was a readier way of tracing it.

One of the most interesting cases was that of a patient suffering from tuberculosis of the right lung, who was under the care of one of my colleagues. . . . After looking at him from behind for a moment, the difference in the amount of rays which passed through the two sides of the chest was very striking, as seen through the fluoroscope. The diseased lung, as I had predicted, being darker throughout than the normal lung. The ribs on the left side were much more distinct than those on the right, and the heart of this patient could be seen more clearly than usual.

Already Williams was applying what was to become one of the hallmarks of his diagnostic approach: a thorough study of the normal, and then a comparison of the pathological with it. "In a patient convalescing from pneumonia," he declared in his April 26 letter, "the part of the lung which was affected was darker as seen through the fluoroscope than normal." Williams concluded with a prediction: "My observations show that the X rays will be serviceable to physicians as well as surgeons, and it will soon be possible to use them to greater advantage than at present."

Dr. Williams's own work during the next few years was one of the major factors in making that prediction come abundantly true.

His studies prior to 1896 had earned him membership in the Association of American Physicians, then as now composed of outstanding clinical investigators, known a bit sardonically as "The Immortals." This august association met in Washington on April 30, 1896, and Dr. Williams there presented his latest findings, which were duly published in the Association's 1896 *Transactions*. He started, as was customary, with some surgical cases.

"My brother, Dr. Charles H. Williams," he reported, "lately brought a patient to me for examination who was thought to have a piece of copper in one of his eyes. I was not very sanguine about the result of the examination, and we therefore first tested the matter in a rough way by placing a piece of bent copper wire . . . on one of Mr. Norton's temples. The Crookes tube was placed near his temple and the photographic plate on the other side of the head, in order to make the test as severe as possible." Williams, in short, was attempting the experiment which had so often balked Edison, an exposure through the human skull. "Finding that the wire could be easily seen in the negative, even though placed far from the plate, we then proceeded to photograph the patient's eye, which we placed near the plate to give it every possible advantage. The position of the eyeball could be distinctly seen in the picture, and in about the center of the eye was a spot corresponding, as we thought, to the piece of copper said to have penetrated it. Dr. [Charles H.] Williams then operated and found and removed a piece of copper $\frac{1}{8}$ by $\frac{1}{4}$ of an inch, which was similar in shape to what we had seen in the negative."

But it was medical rather than surgical X-ray diagnosis which most interested Williams, and he went on to describe both the normal and the pathological states of various organs as viewed through the fluoroscope.

"Below the left lung," he told his fellow Immortals, "is seen the spleen, and by raising and lowering the Crookes tube while looking through the fluoroscope one may so adjust the tube as to follow the outline of the spleen completely, and also to see the lower border of the liver on the right side. By looking through the body from side to side with the fluoroscope, the observer being on the patient's right, the whole outline of the great mass of the liver may, under favorable conditions, be seen hanging in the vault of the diaphragm. On examining one patient, I found that he could move his liver by inspiration and expiration less than an inch [as compared with a normal three inches], and as there was a history of localized peritonitis a year previously, it is possible there were adhesions limiting the movement of the liver. The pulsations of the heart may be followed with the fluoroscope, not only the ventricular, but also the auricular contractions and dilations."

Dr. Williams then reviewed the same cases he had presented in Boston 5 days earlier, including the case of tuberculosis, and cautiously pointed out that with the aid of the fluoroscope, "we may in some cases . . . have an earlier warning of the diseases than by the other physical signs hitherto at our disposal."

For work like this, of course, Williams needed good equipment—and his M.I.T. associates supplied it. A static machine designed by Messrs. Norton and Lawrence was used, and with it, Williams reported, "a photograph of the bones of the hand can be taken . . . after an exposure of five seconds or less, although a longer exposure gives more detail." By May 1896, exposures lasting only $\frac{1}{5}$ second became possible with the Norton-Lawrence apparatus.

Williams, Lawrence, and Norton also seem to have noted that the higher the voltage, the greater the penetrating power of the rays. "It is sometimes of service," Williams reported, "to be able to vary the length of the spark [in modern terminology, the voltage applied to the tube] while observing with the fluoroscope, as the character of the picture changes with the character of the light. For instance, with a long spark [high voltage] the medullary canal of the long bones is distinctly visible, while with a short one this disappears and the bones become darker."

Williams at this early date, it further appears, had already mastered the fundamentals of radiological geometry. "In using the fluoroscope," he explained, "it is important to bear in mind the relative position of this instrument, the Crookes tube, and the organ which is under observation. For example, in examining the heart a good position for the tube is about on a level with the heart in front of the patient, and a little to the right of his median line; the patient should not face the tube squarely, but should be placed with his right side turned a little toward it; the observer, standing behind the patient and holding the fluoroscope to the left back of the latter, thus sees a shadow of the apex projected on the screen of the fluoroscope far to the left, even touching the left posterior axillary line, *thus bringing a large part of the heart into view.*"* The medical profession in New England, and indeed throughout the world, was indebted to Williams for many such detailed clinical "tips."

By the end of 1896, or perhaps early in 1897, Williams was ready to summarize his broad medical experience with the X rays in a classic 57-page paper published in the 1897 *Medical and Surgical Reports of the Boston City Hospital.*

As soon as he had gained some experience with the physics of the Roentgen rays, Williams there explained, "I began to examine my patients by their means, and have done so constantly ever since. The number I have thus far examined amounts to more than 250, and the more extended my experience has become in making these examinations, the more valuable have I found the rays in diagnosis in suitable cases."

Williams described the Norton-Lawrence apparatus in some detail, and noted an important point about the fluoroscope. Although Edison's calcium tungstate was unquestionably brighter than barium platinocyanide, some early experimenters had continued to use the older compound because some samples of calcium tungstate, in addition to fluorescing, *phosphoresced*—that is, continued to glow after the radiation was turned off. This introduced a "lag" in the fluoroscope; the fluorescent view at any moment was blurred by the phosphorescent glow left over from the view a moment or two earlier. But Williams used an improved calcium tungstate screen, "which is the result of the patient and laborious investigation of Mr. T. B. Kinraide, of Jamaica Plains, Boston, Mass." With the Kinraide calcium tungstate screen, "the image disappears as soon as the fluoroscope is removed from the tube. I use three sizes: one 3 by 4 inches, one 7 by 9 inches, and the third 11 by 14 inches."

A diaphragm was used to achieve a sharper image, and perhaps also to protect the patient, "a piece of sheet metal (*e.g.*, brass) six inches wide by twelve inches long, and thick enough to prevent the passage of the X

---

* Italics added.

rays, toward one end of which is cut a rectangular opening—this is preferable to a circular one—about two by three inches being a convenient size. After taking a general survey with the fluoroscope, the part of the body that is to be carefully examined is selected, and the metal plate held . . . in such a position that the X rays coming from the Crookes tube fall directly through the opening, while the surrounding area is shielded by the metal. *The fingers should be protected from the rays while holding the plate,* and to accomplish this object leather straps are fastened onto the plate, so that the fingers may be inserted under them on the upper side; the plate may be moved about and any special part examined."† If a large field were needed, Williams moved the brass plate close to the tube; for a smaller field, he moved it closer to the patient.

Another useful Williams-Norton-Lawrence device was a pencil "made of metal, with a crayon point suitable for marking the skin." Or a strip of lead wire could be fastened with adhesive plaster to an ordinary crayon so that, when it was used, its movements could be followed through the fluoroscope.

Williams now gave his medical readers an introductory lesson in the physics of radiation, a cogent discussion of the relative merits of fluorosscopy *vs.* X-ray photography, a brief review of radiation geometry, and, to illustrate all this concretely, a discussion of the detection of kidney and bladder stones.

"Before attempting to detect any form of calculi in the body," Williams reported, "I first placed several different kinds over a photographic plate, which was enclosed in dark paper to shield it from the light, and exposed them for a few minutes to the X rays. The rays penetrated the calculi made up of uric acid, of cholesterine and biliary salts, very readily, but were obstructed by calculi containing oxalate of calcium in considerable proportion, phosphate of calcium, or other inorganic constituents." It was obvious, he therefore concluded, "that any attempt to detect in the body calculi made up of organic compounds would, so far as our knowledge now goes, be futile, whereas those of inorganic origin might be detected."

To find even inorganic calculi *in situ,* however, another hurdle had to be surmounted. The bony structure in the pelvic area prevented detection. Williams accordingly tried an ingenious tubelike aluminum device, designed for him by his brother-in-law, Dr. William H. Rollins, a Boston dentist, which permitted the rectal insertion of a photographic film. "The rays from the Crookes tube, which is placed over the bladder and some distance from the abdominal wall," Williams reported, "penetrate the tissues and the aluminum wall of the tube and act upon the

---

† Italics added.

film. After an exposure of a few minutes, the instrument is withdrawn and the films taken out in a dark room and developed like any other photographic plate." The presence of inorganic calculi, it was hoped, would be demonstrated. Dr. Williams reported, however, that "in the two cases in which I have used this instrument nothing was found on the films; the calculi were removed and proved on analysis to be made of uric acid." Williams's disappointment—and Dr. Rollins's, too—can be sensed across the years.

Physical experimentation prior to clinical trial, as evidenced by the preliminary X-raying of calculi outside the body, became a standing Williams procedure. He compared X rays through clear water, for example, with X rays through "the various fluids formed in the body in health or disease, such as the blood, ascitic and pleuritic fluid, the urine, pus, fluid from hydrocele, etc." and reported that all were "found to offer about the same resistance to the passage of the rays." Muscle, however, proved a bit denser than water, and so did adipose tissue.

The chief hope for medical diagnosis with the X rays, Williams predicted, lay in the differential opacity of *air* as opposed to water or organic tissue. "... It is readily seen of how much importance is this difference in permeability of air and water by the rays, on account of the great contrast which is thereby afforded in health between the lungs and their adjacent tissues or organs." No doubt this was one of the considerations which persuaded Williams to concentrate so early on radiology of the chest.

After familiarizing himself with the effects of the rays on organic substances in isolation, Williams went on to a radiological study of their appearance under the X rays in normal human anatomy and physiology—a necessary prelude to the study of radiological pathology. He insisted:

> To use the Roentgen rays successfully in practice, it is first essential that the physician become familiar with the appearances in the fluoroscope which present themselves in health. This applies particularly to the thorax, and the picture of this part of the body when seen in the screen of a large fluoroscope presents so much that it should be studied systematically. The trunk appears lighter above than below the diaphragm, and the rise and fall of this muscle, which appears dark in the fluoroscope, are distinctly seen. The chest is divided vertically by an ill-defined dark band which includes the backbone, on each side of which the lungs, forming the brightest part of the picture, are crossed by the darker ribs. The pulsating heart is seen, especially the dark ventricles, and, under favorable conditions, the lighter right auricle, and on the left side above the ventricles the pulmonary artery is made out. A small portion of one side of the arch of the aorta may be observed in the first intercostal space to the left

of the sternum. After this general view has been taken, the outline of the lungs should be noted during full inspiration and expiration.... The lungs usually appear brighter during deep inspiration; in young persons brighter than in older persons, as the tissues of the former are more easily penetrated by the rays. In the thin, the lungs appear lighter than in the heavy, because the outlines are dulled, as it were, by a thicker layer of tissues, which contain much water. It has seemed to me that the right apex is normally darker than the left apex. The normal brightness of the lungs and the normal outlines of the clavicles and ribs should be observed, for as we note different degrees of pallor by reference to our standard of color in health, in the same way is it necessary to know the normal amount of light which should penetrate any given part in order to recognize variations from the normal. The eye must be trained in the use of the X rays as is the ear for auscultation and percussion.

Williams next ventured to introduce *statistics* into radiology. "In six men with healthy lungs," he reported, "the diaphragm moved on an average 2-¾ inches on the right side and 2-½ inches on the left side. In eighteen patients with tuberculous lungs the average excursion of the lungs was 1-¼ inches. In health the diaphragm is less sharply defined in expiration than in inspiration."

Physicians prior to Roentgen had learned much of their pathology at autopsy, and Williams saw that a comparison of X-ray findings with autopsy findings could similarly aid the radiologist. "In order to get further suggestions," he wrote, "... I took a number of radiographs of healthy and diseased lungs just after death. As a specimen of the latter see Fig. 7 [not available], which shows the lungs of a patient who died of pneumonia. The darker was more affected by the process than the lighter; the lightest portion is healthy. These lungs were kindly lent to me for a few moments by Prof. W. T. Councilman. The autopsy of one of my patients showed that he had perfectly healthy lungs. I had examined the chest of this man two days before his death, and found them perfectly clear and the outlines well defined. The outlines shown in the fluoroscope were well seen."

Williams also stressed bilateral examination as a means of comparing normal with diseased tissue—"for example, whether or not one lung is darker than the other. ... When both sides are diseased the opportunity for direct comparison with the normal is lost, and one is obliged to depend upon a recollection of the normal in an individual of the same build."

Williams next proceeded to present 30 cases of tuberculosis, out of more than 50 he had so far examined, comparing in each case the physical findings of the referring physician with his own radiological findings. "At first, in order to make the X-ray examination without bias," he explained, "I examined the patients with the fluoroscope before knowing anything of the physical examination." In a few cases, he conceded, the physical examination told more than the X rays did, "but these were cases that were examined before I had had much experience in the use of the fluoroscope."

Williams summed up the usefulness of the X rays in his tuberculosis series: "Correspondence between the physical signs and the X-ray examination in a considerable number of cases; more extensive disease than was shown by the physical examination in certain cases; an earlier increase in density in the lungs than was detected by the physical examination in still other cases; in one of these no signs in the lungs were detected prior to that found by the fluoroscope, while in some, although one lung was ascertained by the physical examination to be seriously involved, its companion was not suspected until the X-ray examination revealed its increased density; fourth, three cases suggested that increase in density was not present where the physical signs intimated it."

Williams next presented similarly eight cases of pneumonia, but warned, "... The brief description of these cases does not present to the mind how much these examinations conduce to a more accurate estimate of the condition of the lungs in some cases than has hitherto been possible in any other way. This method of examination enables us to judge better than any other way when the lungs have 'cleared up' after an attack of pneumonia, and I am satisfied that it gives us the means of recognizing an increased density in the lungs in pneumonia earlier than has previously been possible."

Williams now proceeded to present "16 cases of pleurisy with effusion, seven on the left and nine on the right side, and one dry pleurisy." He summarized his findings with precision: "In pleurisy with effusion we can estimate the amount of fluid in a general way by the amount of light which passes through the thorax. When the effusion is large no more rays pass through it than through the liver, and the outline of the diaphragm, ribs, and heart are obliterated on the side of the effusion. If there is a smaller amount of fluid the outlines of some of the upper ribs are seen, and with a small effusion the outlines low down in the thorax only are ill-defined. The fluoroscope assists us to distinguish between an effusion and a thickened pleura. In some cases of effusion the fluoroscope shows us displacement to the right, and this displacement is of more frequent occurrence, when the effusion is on the left side. This displacement of the heart to the right may not be recognized by percussion even when it has been pushed much beyond its normal place. In one patient the heart was seen to be displaced more than two inches to the right, but no displacement was detected by percussion. While examining some cases of pleurisy with effusion by the fluoroscope, I have found indications of tuberculosis in the lung where it was not previously suspected."

Next Williams presented five cases of aneurysm (ballooning of an artery due to a weakened wall) and noted: "Aneurysms of the arch of the aorta are most clearly outlined when their borders are nearest the fluoroscope; those on the left when examined from the back, those on the right when examined from the front. It is obvious that aneurysms of the thoracic aorta can sometimes be detected earlier by X-ray examination than in any other way. In obscure thoracic cases where an aneurysm of certain portions of the aorta is suspected, but does not exist, it may probably be excluded by an X-ray examination."

Wherever possible, of course, Williams sought to compare his fluoroscopic findings with the surgeon's observations during a subsequent operation. Here is a dramatic example of surgical confirmation in an aneurysm case:

> C. A., 40 years. Aneurysm. Pulsation seen and felt in the lower part of the neck above and behind the inner end of the right clavicle. There was evidently an aneurysm of the subclavian artery. An operation was advised, but before this was done an X-ray examination was made in order to determine the lower limit of the aneurysm and ascertain if it extended to the larger arteries below, in which case an operation would be more serious, or it might be necessary to abandon it altogether.
>
> *Examination with the fluoroscope:* No indication of any aneurysm extending below the lower border of the clavicle. A radiograph showed the outline of the aneurysm in the neck, but also gave no indication of any below the clavicle. Both sides of the chest were equally clear, thus showing there was no aneurysm there. Operation for ligaturing the innominate artery confirmed the observations made by X-ray examination.

Other diseases were similarly reviewed, and Williams concluded, "The foregoing observations and cases show that by X-ray examinations of the chest we gain assistance in recognizing a density greater than normal in tuberculosis, pneumonia, infarction, edema, congestion of the lungs, in aneurysm, and in new growths; they likewise assist us to recognize fluid in the pericardial and pleural sacs. The distribution, location, and amount of this increase in density which the fluoroscope shows assist us in some cases to differentiate these diseases and conditions. Diminution of the normal density, which is the result of emphysema and pneumothorax, is indicated by the position and movement of the diaphragm; a certain curve of the diaphragm is characteristic of this latter condition. The excursion and position of the diaphragm are of assistance in determining the condition of a lung or lungs in tuberculosis, pneumonia, and other diseases. As is the case with all other observations on which a diagnosis is founded, the conditions which are revealed by the fluoroscope are only to be properly interpreted after experience in making X-ray examinations has enabled the physician to give these observations their due weight."

Radiology had come a long way during the 12 months since Roentgen noticed that glowing screen on November 8, 1895!

Williams devoted an additional dozen pages to a review of his surgical cases, some of them fascinating, but not unlike the work of other pioneers, and he concluded with a modest warning against overenthusiasm: "Interesting, not to say magical, as are the physical phenomena connected with the X rays, we should not be led to assume for them an exaggerated importance in practical medicine. They do unquestionably afford us valuable aid, and through them an advance in our methods of examining patients is obtained. I have thus far found them of especial service in diseases of the chest."

A search of the medical literature reveals no one else in the United States or Canada during 1896 who ranked with Francis H. Williams in breadth of radiological experience, precision of observation, depth of insight, soundness of judgment, ingenuity, and clarity of expression. He was the first to bring to radiology the full range of skills which now characterize it, and can therefore properly be cited as "America's first radiologist."

   # But How Safe Are the Roentgen Rays?

While American researchers from Wright to Williams were busily exploring the beneficent uses of the X rays and reporting their exciting findings, less welcome news was also beginning to trickle in from many parts of the country. The rays, it was learned, do not merely pass through human tissue in the way that light passes through glass. Instead, they may produce undesirable changes in the tissues exposed to radiation.

One of the earliest of these reports came from Professor John Daniel of the Physical Laboratory at Vanderbilt University in Nashville, Tennessee. In February 1896, a child who had been accidentally shot in the head was brought to the laboratory. Could Professor Daniel locate the bullet by means of the new X rays? The newspapers at the time were filled with Edison's unsuccessful efforts to photograph the living brain through the skull. The apparatus available at Vanderbilt was "rather weak." Before attempting to locate the bullet, Professor Daniel and his associate Dr. William L. Dudley decided to make a preliminary test of the feasibility of the undertaking by X-raying some other head. "Accordingly," Professor Daniel wrote on March 23, "Dr. Dudley, with his characteristic devotion to the cause of science, lent himself to the experiment. A plateholder containing the sensitive plate was tied to one side of his head, with a coin between the plate and his head, and the tube was set playing on the opposite side of his head." [1] If an image of the coin could be secured through an adult skull, it would no doubt be quite easy to secure an image of the bullet through the child's skull. To maximize the likelihood of success, the tube was placed only about ½ inch away from Dr. Dudley's hair and was activated for 1 full hour.

No image appeared on the plate. "But yesterday, 21 days after the experiment," Professor Daniel wrote, "all the hair came out over the space under the X-ray discharge. The spot is now perfectly bald, being two inches in diameter. This is the size of the X-ray field close to the tube. We, and especially Dr. Dudley, shall watch with interest the ultimate effect. The skin looks perfectly healthy, and there has been no pain nor other indication of disorder. I called attention to the place before Dr. Dudley had himself noticed it, and we were both for some time at a loss to account for it, as we had no previous intimation of any effect whatever."

Considerable editorial merriment was evoked by this communication;

there were even suggestions in the newspapers and technical journals that the X rays might render daily shaving obsolete.

Numerous mentions of possible damage to the eye of the experimenter from X rays began to appear at about the same time; Edison, Tesla, and Dr. William J. Morton of New York were among those to complain of eye symptoms. It was hard to determine, however, how much of their discomfort was due directly to the X rays and how much to simple eyestrain generated by peering hour after hour at a dimly fluorescing screen.

As the months rolled by and more powerful X-ray equipment was introduced, accounts of more serious damage caused by the rays began to appear. On August 12, 1896, the *Electrical Review* reported:

> Mr. H. D. Hawks, a graduate in the class of 1896, of Columbia College, has for the past few weeks been giving exhibitions in the vicinity of New York with an unusually powerful X-ray outfit. Mr. Hawks, during the afternoon and evening of each day for four days, was working around his apparatus for from two to three hours at a time. At the end of the four days, he was compelled to cease active work, owing to the physical effects of the X rays upon his body. The first thing Mr. Hawks noticed was a drying of the skin, to which he paid no attention, but after a while it became so painful it was necessary to stop all operations. The hands began to swell and assumed the appearance of a very deep sunburn. At the end of two weeks the skin all came off the hands. The knuckles were especially affected, they being the sorest part of the hand. Among other effects were the following: the growth of the fingernails was stopped and the hair on the skin that was exposed to the rays all dropped out, especially on the face and sides of the head. The hair at the temples has entirely disappeared, owing to the fact that Mr. Hawks placed his head in close proximity to the tube to enable spectators to see the bones of the jaw. The eyes were quite bloodshot and the vision considerably impaired. The eyelashes began to fall out and the lids to swell. The chest was also burned through the clothing, the burn resembling sunburn. Mr. Hawks's disabilities were such that he was compelled to suspend work for two weeks. He consulted physicians, who treated the case as one of parboiling.

Incredible as it may seem today, young Hawks thereupon went back to exhibiting his X-ray apparatus! He tried protecting his hand, first with Vaseline and, when that failed to ward off the rays, with a glove, "but the hand was at once burned again, the glove affording no protection whatever. The hand was finally protected by covering it with tin foil."

Within 6 weeks, Hawks had partially recovered and was making light of his injuries. "Summing up," he wrote in the *Electrical Engineer* for September 16, 1896, "I will say that the effects seem to be confined to the skin alone, and consist principally in the drying up of the oils in it, which produces all of the effects on hair and nails as noted, and none of these effects are permanent, but disappear when the skin becomes healthy again."

Hawks also advanced a theory which was to be urged over and over again throughout 1896, and even thereafter: "As to what produces the burn, I think it is purely an electrical effect, and that the ray has [almost] nothing to do with it." Other similar efforts, embraced on occasion even by the rays' victims, to exonerate the rays at all costs are noted below.

The *Electrical Review* concluded its August 12 account of Hawks's X-ray injuries with an invitation; it would be "glad to hear from any of its readers who have experienced similar effects, even in a lesser degree." G. A. Frei of Frei & Co., a Boston manufacturer of X-ray tubes, replied the next day.

"Mr. K., who attends to the testing of the tubes during and after the exhausting process at our work rooms," Frei reported, "complained a few weeks ago of a peculiar itching and burning in his left hand, and thought that it was caused by poisoning with chemicals.... Within a week past the same phenomenon has appeared on my hand. The skin has turned brown and hard, and during last night a blister about three-eighths of an inch in diameter was raised on the little finger. Further developments will be carefully watched and noted." [2]

While he was watching and noting, Frei continued to expose his blistered hand to the X rays. "The swelling increased for several days," he noted in the *Electrical Engineer* for September 16, "till I decided to stop experimenting on my own hands. I had sufficiently demonstrated the effects of the rays as far as I was concerned. Three or four days after I stopped it began to improve. The skin pealed off; I should say I took off three layers. At that stage I was obliged to test three tubes and thoughtlessly I exposed the same hand for about a minute or a minute and a half. This completely stopped all improvement for a number of days. At present my hand is nearly in good condition again. It would undoubtedly be interesting to know what the ultimate result would be, yet I do not care to use my own hands for the experiment, especially as a hand showing the X-ray treatment is not a thing of beauty."

A particularly distressing case was reported in September from Minnesota. It involved William Levy, a resident of Eau Claire, Wisconsin, who had been shot in the head by an escaping bank defaulter 10 years before. The bullet had entered his skull just above the left ear, and had presumably proceeded toward the back of the head. Early in July 1896, having heard about the X rays, Levy decided to have his bullet located, with a view to extraction, and for that purpose he journeyed to see Professor Fred S. Jones at the Physical Laboratory of the University of Minnesota.[3]

Professor Jones was apparently familiar with Dr. Daniel's and Dr. Dudley's experience at Vanderbilt, or with subsequent reports of epilation, for he warned Levy that the experiment might cause him to lose his hair. Levy was undeterred, and the negatives were made on July 8.

"The difficulty of penetrating the skull necessitated prolonged exposures," Jones wrote on September 1.[4] How prolonged he did not say, but a local newspaper, the St. Paul *Dispatch*, reported that Levy sat for the Roentgen-ray plates from 8 o'clock in the morning until 10 o'clock at night. Exposures were made with the tube over his forehead, in front of his open mouth, and just behind his right ear. According to one account, the tube was actually placed inside his mouth. The current to the tube was estimated at 100,000 volts.

"No painful sensations were experienced by the patient during the exposures," Professor Jones reported, "but inside of 24 hours every spot on the head under the tube commenced to blister. In a few days the forehead was an angry sore, in all respects similar to a burn; the lips were badly swollen, cracked and bleeding; the inside of the mouth was so blistered that little food could be taken, and that little was necessarily in liquid form. The right ear was more than doubled in size, and appeared like an ear which had been badly frozen. The hair on the right side of the head is entirely gone."

Treatment was given as for any other serious burn. "The case is being watched with great interest by local physicians," Professor Jones concluded, "and the one feature which is satisfactory to the patient is that two good pictures of the bullet were obtained, showing it about an inch beneath the skull and directly under the occipital process. Of the deleterious effects of the rays there can be no doubt." [3]

This report was alarming, of course, but a follow-up story indicated that the "deleterious effects" were only temporary. The *Electrical Review* was able to reassure its readers on October 21, "Mr. Levy has recovered from the effects of his burns, but he still has half a bald head. He is a plucky man, about 30 years of age, and intends to have the investigations carried further and the bullet removed. He has already written to Professor Jones, asking for another sitting. It is necessary now to have a negative showing just how far below the surface the bullet is located before the doctors decide whether the operation can be safely performed."

The X-ray burns did not always heal that promptly, as Professor R. B. Owens of the University of Nebraska found out. A prominent Lincoln, Nebraska, attorney had had two X-ray negatives made of his shoulder in the latter part of June. The first exposure was for 1 hour; the second, on the following day, was for 2½ hours. About 1 week later there was slight redness, accompanied by much pain. This gradually increased until the area exposed to the rays looked like a severe burn, about 12 to 15 square inches in size. "Since this time," Professor Owens reported in the *Electrical World* nearly 6 months later, on December 19, "every attempt to control the inflammatory action has failed." Professor Owens was concerned, moreover, by the fact that X rays pass so readily through human tissue and might, therefore, in addition to the visible skin effects, do unsuspected damage "within the tissue itself . . . far from the surface of the skin."

A similar slow-to-heal case which might involve damage far deeper than the skin was reported by a Dr. Stickney in Boston in December:

> The patient, Mrs. Q., came under my care last August, at which time she was suffering from some obscure abdominal trouble. She wished to have the X ray used on her as a possible means of diagnosis, and with that purpose in view made her arrangements with an expert in skiagraphy, and requested me to be present. The whole abdominal region was exposed to the X ray, but the force of the ray was focused more to the region of the liver, as that was where she complained of her trouble. There were three exposures made—one of 20 minutes, one of 30 minutes, and the last of 35 minutes. The Crookes tube was not brought nearer than 18 inches to the parts exposed.
>
> She experienced no discomfort at the time, but some two days after called at my office, complaining that the region exposed to the X ray felt as though it had been burned by the sun. Upon examination I found the appearance of the parts exposed to be similar to that seen in severe forms of sunburn. The condition of the parts from this time grew rapidly worse, until a surface some eight inches in diameter had sloughed. The slough was very slow in separating, and the surface has been very slow in filling in, *the vitality of the parts seeming to have been affected much deeper than the slough would indicate.* All the different treatments for burn and ordinary lesions of like nature have been adopted, together with a thorough curetting, but nothing seems to be of much assistance. The lesion has been very painful from the first.
>
> At the present time . . . a surface of four inches in diameter is still left unhealed.[5] *

Serious damage from the rays was also reported from Edison's laboratory. Elihu Thomson of General Electric cited two Edison cases in a letter to Dr. E. A. Codman of Boston dated December 1. Thomson called these cases "severe, since they took place over the hands and arms of the

---

* Italics added.

victims, and made it necessary for them to stop work altogether in connection with X rays. The story goes that one of them was told by his physician that if he continued to work it would be necessary to amputate his hands." [6]

The worker threatened with amputation was in all probability Edison's glassblower, Clarence Dally; the sequel to his burns is noted below (page 162). In later years Edison cited these injuries to his "boys" as his reason for abandoning X-ray research.

Not all experimenters, it should be noted, had such experiences. Thus, Dr. Williams was able to report at the end of 1896 or early in 1897, "No harmful effects have been received in any way by the patients, more than 250 in number, whom I have thus far examined by the X rays at this hospital, and there need not be the slightest anxiety on the part of the patient *if the examinations are made by someone who has had experience and has suitable apparatus.*" [7]†

Professor W. M. Stine of the Armour Institute of Technology reported a further case—not his own, it appears, but one which had "just come under the observation of the writer." The patient had been exposed to a focus tube "for periods of about two hours each on two successive days. During most of this time the tube had been placed within a few inches of the back, at the base of the dorsal region. In a few days an irritation and itching sensation were noticed. The skin over a considerable area had turned to a dark brown, or mahogany, color. A few days later the area had increased, and the skin grew very red and inflamed, but no blisters were noted. Other portions of the skin which had been exposed to the tube for only a short time were slightly tanned and somewhat hard and dry. In due time the skin peeled off where the burn had been most pronounced. The whole occurrence resembled a bad sunburn." [8] Professor Stine's own hands, he added, had become tanned while working constantly with the focus tube.

Professor Stine concluded, however, that "the effects are not due to the X rays, but rather to ultra-violet rays, which are always present to a greater or less extent." He added, "It is noteworthy that such effects only result from exposure to the focusing tubes, when, owing to the concentration of energy, ultra-violet rays of considerable intensity must be produced."

Finally, Professor Stine suggested a simple way of forestalling X-ray burns. "When pear-shaped tubes are used, in which the impact is extended over a large area of glass, no burns seem to result from even long exposure to powerfully excited tubes." Then he hedged a bit. "This, however, is only stated as a matter of personal experience and observa-

---

† Italics added.

tion. There may be other investigators who can state results to the contrary."

A much more dogmatic effort to explain away the X-ray burn was written by Nikola Tesla on November 30, 1896.[9] "As to the hurtful actions on the skin, which have been variously reported," Tesla declared, "I note that they are misinterpreted. These effects have been known to me for some time, but I have been unable, on account of pressing matters, to dwell on the subject. They are not due to the Roentgen rays, but merely to the ozone generated in contact with the skin. Nitrous acid may also be responsible, to a small extent. The ozone, when abundantly produced, attacks the skin and many organic substances most energetically."

Apparently Tesla was unaware of Hawks's report that Vaseline would not protect the skin, for he recommended such a procedure. "The radical means . . . of preventing such actions is to make impossible the access of the air to the skin while exposing, as, for instance, by immersing in oil." Tesla himself, however, used another sovereign preventive. "I have always taken the precaution when getting impressions with the rays, to guard the person by a screen made of aluminum wires which is connected to the ground, preferably through a condenser." Just how such a grounded aluminum screen would ward off the deleterious ozone, Tesla did not make clear.

The Boston tubemaker Frei, meanwhile, had also developed a new theory of how to avoid such burns. In addition to making tubes he had begun manufacturing static machines. Back on August 19, he had had no doubt that the burns "must be the effect of the rays," [10] and in early September he was still attributing his own blistered hands to "the effects of the rays." [11] But in December he wrote, ". . . I have persistently kept on with my experiments in that line and finally came to the conclusion that the effects which we perceive on the skin, the hair or nails, are not caused by the action of the X rays in any way." [12]

His earlier experiments, Frei went on to explain, had been performed with a Ruhmkorff coil, reinforced at times by a "step-up coil." The coil was what caused the burns, he now affirmed. Frei's later experiments were conducted with one of his static machines instead—a machine giving an 8-inch spark, or roughly 90,000 volts. He spent more time with the X rays, and the equipment was more powerful; yet when using the static machine, he reported, "neither myself nor any of the persons I ever experimented upon . . . have ever felt any ill effects."

It was possible, someone had suggested to Frei, that his hands had become "X-rayproof" as a result of the earlier burns. But Frei (quite rightly, of course) did not accept this explanation. To disprove it, he launched a new set of experiments on his previously unexposed left foot. "For several weeks I subjected it to the action of the rays every four days from half an hour to an hour at a time. The tube was brought as near the foot as possible without touching it, but up to the present time there is neither discoloration nor any of the other now well-known effects to be seen or felt. This proves conclusively, at least as far as my own observation goes, that whatever ill-effects we get on our skins are caused only when we use induction coils in one form or another, while no such effects are perceived when we use the static machine."

As further evidence that static machines were safe, Frei could point to the experience of Dr. Walter James Dodd of the Massachusetts General Hospital, who had been experimenting with X rays there for several months without apparent harm. Then, in October 1896, a General Electric physicist (probably Elihu Thomson) had lent Dodd an induction coil—whereupon, in November, Dodd had developed a severe dermatitis.[13]

Physicians throughout the country were becoming increasingly worried about X rays during the second half of 1896. Dr. D. W. Gage of McCook, Nebraska, had sounded the alarm in the *Medical Record* (New York) as early as August 29: "I wish to suggest that more be understood regarding the action of the X rays before the general practitioner adopts them in his daily work. Several cases of alopecia [loss of hair] and erythema [skin reddening] have followed its use in Omaha and Lincoln, and in one case of my own, when the rays were utilized in trying to determine the presence of a foreign body in the stomach of a child, erythema and finally sloughing took place, leaving a lesion over the region penetrated by the rays, which is at present the size of a hand."

Frei, as an equipment manufacturer, must have been familiar with this growing concern among doctors. He thought that their anxiety should be allayed and that the induction coil rather than the X rays should be made to shoulder the blame. "Many physicians," he wrote, "bring forth the argument that the application of the X rays might prove dangerous to their patients, that here a foot had to be amputated, there someone's finger nails dropped off, another has a sore of three months' standing, etc. Such arguments can be met with the above fact that the X rays are not the direct cause of the trouble and with this fact established remedies could undoubtedly be found to reduce, if not entirely eliminate, the effect on the skin when coils are to be employed."[12] Frei's communication was headed:

X RAYS HARMLESS WITH THE STATIC MACHINE.

But this opinion was nonsense—and dangerous nonsense, too, for it gave experimenters, physicians, and patients alike a false sense of security. Credit for refuting the claims of the static machine manufacturers and other enthusiasts, by an experiment on his own body, belongs to Elihu Thomson of General Electric.

Thomson had developed the "Thomson Inductorium," an induction coil adapted especially for X-ray use and sold by General Electric in competition with Frei's static machine. His experiments on himself, in addition to establishing that the X rays themselves caused the burns, also served to clear the reputation of his device.

"There were two serious misconceptions in the early days," Thomson later wrote, "which tended to do harm and to need emphatic correction. It was claimed by some that the Roentgen rays themselves were innocuous and that any injury by them was to be laid to the electrical discharges or changes of electrical conditions affecting the skin and tissues." (This allegation, of course, placed the entire electrical industry under a cloud.) "It was also claimed and believed by many that tubes excited by static machines ... would not produce injury, while those operated from induction coils were far more likely to do so. These ideas were shared by some authorities who should have known better." Accordingly, Thomson continued, "I deliberately determined to make some crucial experiments upon myself and publish the results. I asked myself what part of my body I could best afford to lose and decided it was the last joint on my left little finger." [14]

This fingertip Thomson exposed "for half an hour to the radiation of a strongly excited tube (single focus)," he reported in the *Electrical World* for November 28, 1896. A static machine was used to activate the tubes. "The back of the finger was placed almost in contact with the glass.... It was thought that an effect equal to four or five hours' exposure at ordinary distances might in this way be produced in half an hour. For several days after the exposure no noticeable effect was produced, and the matter was given no further thought; but at present writing, eleven days after the exposure, the skin of the back of the finger is red, swollen, and painful to the touch, and the finger feels somewhat stiff. It has begun to blister." More than 6 weeks later, on December 16, the finger still required a bandage.[15]

Thomson's point was clearly made. Such burns were due to the rays themselves, regardless of whether a static machine or an induction coil was used to generate them. Thomson also treated another finger with a series of short exposures over a period of many days to demonstrate that the effect was cumulative—but that was the following year.

Thus, by the close of 1896, at least some of the basic facts about X-ray burns were known, although as yet not universally accepted as being due to the rays themselves. That subtler but far more disastrous effects might follow overexposure after a delay of many years was as yet barely suspected by a few Jeremiahs like Owens out in Nebraska and Stickney in Boston.

REFERENCES

1. *Science (n.s.)*, *3:* 562–563, 1896.
2. *Electrical Rev. 29:* 95, 1896.
3. *Ibid.*, p. 202.
4. *Ibid.*, p. 127.
5. *Boston Med. Surg. J., 135:* 719, 1896.
6. *Boston Med. Surg. J., 135:* 610–611, 1896.
7. *Med. Surg. Rep. Boston City Hosp.*, 8th series: 190, 1897.
8. *Electrical Rev., 29:* 250, 1896.
9. *Ibid.*, p. 277.
10. *Electrical Engineer, 22:* 259–260, 1896.
11. *Ibid.*, p. 276.
12. *Ibid.*, p. 651.
13. MACY, J., *Walter James Dodd—A Biographical Sketch*, pp. 19–21. Houghton Mifflin Company, Boston 1918.
14. WOODBURY, D. O., *Beloved Scientist*, pp. 225–227. Whittlesey House, Division of McGraw-Hill Book Company, New York, 1944.
15. *Electrical Engineer, 22:* 653, 1896.

8 Postscript: The Curious Case of Emil H. Grubbé

In later years, a number of Americans claimed to have worked with the X rays before Arthur W. Wright of Yale exposed his first plate on January 27, 1896. Their claims can in most cases be dismissed for lack of contemporary evidence, and in some cases they can be proved mistaken. In his 1930 autobiography, for example, Professor Michael I. Pupin of Columbia claimed to have exposed his first plate on January 2, 1896, but in April 1896 he stated that he had begun his work on February 7,[1] and contemporary evidence supports the later date.

The claims of Dr. Emil Herman Grubbé (1875–1960) of Chicago, however, cannot be so lightly dismissed, for they are buttressed by two documents which, if they are what they purport to be, establish the truth of at least some of his allegations. Grubbé claimed to have worked with the X rays long before Wright. He said he was the first person in the world to use the new rays in the treatment of disease, the first to manufacture focus tubes for X-ray use, the inventor of the fluoroscope, the first to protect patients from the deleterious effects of the rays—and the first to be injured by the rays. Because his claims have been taken seriously by a number of earlier writers on the history of radiology, and because, if true, they would require a substantial recasting of several chapters in Part I of this book, his story must be scrutinized here at some length.

According to his own account,[2] which varies from the surviving record, Grubbé entered college in 1891 at the age of 16, took a pharmacy degree at 18, a B.S. at 19, and an A.M. at 20, in 1895. In addition, this remarkable 20-year-old was (according, once more, to his own account) busy with many other activities in Chicago. He was teaching physics and chemistry at a Chicago homeopathic medical school, the Hahnemann Medical College; he was taking a medical course at the Hahnemann, looking toward an M.D.; and he was in business as an assayer and refiner of rare metals, specializing in platinum.

In the course of his work, Grubbé later alleged, he accumulated a considerable amount of platinum, paid him as fees by an Idaho mining company. There was no ready market for this metal, but Grubbé knew that, since it had the same coefficient of expansion as glass, it could be used in the manufacture of lead-in wires for vacuum tubes. He accordingly "came to the decision that I would go into another business, that of manufacturing vacuum tubes, and thus find a profitable use for my platinum."

Luck, according to Grubbé, favored this enterprise immediately. "One warm morning, in August 1895, a man, in passing through the court, was attracted by the sight of beakers, Florence flasks, thistle tubes, test tubes, and retorts which he saw through the open door of my workshop. . . . He walked up to where I was sitting at my desk, and asked, in broken English, if I could speak German. When I told him yes, he introduced himself as Albert Schmidt. . . . He told me he was a glassblower and had made many such glass articles as we were working with. He was looking for work. . . ."

Grubbé asked Schmidt if he were familiar with the manufacture of vacuum tubes. "Yes," he quoted Schmidt as replying, "I worked for the Allgemeine Elektrizitäts-Gesellschaft in Germany and made several kinds of illuminating or light bulbs and also several different types of high vacuum tubes."

Grubbé reported that he was "dumbfounded when I heard these answers from the lips of Schmidt. I could scarcely believe it. Either fate or fortune [Grubbé was a confirmed atheist] must have had something to do with sending him to my place on that particular morning." Grubbé hired Schmidt immediately.

The two men took up the manufacture of incandescent lights, Grubbé stated, and all their spare time was "devoted to experiments with Crookes or high vacuum tubes. . . . Both of us became completely absorbed in the subject. It was fascinating. Often we would be so engrossed with some particularly interesting problem that we would forget to take time to eat." Schmidt had brought technical books and journals with him from Germany; Grubbé read them. Thereafter, "we not only duplicated Lenard's experiments but also the work of Crookes, Jackson, and Hertz, as recorded in Schmidt's books."

Lenard had used potassium platinocyanide crystals in some of his experiments, Grubbé stated, and so "having much platinum on hand I decided to make some of these crystals." In the course of duplicating the experiments of Crookes, Hertz, Jackson, and Lenard before Roentgen made his announcement, Grubbé was, he declared in 1949, "one of the very few individuals, living or dead, who actually worked with X rays before they were discovered." When the announcement did reach him, of course, Grubbé promptly launched a program of X-ray research.

Grubbé did not state the day on which this research began, but he indicated that it was very early. "Because I was a manufacturer of vacuum tubes as well as a practical user of them," he wrote, ". . . I was, probably, the only person in the United States who had available all the facilities needed to duplicate the experiments which made possible this amazing revolution. I did not have to go out of my shop. . . ."

Each tube that Grubbé and Schmidt manufactured, of course, had to be tested for X-ray production. The procedure usual at the time was followed. ". . . In testing Crookes tubes, my hands (usually the left one) were exposed between the fluorescent crystals and the electrically excited tube while it was still attached to the mercury pump. This test had to be made in order to judge whether a tube was sufficiently exhausted or had a high enough vacuum to produce X rays for practical work. Such tests were made many times daily and for many days in succession. Often my hand was almost in contact with the electrically excited Crookes tubes during most of the testing periods." In all, Grubbé estimated, his left hand "was exposed to the X rays for a total of one hundred and fifty to two hundred hours."

The inevitable, he averred, followed. "During the latter part of January 1896, the back of my left hand developed symptoms of acute dermatitis. At first there was intolerable itching on the back of the hand. Later the hand became so inflamed, swollen, red, and painful that I had to put on a bandage. A few days later, blebs and blisters began to form on the back of the hand. At a still later period there was desquamation of the skin and epilation of hairs." The pain and injury were so acute, Grubbé reports, that he consulted a physician about it on January 27, 1896—the day on which Wright at Yale exposed his first X-ray plate.

". . . I believe," he wrote, "I happened to be the first person detrimentally affected by these new rays.

"Viewing the whole subject in retrospect, I am sure that fate was cruel to me when she selected my body to be the first to be burned by X rays, for, unlike those who followed me in this work, I had no one to teach me the dangers incident to exposure of the human body to the luminous hemisphere of the electrically activated Crookes tube."

But Grubbé did not rest upon a mere claim that he was the first to be injured. His pretensions went much further.

When he took his burned hand to a physician, Dr. J. P. Cobb, in the faculty room of the Hahnemann Medical College on Monday, January 27, Grubbé affirmed, "several other members of the faculty entered the room. Among them were Dr. J. E. Gilman, Dr. A. C. Halphide, and Dr. R. Ludlam, Sr. My ailment being a new one, Dr. Cobb used me as a clinical subject. He explained my symptoms and had me explain the nature of the agent which produced the dermatitis. . . . At this time my hand looked as though it had been scalded. It was swollen to twice its normal size and was very painful."

Each of the doctors present, Grubbé continued, offered remedial suggestions, except Dr. Gilman. His mind was roving far beyond the immediate problem. "Dr. Gilman, after thinking over the origin of the dermatitis, said that although he would not suggest a remedy for the treatment of my burned hand, he was very much impressed with the power of these new rays, and he concluded with the statement that 'any physical agent capable of doing so much damage to normal or healthy cells and tissues might offer possibilities, if used as a therapeutic measure, in the treatment of pathological conditions. . . . ' As examples of such lesions he mentioned cancer, lupus, and indolent ulcers."

Here, according to Grubbé, was the first suggestion in history that the X rays might have therapeutic value. It was a solemn moment. "This statement of Dr. Gilman's made a profound impression upon all those present. Dr. Ludlam and Dr. Halphide were especially impressed."

Grubbé gave in intimate detail the aftermath of this January 27 consultation. On the morning of Wednesday, January 29, he reported, he was sitting in his laboratory meditating. "Think of it," he recalled saying to himself. "Up to the present time the X ray has been used only to *find* disease . . . but now it might also offer possibilities in the *cure* of disease." Sure enough, at 10 a.m., a woman with cancer of the breast opened the door of his laboratory and walked in. She asked for Grubbé and, when he had identified himself, she handed him a letter which read:

E. H. GRUBBÉ
12 PACIFIC AVENUE
DEAR SIR:
   This will introduce Mrs. Rose Lee who has carcinoma of the left breast.
   She is willing to have you make X-ray applications.
   I hope you can help her.
Yours truly,
R. LUDLAM, M.D.
January 28, 1896.

Dr. Grubbé later deposited the original in the Smithsonian Institution, where it is now preserved.

Dr. Grubbé reported that he explained to Mrs. Lee the nature of the treatment, exhibited his X-ray apparatus, and assured her that none of the electrically activated parts would touch her body and that she would experience no pain. Mrs. Lee consented to the treatment.

"She was placed on her back," Dr. Grubbé wrote, "on an improvised operating table, and made as comfortable as could be. . . . The diseased breast was bared. Next, since the development of dermatitis on my hand had suggested that, if X rays were to be directed to a diseased area, the healthy adjacent tissues must be protected from these rays, and since at that time, lead was known to offer the most resistance to the X-ray, I had provided a number of pieces of sheet lead, taken from the inside of China tea chests, to use for this purpose. These pieces of lead were placed on the healthy parts adjacent to the diseased area."

If it occurred on January 29, this was beyond doubt the first occasion in history on which such precautions for the protection of a patient were taken.

The Crookes tube, activated by a Ruhmkorff coil, was now suspended 3 inches over the cancerous breast and turned on. The exposure continued for 1 hour. "Similar applications were to be given daily," Dr. Grubbé explained, "until cumulative effects, as would be shown in the development of dermatitis, made their appearance."

"Thus, for the first time in history," Dr. Grubbé concluded his account of the day's happenings, "X rays had been used for *treatment*, not diagnostic purposes.... That was the beginning of the treatment of diseases with X rays; that was the origin of X ray therapy. It occurred on Wednesday, January 29, 1896.... Without the blaring of trumpets or the beating of drums, a new therapeutic agent had arrived.

"X-ray therapy was born."

But the next day was to be an eventful one too. A second patient walked into Dr. Grubbé's office, a man of 80 bearing a very similar note:

E. H. GRUBBÉ
12 PACIFIC AVENUE   CHICAGO, January 29, 1896
MY DEAR SIR:
    The bearer, Mr. A. Carr, is the patient of whom I spoke the other day. He has had lupus for twelve years. He will come for X ray treatment as often as you think necessary.
                                    Yours truly,
                                    DR. A. C. HALPHIDE

The original of this note, too, Dr. Grubbé presented to the Smithsonian Institution.

During the weeks which followed, Dr. Grubbé wrote, he gave Mrs. Lee 18 treatments and Mr. Carr 21. He did not claim to have cured them, or even to have lengthened their lives. On the contrary, he frankly confessed that "no dramatic results were obtained. Neither case was reported clinically by the physicians who sent them to me because both parties died within a month after commencing X-ray treatment, and before sufficient cumulative effects had been obtained in either case to warrant any conclusions as to the value of the new therapeutic agent." Dr. Grubbé concluded, "This, briefly, is the story of the origin and birth of the treatment of diseases with X rays."

Is it a true story? Was Dr. Grubbé of Chicago in fact working with X rays before Wright at Yale (January 27), Trowbridge at Harvard (January 31), Cox at McGill (February 3), Goodspeed of Pennsylvania (February 5), Grubbé's fellow Chicagoan Dr. Burry (February 6), and many others whose stories have been reviewed above?

It would be generous to be able to accept Dr. Grubbé's account precisely as he wrote it, for he was beyond doubt truly an X-ray martyr.

During the 1900's and thereafter, his surgeon and others agree, he suffered a total of at least 83 surgical operations to relieve his discomfort and to retard the progress of gangrene from his left hand up his left arm to the elbow and then to the shoulder joint. His face was grossly disfigured with cancer. He was sterile, and his marriage was without issue, a misfortune he attributed to the X rays. He lived in agony for many years, yet, almost until the end, he continued to work with the rays.

"My courage is maintained by my work," he wrote in 1949. "Every day I treat patients who suffer more or are encumbered more than I, and so I go on. By helping others, I help myself." And he saw where his X-ray injuries were leading. "Eventually, in all probability," he wrote, "I will die from the effects of these early uncontrolled exposures to X rays. And like many of the early pioneers, I, too, will die a victim of natural science, a martyr to the X ray."

Grubbé's prediction came true. He died, of metastatic cancer, on March 26, 1960.

He concluded his chapter entitled "The Effects of the X Rays on the Author's Body" on a noble note: "I have lived long enough to see the child that I fathered develop into a sturdy, mature, and, worthwhile product; and I hope, as I approach the evening of my day, to see even more uses for X-ray therapy in the alleviation of the ills of mankind."

Thus, Grubbé's account of Grubbé. Further details can be found in Dr. Paul C. Hodges's 1964 biography of Grubbé.[3]

Dr. Hodges's meticulous research establishes beyond doubt that Emil Grubbé was a publicity seeker, "vain, boastful, incompletely truthful," and an unreliable witness concerning his own accomplishments. Dr. Hodges also reports that, except for the two letters dated January 28 and January 29, 1896, now in the Smithsonian and reproduced in his book, there is not a shred of contemporary support for Grubbé's story. On the contrary, all of the circumstantial evidence argues against the acceptance of Grubbé's claims. For example:

1. Grubbé first published his claims in 1933, after the witnesses to his alleged 1896 achievements—Cobb, Gilman, Halphide, Ludlam, and others—were already dead.

2. Grubbé's explanation for the delay is that he thought the crucial documents—the two notes now in the Smithsonian—had been de-

stroyed, and that he published when they unexpectedly came to light again. But this is hardly convincing. If he had published at any time during the first few years after 1896, he would not have needed documentary verification; Cobb, Gilman, Halphide, Ludlam, and no doubt others could have corroborated his story if it were true.

3. Grubbé published frequently on the X rays between 1898 and 1933, including long, rambling articles in which he recounted his own work with the rays. His 1896 priority claims are conspicuous by their absence from these earlier Grubbé papers. Indeed, in the course of discussing a paper by Dr. Gilman in 1901, Dr. Grubbé came close to *denying* any early experience with X-ray therapy. "I have not had very much experience with the application of the X rays to cancer," Grubbé stated in 1901. "However, I have treated several cases by the electrolytic method." Grubbé then described two cases treated with X rays; neither of them was Mrs. Rose Lee, whom Grubbé 31 years later claimed to have treated in 1896. Grubbé's failure to make his claim at this meeting, with Dr. Gilman present to confirm it and with the early history of X-ray therapy for cancer the topic under discussion, is an eloquent silence indeed.

4. Even if it is conceded that Grubbé, for reasons of his own which he never revealed, chose to keep his 1896 achievements a secret from 1896 to 1933, how can the silence of Drs. Cobb, Gilman, Halphide, and Ludlam be explained? Dr. Cobb, if Grubbé's story is true, was the first man to treat an X-ray burn. Dr. Gilman was the first to suggest that the X rays might be used to cure cancer, lupus, and indolent ulcers. Dr. Ludlam was the first to refer a patient for X-ray therapy, and Dr. Halphide was the first to refer a lupus patient. It is hard to believe that these men were as reticent as Grubbé, and maintained their conspiracy of silence with him throughout their lives.

5. Grubbé explained the silence of the other physicians by saying that the treatment of the two patients was not successful, and therefore no clinical report was warranted. But this, like his explanation of his own silence, carries no conviction whatever, for during the first weeks of February 1896, when Mrs. Lee and Mr. Carr were allegedly still under treatment by Grubbé, the Chicago newspapers were filled with almost daily accounts of the far less newsworth X-ray exploits of other Chicagoans—men such as Burry, Scribner, McBerty, Michelson, and Father Meiner. The Chicago *Tribune* ran X-ray stories on February 7, 9, 11, 13, 14, 15, 16, 18, 19, and 23, as noted above; other papers also covered local X-ray developments. Reporters swarmed through the cities. As Professor Dolbear remarked in March, "Experimenters are daily besieged by the multitude of reporters from the daily press, anxious to be the first to describe whatever is done." That the reporters missed not only

Grubbé but also his associates Cobb, Gilman, Halphide, and Ludlam seems in retrospect curious indeed. The doctors could hardly have known *in advance* that Grubbé's X-ray treatments would later prove unsuccessful. Indeed, the mere fact that X-ray equipment was in use in Chicago in January 1896, well in advance of Dr. Burry's February work (see page 22), would have made sensational headlines even if no patients were mentioned or cures claimed.

6. Next, consider the German glassblower, Schmidt—if, indeed, there was such a glassblower. Why did he, allegedly a key participant in those exciting events, hold his tongue?

7. Further, consider the patients, Mrs. Lee and Mr. Carr, and their families and friends. Why did they not reveal the facts to the Chicago reporters?

8. Fortunately, we need not rest on such a general absence of evidence. One of the key participants in the story as Grubbé told it actually did record his personal recollections of the beginnings of radiology in Chicago. In a paper entitled "The Roentgen Ray in Carcinoma," published in the January 15, 1901, issue of an obscure electrotherapeutic journal called *The Clinique*, Dr. J. E. Gilman—the man who, according to Grubbé, suggested on January 27, 1896, that the rays might be therapeutic—began his story as follows: "On the sixth day of February, 1896, the discovery of the Roentgen ray was given to the scientific world; the Crookes tubes were no novelty to the electricians but this new use of them excited the liveliest interest and some of the practical electricians at once set to work to experiment with them. [In Chicago,] Profs. [W. P.] Pratt and [Hugh] Wightman the next day (the 7th of February) began to organize a laboratory for work with the new application of force and by the thirteenth of April, 1896, had made a series of experiments on bacterial life and development as influenced by the X ray. These experiments were duly reported in the daily journals as witness this from the *Times-Herald* of April 19, 1896...."

With respect to cancer, which Grubbé alleged that he treated with X rays in January 1896, Dr. Gilman had this to report: "In April 1896, Dr. Pratt reported two cases of cancer of the stomach in which hemorrhage was controlled and the pain materially lessened [by X-ray therapy]. These cases drifted out of sight and I have been unable to follow up the results."

Concerning his own contribution to X-ray therapy, Dr. Gilman was not at all modest: "Early in the history of the therapeutic use of the X ray, I was personally interested in the use of it for a great variety of disease conditions. I tested in Dr. Pratt's laboratory the influence it possessed of controlling diseased actions in many different forms. I had the honor to report to this society, in June 1897, a paper on the X ray in therapeutics, giving in detail a cure of tubercular disease of an advanced stage." That this man who, according to Grubbé, first suggested the therapeutic use of the X rays in 1896, should have failed to mention his own perspicacity when detailing his later and lesser contributions exceeds the bounds of credibility.

Only two conclusions are possible: either Emil Grubbé was ignorant of this paper by Dr. Gilman when he gave Dr. Gilman a central role in his mythical account of the events of January 27, 1896, or else he failed to anticipate that, although dead men tell no tales, their published writings do, and that Gilman's obscure publication might later be unearthed to discredit an otherwise shrewdly fabricated tale.

This leaves unexplained the two letters now in the Smithsonian. Dr. Hodges, in his biography of Grubbé, agrees that these letters are the heart of the matter, for "it is they alone which bolster Dr. Grubbé's claim to have applied X rays therapeutically in January 1896." Dr. Hodges accepts them as authentic.

"At the outset," he writes, "I assumed that the letters were at worst frank forgeries, at best genuine but with altered dates; but I was wrong. At my urging, the Smithsonian submitted them to one of the nation's most respected crime detection laboratories, where it was established that there was no evidence of erasures; that paper, ink, style of writing, and other details were in keeping with the purported date of writing; and that the Ludlam signature appeared to have been written by the same hand that penned other unquestionably genuine Ludlam signatures I was able to submit for comparison."

Any number of hypotheses, however, can be framed to reconcile the report of the crime-detection laboratory—the F.B.I.—with the fact that Grubbé did not use X rays in January 1896.

With respect to paper, ink, style of writing, and similar details, for example, the absence of anachronistic flaws suggests that the letters were fabricated reasonably soon after their purported date. Grubbé during the late 1890's and early 1900's was closely associated with the group of dissident Chicago physicians known as electrotherapeutists, who were at odds with the American Medical Association and who quarreled among themselves over claims to priority in the use of X rays. One such priority dispute among the electrotherapeutists raged during the summer of 1896; another broke out in 1902. If the two letters now in the Smithsonian were fabricated during one of these early disputes, the appropriateness of the paper, ink, style of writing and other details would be readily understandable—and of no probative value whatever. Having fabricated the letters at an early date, Grubbé may then have decided that to use them would be too risky, and put them away. In 1933 he averred that he had thought they were destroyed and had only recently come upon them again; this may well have been true—but irrelevant to the authenticity of the letters.

The similarity between the Ludlam signature on the letter now in the Smithsonian and other unquestioned Ludlam signatures can also be explained without conceding the authenticity of the letters. Dr. Ludlam, too, was a member of the electrotherapeutist group which quarreled over X-ray priorities. If he and Grubbé concocted the letter together, the apparent authenticity of the Ludlam signature would be readily understandable. These possibilities are not offered as the true explanations of the letters, but as illustrations of how the crime-detection laboratory findings can be reconciled with the falsity of Grubbé's priority claims. Ingenious readers should not find it difficult to concoct other reconciliations of the same kind.

A distinction must be drawn, moreover, between the positive and negative use of crime-detection laboratory findings. The discovery of a watermark inconsistent with the alleged date on a document, or of an ink not available on that date, or of an incongruity in handwriting, may in some cases quite conclusively prove the falsity of the document. But *failure* to find flaws is never conclusive proof of authenticity. It may instead be a tribute to the skill and thoroughness of the forger, or a revelation of the inadequacies of the crime-detection laboratory.

Whether the two letters now in the Smithsonian were forged, or were written soon after their purported dates by the men who signed them, or whether there is some other explanation, may never be known. However, Grubbé's story is so implausible, so lacking in contemporary corroboration, and in such irreconcilable conflict with readily provable facts, and Grubbé's untruthfulness in other respects is so readily demonstrable, as to warrant the inclusion of his claims in this postscript rather than in the body of a history of American radiology.

REFERENCES

1. *Electricity (New York), 10:* no. 14, April 15, 1896.
2. GRUBBÉ, E. H., *X-Ray Treatment, Its Origin, Birth and Early History.* The Bruce Publishing Company, St. Paul, 1949.
3. HODGES, P. C., *The Life and Times of Emil H. Grubbé.* University of Chicago Press, Chicago, 1964.

PART II. THE GAS-TUBE YEARS (1897–1913)

9   Enter the Radiologist

During the years after 1896, X-ray tubes were sometimes called "vacuum tubes," but the amount of gas remaining in the tubes after evacuation was by modern standards substantial. Without this gas residue, the pre-1913 tubes would not work. Hence, the early tubes came later to be known as "gas tubes" (to distinguish them from the much more highly evacuated tubes available after 1913), and the years from 1896 through 1913 or 1914 came to be known as the "gas-tube era."

Among the major advances of the gas-tube era was the emergence of a new scientific breed—a small but influential group of physicians, well-versed in the physics of radiation as well as in medical practice, who called themselves "radiologists" or "roentgenologists," and who raised the use of the X ray for diagnosis and for therapy to the status of a new medical specialty.

Dr. Percy Brown of Boston, at the December 1908 meeting of the American Roentgen Ray Society, described the trials and tribulations which brought this new specialty into being[1]:

> The throat mirror needed the practiced eye, the stethoscope an acute ear, and the scalpel trained fingers, but [in the early days] this new affair, these X rays, their very name a confession of inexactitude, could be managed by any hospital photographer, ward orderly or nurse. The one thing needful ... was a hand to start the machine and then—to stop it. A process purely mechanical; no brains necessary. I heard it said, about ten years ago, that any high-school boy, given a smattering knowledge of human anatomy, should be able to 'take X-ray pictures,' to borrow the expression used. ...
>
> Clumsy apparatus and tiresome details made private office practice with the new rays undesirable, and patients were often sent for a diagnosis to the larger hospitals or to the laboratories of the technical schools. ... In isolated communities Dr. Thomas, Dr. Richard, and Dr. Henry struggled manfully to determine the position of fracture fragments with complete disregard of certain fundamental laws of optics; or, in blissful ignorance of the phenomena of a Roentgen dermatitis, continued to produce sloughs where often a simple dermic lesion formerly existed. It is not surprising that the patient regarded the cure as worse than the disease; and as a consequence, not to speak of the additional effect of frequent fantastic diagnoses, the Roentgen rays received a series of blows in the eye, of which the ecchymosis has not yet disappeared.

What was the reason for this state of things? It is not hard to find. The practice of using the Roentgen rays for the purposes of medicine was not placed on a stable basis. It was a piebald proceeding, a sort of Joseph's coat of many colors, which fitted no one. The attendant wires and sparks suggested an electrician's work, surely; . . . but there were the plates, dark room and chemicals, considered usually the accessories of the photographer. Neither of these artisans, on the other hand, could be expected to intrude themselves so far into the realms of medicine as to offer a diagnostic verdict. . . .

The electrician, after dallying in the dark room with the chemicals, produced photographic results of no higher quality than might be expected of an electrician; the photographer, after producing a generous display of pyrotechnics in the immediate vicinity of the patient, finally met with a practical electric problem quite beyond his depth; while the surgeon, albeit well versed in all heretofore employed methods of diagnosis, skillfully cut for renal stone in an endeavor to find what was, in reality, the elusive suspender button. . . .

When, therefore, there appeared at this juncture the one so long needed, an individual who foresaw the importance of roentgenology as a medical specialty, and was prepared to declare himself a devotee thereof, his arrival was as opportune as Sheridan's at Winchester. . . .

As a result of his efforts, first, certain technical features of the work have been exalted from the mere connecting of wires and rule-of-thumb manipulation to an involved study of electrostatics and the management of electrical discharges *in vacuo*. Second, by demonstrating that roentgenology, the science, and photography, as a calling or a trade, have nothing in common, he has established the fact that his diagnostic plates are merely a means to fortify his opinion as a diagnostician, and are not to be "struck off" at so much the dozen. . . .

The consulting practitioner, weighted down with the responsibility of his patient's welfare, has learned to demand the type of diagnostic and therapeutic result which only true work can produce. . . .

At the same 1908 meeting of the American Roentgen Ray Society, a prominent New York surgeon, Dr. Reginald H. Sayre, explained why many physicians who had formerly used X rays themselves had now abandoned them and were referring their patients to specialists like Dr. Brown.[2]

"I was one of those who early tried the Roentgen rays," Dr. Sayre told the radiologists. Indeed, he had begun to experiment back in 1896, and had continued to use X rays in his practice for several years thereafter. But, he declared, "I found, before the lapse of many years, that if I was to do as good X-ray work as was being done by others, I could not practice surgery. I had no time to develop my plates except at night, when I required sleep. The demands of my surgical practice were too exacting to permit me to do justice to the X-ray work."

Some physicians who found themselves in this position dropped their other specialty and became radiologists. Dr. Sayre chose the opposite course. "I . . . concluded that I would cease taking pictures with the ray, and would let somebody who had become more competent than I carry on the work, and that I would seek his advice when I wanted a skiagram made.

"That method has been vastly more . . . satisfactory to me and to my patients. If you want an examination made of the blood, you get a better one made by a man who makes a specialty of blood examinations than by the ordinary clinical observer. The latter ought to associate himself with the laboratory worker who has perfected himself in the technique. If you want a proper examination of the body by X ray, call in the assistance of a competent radiologist who will give you satisfactory interpretations on the points on which you are in doubt. We must work hand in hand if we expect to get good results and accurate results. This is the day for specialism, and I believe that the work that is being done by the society in placing radiography on a firm, broad, scientific foundation cannot be overestimated."

Dr. Russell D. Carman of St. Louis echoed these sentiments 2 years later in a paper entitled "Medical Roentgenology as a Specialty." "The right of a specialty to existence has only this test," Dr. Carman declared, "that it employ the specialist's entire time and attention with increased benefit to himself, to the profession, and to the public. Judged by this test, roentgenology is and of right ought to be a legitimate specialty." [3]

Efforts had been made, Dr. Carman conceded, to reduce the specialty to a set of rules which anyone could apply—"to establish a definite length of exposure, given a certain tube, plate, current, weight of patient and purpose of radiography; but the rule thus derived is not sufficiently approximate to be practically helpful. To ask how long a plate should be exposed for a given case is comparable to asking a locomotive engineer how far it is necessary to open the throttle in order to run at the rate of forty miles an hour."

Successful employment of the X rays, Dr. Carman continued, "demands an intimate knowledge of a highly complex apparatus, practical acquaintance with the essentials of a good radiogram, ability to interpret a radiograph properly, detailed instruction in the art of localizing foreign bodies, familiarity with the therapeutic use of the rays, and an appreciation of the dangers which may attend their careless or unskilled application." Indeed, Dr. Carman considered the requirements so difficult as to warrant a startling conclusion: ". . . There are in the United States today [1910] barely a dozen roentgenologists who are capable of performing really expert service."

Typical of the general practitioners who gradually became radiologists was Dr. J. Grosvenor Cross of Rochester, Minnesota. He secured X-ray equipment very early, in February 1896, and he demonstrated its usefulness to his neighboring physicians at local medical society meetings in August 1896 and again early in 1897. Among those who thus learned of Dr. Cross's X-ray machine were two young Rochester surgeons, Dr. William Mayo and Dr. Charles J. Mayo. Helen Clapesattle has told the story of Dr. Cross and the Mayo brothers in her definitive biography, *The Doctors Mayo*. A week after Dr. Cross demonstrated his X-ray machine in 1897, Miss Clapesattle states,

> the Mayo brothers had an occasion to test the machine for themselves. A little boy who had swallowed a vest buckle was brought to the office. It would help in deciding how best to remove it if the doctors could know just where in the esophagus it was lodged, whether it was open or closed, and if open in what direction its prongs were pointing, so they went over to see whether Cross's X-ray machine could tell them.
>
> Dr. Cross made two pictures, one of which showed the buckle in remarkably clear outline, with the prongs pointing upward, so that drawing it out through the mouth would punch them into the esophagus walls. Consequently Dr. Charlie made an incision into the esophagus and pulled the buckle out blunt end first. His subsequent report of the case, written quite uncharacteristically without any reference to Dr. Cross's part in it, was one of the first on the use of the skiagraph, as an X-ray picture was called, to appear in the Northwest.
>
> During the next three years Dr. Cross did a considerable amount of X-ray diagnosis for the Mayos, most of it to locate foreign bodies such as needles, bullets, and bits of glass or steel so the surgeons could remove them more easily. In defining the position and extent of fractures also they found the Roentgen ray a marvel, but it was still of little use in the diagnosis of organic disease, for techniques and substances to render the organs of the body opaque to the ray had yet to be found.
>
> In those early stages the X ray could be dangerous. Manufacturers, eager to make the apparatus as simple as possible, did not provide sufficient protection and enthusiastic operators did not exercise sufficient care, so that severe burns and skin affections [followed]. . . . Word of this possibility spread among laymen, and unscrupulous persons found a new racket in suing the X-ray specialist for damages.
>
> One of the patients Dr. Cross handled for the Mayos sued him for ten thousand dollars, claiming severe injury as the result of the X ray. His bill of particulars set forth a convincing case, and Burt Eaton, the lawyer defending Dr. Cross, was worried and went to Dr. Will for advice. When he finished reading the particulars, Dr. Will said the man had listed the very same complaints in a letter he wrote them before he ever appeared for examination. A long search finally

turned up the letter, and that was the end of the case against Dr. Cross.

Before long even Twin City doctors were referring patients to Dr. Cross for X-ray diagnosis, and early in the 1900's he moved to Minneapolis to continue his practice there.

Thus another general practitioner joined the ranks of the radiologists. Who were these pioneer radiologists? A survey made by Dr. Brown provides several interesting answers. He sent a questionnaire to all members of the American Roentgen Ray Society in the summer of

Date of Medical Degree

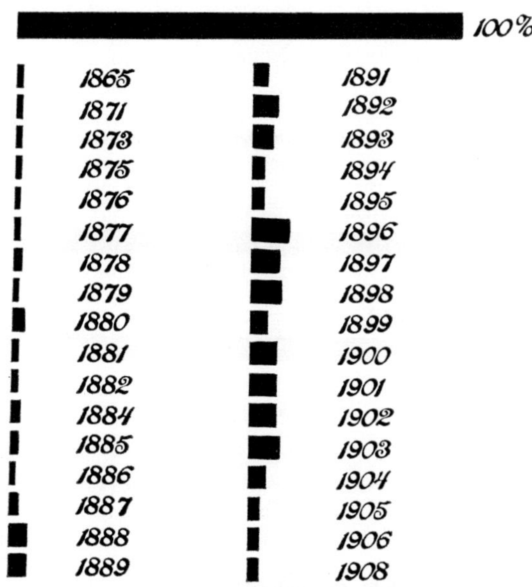

FIG. 19. From *American Quarterly of Roentgenology*, 2: 249, December 1910.

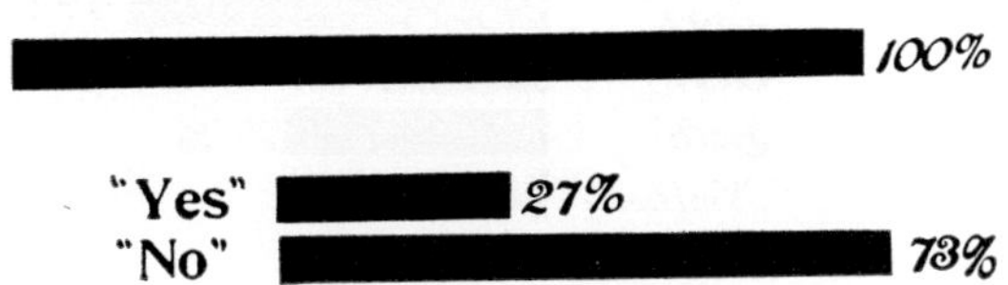

FIG. 20. From *American Quarterly of Roentgenology*, 2: 253, December 1910.

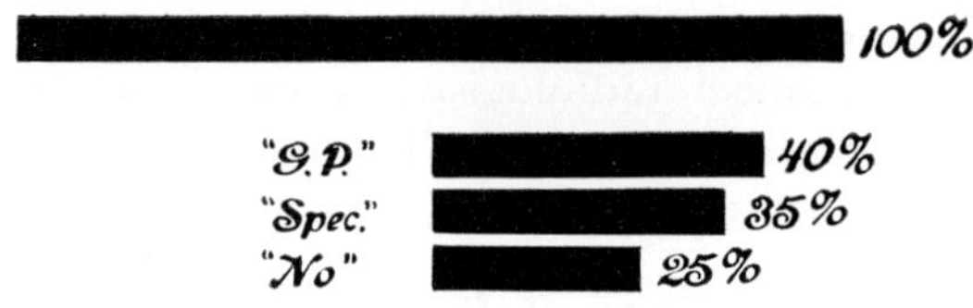

FIG. 21. From *American Quarterly of Roentgenology*, 2: 253, December 1910.

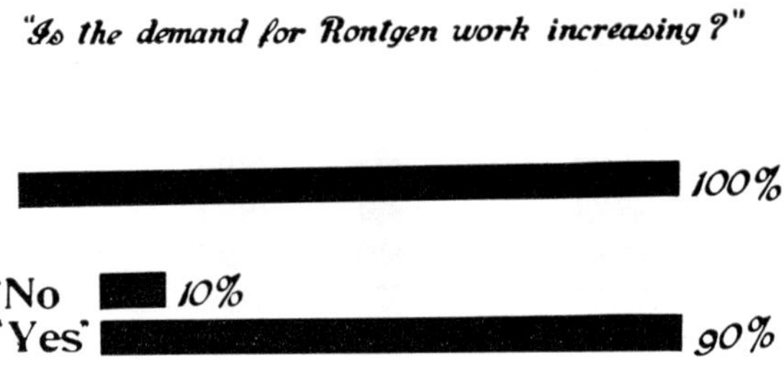

FIG. 22. From *American Quarterly of Roentgenology*, 2: 256, December 1910.

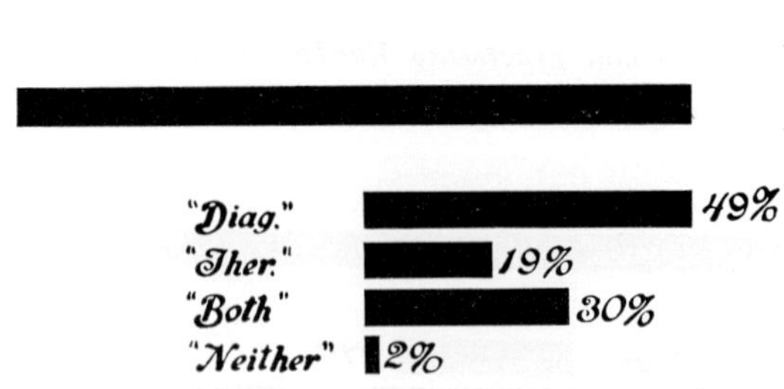

FIG. 23. From *American Quarterly of Roentgenology*, 2: 260, December 1910.

1910. About half of the members replied, and Dr. Brown summarized the returns at the September 1910 meeting of the society.

The great majority of those responding had received their medical degree during the years 1896 through 1903 (Fig. 19). Thus the specialty in 1910 was staffed primarily with younger men, most of whom were still in school or in medical school when Roentgen's discovery was announced. Among those receiving their degrees between 1900 and 1903, however, a considerable number had begun working with X rays in 1896 or 1897 as physicists, engineers, electricians, photographers, or in other technical capacities, and had thereafter gone back to school and earned their M.D. degrees specifically for the purpose of qualifying as radiologists. Several leaders of the profession—Dr. Mihran Krikor Kassabian of Philadelphia, Dr. Eugene Wilson Caldwell of New York City, and Dr. Walter James Dodd of Boston, to cite only a few examples—were included in this category.

Only 27 per cent of the ARRS members in 1910, Dr. Brown's survey indicated, were limiting their practice to radiology (Fig. 20). The remainder were about equally divided between general practice and some other specialty (Fig. 21). Almost all the members agreed that the demand for their X-ray services was increasing (Fig. 22).

Finally, Dr. Brown's survey throws a rather surprising light on an important current issue. During the 1950's and 1960's some radiologists and medical educators were arguing that radiology should be divided into two independent specialties, one concerned with radiation in the diagnosis of disease and the other concerned with radiation as a form of treatment. In 1910, it appears, a considerable cleavage had already developed. Only 30 per cent of the ARRS members responding stated that they were using the rays in both ways; about half were concerned solely with diagnosis, and there was a significant minority specializing solely in therapy (Fig. 23).

In the chapters which follow, these specialties are considered separately.

REFERENCES

1. *Trans. Amer. Roentgen Ray Soc.*, 232–237, 1908.
2. *Ibid.*, pp. 238–239.
3. *J. Missouri Med. Ass.*, 7: 121–123, 1910–1911.

10   Learning to See with the X Rays

During the first few years of the "gas-tube era," most of the practical diagnostic work with the X rays was concerned with broken bones and with the localization of foreign objects lodged in the body. Then the field gradually broadened. More and more X-ray workers adopted and extended the technique of chest fluoroscopy pioneered in 1896 by Dr. Williams of Harvard at the Boston City Hospital. The X-ray study of bone fractures inevitably led to the study of diseases of the bone, and then to diagnosis of the diseases of the joints. Orthopedic surgery was revolutionized by this work. In 1895, a leg which was shortened only 1 or 2 inches following a fracture was considered an "excellent result"; not so many years later, with X-ray visualization available, the same result might lead to a suit for malpractice. From such relatively simple chores as localizing gunshot in the hand or foot, radiologists proceeded to develop far subtler methods of localization—capable, as noted above (page 72), of localizing slivers of metal or glass lodged in or near the eyeball.

All this, gratifying though it might be, soon became commonplace. The far more fascinating challenge which the early radiologists faced was how to extend the boundaries of their art into wholly new regions— the brain, for example, and the gastrointestinal tract. To meet this challenge, they had to devise new techniques. Equally important, they had to learn to decode the meanings implicit in the images recorded on their plates or projected on their fluoroscopic screens. The challenge was to discover in those images diagnostic signs or clues which had never before been perceived.

Thus, the gas-tube era was the golden age of a procedure which later came to be known as "retrospectoscopy." A radiologist made his negatives, examined them, and failed to reach a sound diagnosis. Then the patient was operated on, or died and was examined at autopsy. The radiologist attended the operation or the autopsy and learned the true diagnosis. Thereafter, in retrospect, he re-examined his plates and searched, with whatever embarrassment, for the clues that he had missed before. The rewards of retrospectoscopy came later, when another patient revealed similar indications on his X-ray plates, and the radiologist could this time diagnose with confidence. Dr. Leo Rigler of the University of Minnesota Medical School captured the essence of retrospectoscopy in a pair of sketches drawn many years later (Fig. 24).

Dr. Pfahler Examines the Brain

Typical of the gas-tube era pioneers who mastered the art of retrospectoscopy was Dr. George Edward Pfahler (1874–1957) of Philadelphia. Young Pfahler was a freshman medical student at the University of Pennsylvania in 1895 when Roentgen made his discovery, and he was just completing his internship at the Philadelphia General Hospital when he was introduced to roentgenology. The hospital's chief resident physician, Dr. Daniel E. Hughes, turned to him one morning and announced, "Dr. Pfahler, the Board of Directors have decided to install an X-ray machine and they want you to operate it." [1]

During moments of reminiscence many decades later, when he was recognized as one of America's foremost radiologists, Dr. Pfahler liked to quote his reply: "Dr. Hughes, I can see no future in this field. All of the bones of the body and foreign bodies have been demonstrated. But I am here to do what I am told."

The "X-ray laboratory" established for Dr. Pfahler in 1899 was typical of many others during the gas-tube era. A room 12 by 15 feet was assigned him, but it soon had to be cut down to 12 by 12 feet in order to make space for a photographic darkroom where Dr. Pfahler could develop his plates. His equipment consisted of a Ruhmkorff induction coil plus a tube stand and a Sayen self-regulating tube, manufactured by Queen & Co. of Philadelphia. A stretcher mounted on a carriage completed the meagre laboratory furnishings.

Yet Dr. Pfahler considered himself fortunate, for at Philadelphia General "there was an unlimited amount of pathological material, permitting much experience . . . in the diagnosis of what were formerly obscure conditions. We had the very great advantage of autopsy study and confirmation of diagnoses because during that period, Dr. John V. Shoemaker, who was Director of Health, issued an order for the City of Philadelphia that there should be an autopsy on all patients dying in the . . . hospital. This gave great opportunities for us to study the body during life and . . . then permitted observations at autopsy."

Dr. Pfahler made good use of these rich opportunities, and in 1901 he decided to try his hand at X-ray examination of the brain. Interest in brain radiography had continued high ever since Edison in 1896 had sought without success to produce a brain negative. Would a brain tumor, Dr. Pfahler wondered, show up on an X-ray plate? He discussed the matter with Dr. Charles K. Mills, the neurologist at Phila-

CONVENTIONAL VIEWING

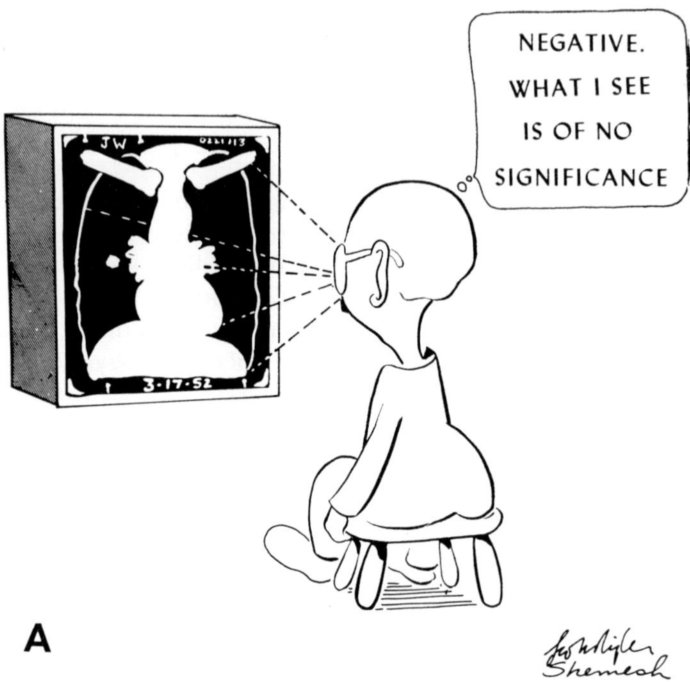

'RETROSPECTOSCOPIC' VIEWING

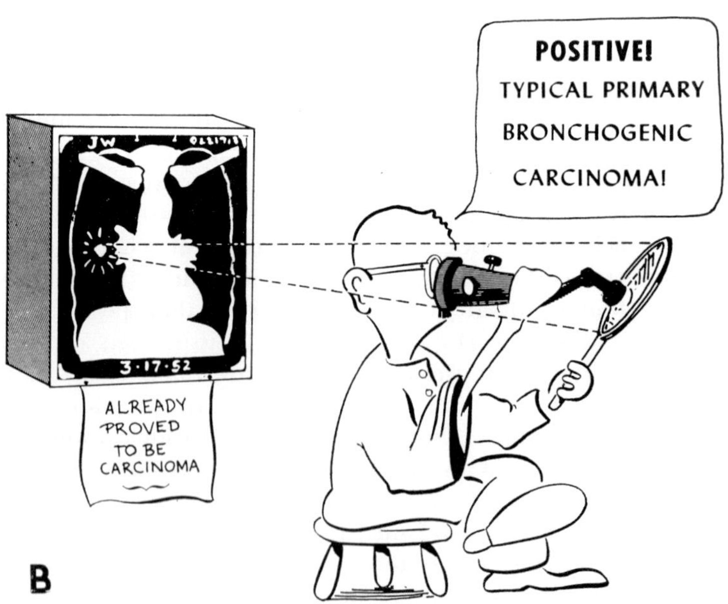

FIG. 24. Two unpublished drawings supplied by Dr. Leo Rigler.

delphia General Hospital and clinical professor of nervous diseases at the University of Pennsylvania.

"My previous experience with the rays in attempted localization of tumors had not been successful," Dr. Mills later noted. "In 1900 I called in Professor Arthur W. Goodspeed of the University of Pennsylvania to assist in the localization of a suspected cerebellar tumor in the case of a child. The investigation was carried out with great care, but the skiagraph did not show any shadow indicating the presence of a tumor. On two occasions I have had efforts made to locate tumors in the pelvis by means of the X rays—once by Professor Goodspeed, and in another instance at the Pennsylvania Hospital. . . . In the latter case a doubtful shadow was obtained, in the former the result was negative." [2]

Nor did a review of the published medical literature suggest to Dr. Mills that an effort by Dr. Pfahler to visualize a brain tumor was likely to produce results. "The only case . . . in which a brain tumor has been clearly localized by means of the X rays in the living subject," Dr. Mills told a meeting of the College of Physicians of Philadelphia in February 1902, "is one reported by [Archibald] Church, of Chicago."

Dr. Church had published his case in the *American Journal of the Medical Sciences* for February 1899. His patient was a 15-year-old boy with symptoms suggesting a tumor of the cerebellum. Dr. Church had sent his patient to the laboratory of Wolfram Fuchs (see above, page 64). The skiagrams made by Fuchs showed a clearly distinguishable outline of what appeared to be a nodulated tumor, but the tumor appeared to be inoperable. Subsequently the boy died, and at autopsy a tumor of precisely the kind suggested by the outline was found where the X-ray plate suggested that it would be found. With the exception of this solitary case, Dr. Mills could find no previous successful use of the X rays in localizing a brain tumor.

Still, Dr. Mills knew that Dr. Pfahler had been "doing much extremely valuable work with the X rays at the Philadelphia Hospital," so when Dr. Pfahler made a request to try his hand at X-raying the brain, "I was glad to accede. . . ."

A patient willing to cooperate was soon found. She was a 32-year-old laundress, admitted to Philadelphia General in October 1901 with paralysis of the right arm, splitting headaches which caused her the greatest misery, and other neurological symptoms suggesting a large brain tumor. With Dr. Mills's consent, Dr. Pfahler went to work.

The laundress "was placed in the proper position," Dr. Pfahler recorded, "and an exposure of four minutes was made with a moderately hard vacuum. I placed the anode of the tube directly opposite to the area in which Dr. Mills had [by clinical inference] located the tumor, and at a distance of 18 inches from the plate, for the reason that at this distance the shadows of the upper side of the skull would be dissipated by the divergence of the rays, and yet good definition of the structure on the opposite side of the skull would be obtained."

The plate far exceeded Dr. Pfahler's fondest hopes. It "showed good detail of all the structures, namely, the scalp, the outer table of the skull, the diploe, and the inner table, the frontal sinuses, the ethmoidal, sphenoidal, and mastoid cells, the coronal suture, the groove of the posterior meningeal artery, the outline of the base of the skull, and shadows corresponding to the depressions of the frontal convolutions."

Within this mass of shadowy data, Dr. Pfahler's eye was able to isolate the image that he was seeking—"a large shadow lying between the coronal suture and the posterior meningeal artery. . . ."

But was this "large shadow" in fact the outline of a tumor, or an artifact of some kind? To confirm his findings, Dr. Pfahler next made a similar plate of the brain of another woman of the same age and weight. This "normal comparison negative" was also a very good one, "as shown by the fact that good definition was obtained of the base of the skull and mastoid cells." It "did not show the shadow of the tumor as seen in the first plate. . . . I then repeated the exposure upon the patient with the tumor and obtained the same shadows as before." The tumor appeared to be dumbbell-shaped, with two clearly distinguishable lobes.

Dr. Pfahler accordingly presented his plates and opinion to Dr. Mills, who "agreed with me that the shadow obtained in the case of his patient was probably that of the tumor. Its definite outline in the upper portion seemed to indicate that it was superficial and therefore removable."

An operation was performed on December 11, 1901, by Drs. W. J. Hearn and John Chalmers DaCosta. Both Dr. Mills and Dr. Pfahler were present, along with other surgeons and neurologists, no doubt attracted by this opportunity to practice X-ray retrospectoscopy. The physicians were loud in their praise of Dr. Pfahler when the tumor was located in precisely the place which the X-ray shadow suggested, but Dr. Pfahler was disappointed, for the tumor excised by the surgeons was much smaller than the one shown on his plate, and was not dumbbell-shaped. "If I have demonstrated the tumor, then only half of the tumor has been removed," he remarked as the scalp was being closed.[1]

The patient survived the operation by only a few hours. Dr. Pfahler attended the autopsy, and, as he had anticipated, "a large remaining subcortical portion of the tumor . . . corresponding to the remainder and less definite part of the shadow" was found.[2]

Dr. Pfahler continued his studies of brain tumors thereafter, and at the September 1904 meeting of the American Roentgen Ray Society he was able to report further progress based on a series of 100 brain examinations.[3]

Following the case of the laundress, Dr. Pfahler explained, he had begun, at the suggestion of Dr. Mills, to experiment with the brains and skulls of cadavers. First he made plates of the head of a 63-year-old man. He then opened the skull, removed a portion of the brain, and replaced it with an embalmed tumor. Then he replaced the section of the skull and sutured the scalp, "so as to preserve as nearly as possible the conditions that would be found in the living subject. *The negative made showed a very distinct shadow of the tumor."* * A whole series of further experiments, using other types of tumor lodged in other regions within the skull, produced equally positive results.

During these cadaver experiments, Dr. Pfahler noted one of the commonest radiological pitfalls of the gas-tube era—a lack of sufficient "latitude." The radiologist had to guess the precise duration of exposure which would produce a detail-rich plate under the prevailing conditions. For a given view, for example, 3 minutes might be too short, but 4 minutes might prove too long. Dr. Pfahler met this problem by linking the duration of exposure to the other variables in the situation. He continued in his 1904 report:

> Realizing that much of the success in skiagraphy of the brain must of necessity depend upon accurate technique, I . . . conducted a series of experiments to find the best possible technique. In skiagraphy we have five principal varying factors. These are the distance of the anode from the plate, the time of exposure, the vacuum of the tube, the amount of current, and the thickness and density of the part examined. The first four are more or less under our control. The fifth is always variable, and, therefore, the other four must be judged and regulated in proportion to the fifth. Fortunately, the . . . thickness of the adult skull is not very variable, but must not be entirely ignored.
>
> In this series of experiments I used at one and the same time three different tumors, one a spindle-celled sarcoma, one an epithelioma, and one a perithelioma. One was placed in the prefrontal region, one in the motor region, and one between the two halves of the cerebellum. My first series of plates was made to determine the best time of exposure. In this test I used a tube the vacuum of which was equal to two and a half inches of parallel air spark at a distance of 18 inches and as the subject, I had the body of a woman, aged 42. The times of my exposures were two, two and a half, three, three and a half, and four minutes, respectively.
>
> My best results were obtained with an exposure of three and a half minutes.

---

* Italics added.

I then made a series of negatives in which the distances of the anode from the plate were twelve, fifteen, eighteen, and twenty-one inches, respectively. My best results were obtained at a distance of eighteen inches. At this distance the shadows of the proximal side of the skull will be more or less diffused, and yet sufficient detail of the opposite half of the brain be obtained.

The degree of vacuum is our most variable factor and the one that is least under our control, and, therefore, experience and judgment in varying the other factors accordingly will have an important bearing upon the results in each case. I used a self-regulating tube and used as nearly as I could vacuums corresponding to two, two and a half, three, and three and a half inches of parallel air spark.

My best results were obtained with a vacuum of two and a half inches.

Having performed this experimental work, Dr. Pfahler was in a position to offer his services to clinicians with greater self-confidence, and clinicians sent him their patients with greater willingness. Dr. Mills, for example, sent him several more patients. In one, Dr. Pfahler found the shadow of something "2½ inches in length, 1½ inches in width at its widest portion, irregular in outline, and from its density...I estimated it to be about a half inch in thickness." In the light of the case history, Dr. Pfahler interpreted the object casting the X-ray shadow to be a *gumma*, that is, a late syphilitic lesion. Drs. Hearn and DaCosta operated, and indeed found a gumma which "corresponded exactly to the location and dimensions given in the skiagraphic examination." In several cases of "softening of the brain," too, Dr. Pfahler was able to demonstrate "transparent areas" in the negative "which corresponded exactly with the area of degeneration" subsequently found at autopsy.

"In addition to the tumors and cases of softening," Dr. Pfahler reported in 1904, "I have had a case in which the skiagraph seemed to show thickening of the membranes to a considerable extent. This corresponded to the clinical symptoms. No autopsy has been obtained, and, therefore, I can draw no definite conclusion."

Dr. Pfahler continued his report on an optimistic note: "I believe that we should be able to show in the skiagraph most large lesions, such as new growths, softening, hemorrhage, and abscess." In this he was mistaken. Later studies were to show that the great majority of tumors do not cast a shadow directly visible on the X-ray plate, and subtle means were therefore developed to identify and locate them indirectly (see below, pp. 219–229). Dr. Pfahler himself concluded on a word of caution: "I would never take the responsibility of an operation upon the brain *purely* upon skiagraphic evidence." Rather, the X-ray findings should be used for "confirming or adding to the clinical evidence." [3]

"Diagnosticating" the Gastrointestinal Tract

The one medical specialist for whom the X rays seemed at first to have no value was the gastroenterologist. The organs with which he was concerned—the stomach, duodenum, and intestines, for example—cast almost no detectable X-ray shadow. Hence, it seemed that the X-ray diagnosis of gastrointestinal conditions lay forever out of reach. Yet, before the end of the gas-tube era, gastrointestinal radiography and fluoroscopy were firmly established. As early as the December 1908 meeting of the American Roentgen Ray Society, papers were read by Dr. Augustus W. Crane of Kalamazoo, Michigan, on "X-Ray Evidence in Gastric Ulcer," by Dr. Pfahler of Philadelphia on "The Roentgen Rays as an Aid in the Diagnosis of Carcinoma of the Stomach," by Dr. Charles Lester Leonard of Philadelphia on "The Roentgenographic Study of Motion in the Viscera," and by Dr. Henry K. Pancoast of Philadelphia on "Radiographic Examination of the Gastro-Intestinal Tract." [4]

The enthusiastic tone of this 1908 meeting was set by Dr. Pancoast, who reported, "It has been a comparatively short time since the first pioneers in gastro-intestinal radiography demonstrated the practicability and simplicity of X-ray examinations of the stomach and large bowel, but in that short space of time most extraordinary progress has been made, because this work was at once taken up and has been developed by a large number of radiographers, working both individually and collectively, who immediately realized its importance and its wide range of application and usefulness. At the present time gastrointestinal radiography takes equal rank in importance with X-ray diagnosis in connection with diseases and injuries of bones and joints, urinary calculus, and the location of foreign bodies."

The secret of this success was the use of a "contrast medium"—that is, a substance opaque to the X rays which could be mixed with food and swallowed to display the upper gastrointestinal tract, or introduced by enema for study of the lower tract. As Dr. Russell D. Carman of the Mayo Clinic subsequently wrote, "The fundamental principle of roentgen-ray examinations of the stomach and intestine is the visualization of their outline by filling them with substances opaque to the ray, a principle which we owe to [Hermann] Rieder of Munich, who, in 1904, first used bismuth subnitrate for the purpose." [5]

Dr. Carman's "fundamental principle" was sound, but his history was far from the mark. The principle was in fact established long before 1904, and not by Rieder of Munich. Many others in the United States, France, Germany, and perhaps in other countries had worked with contrast media before Rieder, some as early as 1896. Their remarkable findings were almost completely overlooked, not only by Dr. Carman but by most of his contemporaries.

Walter B. Cannon

Among the forgotten pioneers was Dr. Walter B. Cannon (1871–1945) of Harvard. His studies deserve detailed consideration, for, in addition to demonstrating the usefulness of contrast media, they elucidated the basic physiology of the gastrointestinal tract. In 1913 he recalled[6]:

> In the fall of 1896, when I was a first-year student in the Harvard Medical School, and Dr. Albert Moser, a Cambridge acquaintance, was a second-year student, we went to Prof. H. P. Bowditch and asked for an opportunity to undertake a physiologic investigation. He suggested that we test by means of the newly discovered Roentgen rays the ... view ... that substances when swallowed are shot down the esophagus by pressure developed in the mouth, and are not pushed down by a peristaltic wave. A small static machine and some simple tubes were secured, and we set to work.
>
> Our first observation was made on Dec. 9, 1896, when we watched globular pearl buttons pass down the esophagus of a dog.
>
> ... Then we procured a goose and made for it a box so arranged that the long neck reached up through the cover. A high cardboard collar was then attached to the top of the box in such a way that it could be closed in front when surrounding the goose's neck. Thus the goose, with the appearance of using the most stylish neckwear, presented to the fluorescent screen a very satisfactory extent of esophagus. At the meeting of the American Physiological Society in Boston, December 29, 1896, the phenomena of deglutition [swallowing] as exhibited by the goose when swallowing capsules containing bismuth subnitrate was informally demonstrated to the members by means of the Roentgen rays. This was, I think, the first public demonstration of movements of the alimentary canal by use of the new method.

Ten days later, Cannon and his fellow medical student went on to employ "bismuth subnitrate mixed with the food (in this case a bread mush) to render the swallowed mass visible." After completing their studies of the esophagus, moreover, they went on to study the action of the stomach with the same bismuth meal.

On April 23, 1897, for example, they fed bread, soaked in warm water and mixed with bismuth subnitrate, to a cat, and noted with fascination the series of wavelike contractions known as *peristalsis* passing along the muscular coating of the stomach. Each contraction started at about the middle of the stomach and moved downward toward the pyloric valve at the stomach exit. These results were reported in *Science* for June 11, 1897. During the months that followed, the two students found time, despite their medical classwork, to make many additional studies of these peristaltic stomach waves.

In the fall of 1897, Cannon and Moser extended their studies to a human patient, "a seven-year-old girl placed in the sitting posture. Gelatin capsules containing bismuth were used for solids, and were traced to a point below the heart. The motion was very regular. . . . Semi-solids—a mush of bread and milk—could be seen about as far as solids, *i.e.,* to just below the heart. The motion of the mushy bolus was the same as with solids, except that the rapidity was perhaps slightly greater." [7]

Now Dr. Francis H. Williams of the Harvard Medical School joined forces with the two students. Observations were made on three children: James W., aged 10; M. W., a girl of 7; and K. A., a boy of 5. The children lay stretched out on their backs on a canvas stretcher. "The target of the vacuum tube was 45 to 60 centimeters from the under surface of the body at a point under the umbilicus; and the fluorescent screen was placed over the abdomen." Periodically, as digestion continued, tracings were made of the shape and position of the stomach (Fig. 25).

"Thus we see that if bismuth is given as described above," Dr. Williams wrote, "an outline of part of the stomach, its position in inspiration and expiration, and some peculiarities of shape may be noted; likewise that its changes in size during the process of digestion may be observed; further, the respective rapidity with which digestion proceeds in different individuals may be watched. After the various characteristics belonging to the stomach in health have been established, the presence of abnormal conditions of this organ, such as some cases of malignant disease, will perhaps be more readily recognized than at present. The constant presence of a darkened area in the stomach, for example, may suggest the thickening of its walls due to a malignant disease; some displacements or adhesions may be recognized, as well as hour-glass contractions, or an unusual delay in the digestive process."

Dr. Williams was modest. "These observations are preliminary in character," he wrote, "and merely suggest some of the ways in which this problem may be approached." [8] Yet, with his customary acuity, he had in that single paragraph placed his finger on many of the diagnostic signs which are still proving useful today.

Young Cannon continued his stomach studies with the bismuth meal through 1897 and 1898, and reported at length on "The Movements of the Stomach Studied by Means of the Roentgen Rays" in the *American Journal of Physiology* for May 1, 1898:

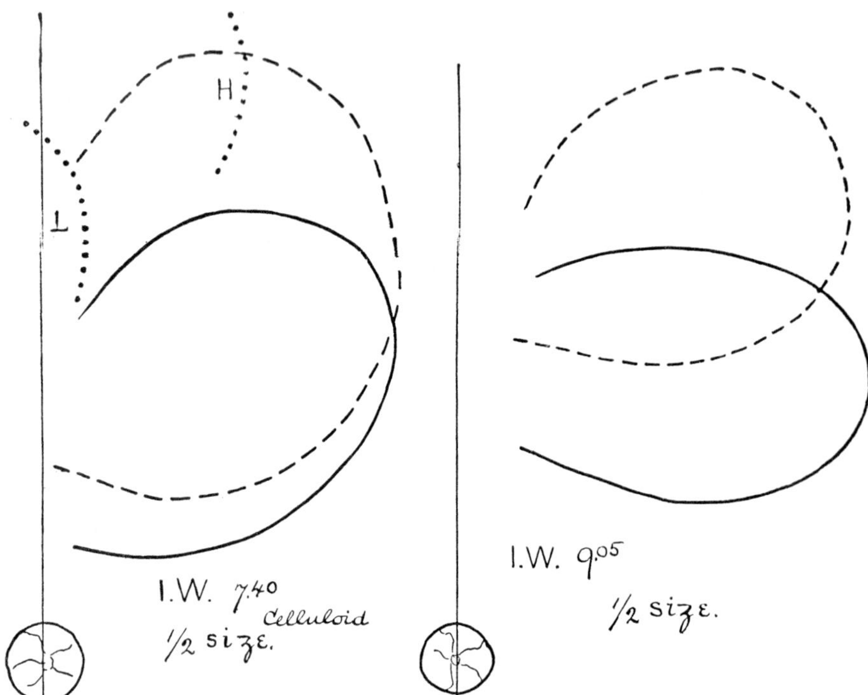

Fig. 25. From Williams, Francis, *The Roentgen Rays in Medicine and Surgery*, Ed. 3, p. 364, The Macmillan Company, New York, 1903.

Within five minutes after a cat has finished a meal of bread, there is visible near the duodenal end of the antrum a slight annular contraction which moves peristaltically to the pylorus; this is followed by several waves recurring at regular intervals. Two or three minutes after the first movement is seen, very slight constrictions appear near the middle of the stomach, and, pressing deeper into the greater curvature, course slowly toward the pyloric end. As new regions enter into constriction, the fibers just previously contracted become relaxed, so that there is a true moving wave, with a trough between two crests. When a wave swings round the bend in the pyloric part the indentation made by it deepens; and as digestion goes on the antrum elongates and the constrictions running over it grow stronger, but, until the stomach is nearly empty, they do not entirely divide the cavity.

After the antrum has lengthened, a wave takes about thirty-six seconds to move from the middle of the stomach to the pylorus. At all periods of digestion the waves recur at intervals of almost exactly ten seconds. So regular is this rhythm that many times I have been able to determine within two or three seconds when a minute had elapsed simply by counting six similar phases of the undulations as they passed a given point. It results from this rhythm that when one wave is just beginning, several others are already running in order before it. . . .

The number of waves during a single period of digestion is larger than might possibly at first be supposed. In a cat that finished eating fifteen grams of bread at 10:52 a.m., the waves were running regularly at 11 o'clock. The stomach was not free from food until 6:12 p.m. During that time the cat was fastened to the holder at intervals of half an hour and the waves were always observed, following one another in slow and monotonous succession. At the rate of 360 an hour, approximately 2,600 waves passed over the antrum during that single digestive period.

Earlier researchers knew, of course, that in order to leave the antrum of the stomach, food had to pass through the pyloric valve or sphincter into the duodenum. But precisely how did this valve work? And was the food ejected, or did it merely drop through the pyloric valve in response to gravitational forces? Cannon learned by means of his X-ray studies that the food was in fact ejected with considerable force, and that the function of the pyloric valve was far more selective than had been anticipated.

In cats fed with bread mixed with subnitrate of bismuth, ten or fifteen minutes elapse after the first constriction in the antrum before any food can be seen in the duodenum. When food does appear it is spurted through the pylorus and shoots along the intestine for two or three centimeters.

Not every constriction-wave forces food from the antrum. On one occasion, about an hour after the movements began, three consecutive waves were seen, each of which squirted food into the duodenum. The pylorus remained closed against the next eight waves, opened for the ninth, but closed once more against the tenth and eleventh. . . . In this irregular way the food continued passing from the stomach. . . .

When a hard bit of food reaches the pylorus, the sphincter closes tightly and remains closed longer than when the food is soft. . . . On one occasion, the sphincter was seen to open only seven times in twenty minutes following the arrival of a hard particle of food at the pylorus. The conclusion may therefore be drawn that hard morsels keep the pylorus closed and hinder the passage of the food into the duodenum.

The wavelike constrictions of the stomach, Cannon noted in conclusion, are amazingly sensitive to emotional states. On one occasion, for example, Cannon was watching the rhythmic undulations coursing regularly over the stomach when the cat "suddenly changed from her peaceful sleepiness, began to breathe quickly and struggled to get loose. As soon as the change took place, the movements in the stomach entirely disappeared; the pyloric portion relaxed and presented a smooth rounded outline. I continued observing, and stroked the cat reassuringly. In a moment she became quiet and began to purr. As soon as this happened, the movements commenced again in the stomach; first a few constrictions were visible near the end of the antrum, then a few near the sharp bend in the lesser curvature, and finally the waves were running normally from their habitual starting place.

"By holding the cat's mouth closed between the thumb and last three fingers and covering her nostrils with the index finger, she could be kept from breathing. At the first sign of discomfort the fingers were removed. This experiment was repeated a great many times on different cats, and invariably the evidence of distress was accompanied by a total suspension of the motor activities of the stomach.... It has long been common knowledge that violent emotions interfere with the digestive process, but that the gastric motor activities should manifest such extreme sensitiveness to nervous conditions is surprising."

Like Dr. Williams, young Cannon had, from the very beginning, intuitively concentrated on the essentials. His studies of anxious cats, for example, remain directly relevant to the problem radiologists face today, distinguishing between functional disorders of the stomach and organic pathology in that organ.

Cannon continued his pioneering researches on both cats and humans after 1898 and published his findings in a series of notable papers as well as in his 1911 book, *Mechanical Factors of Digestion*. Yet even after the book appeared, leading radiologists remained ignorant of the role he had played in developing contrast media while still a Harvard medical freshman.

Other Experimenters

The roles of other pioneers have been similarly ignored. In 1897, for example, Dr. Charles Lester Leonard of Philadelphia reported in the *Journal of the American Medical Association* that he had washed out the stomach of a patient, instilled an emulsion of bismuth, and thus diagnosed a case of gastroptosis—drooping of the stomach. Indeed, the bismuth-laden stomach had dropped so low that the X-ray plate showed "the area of the stomach through the bones of the pelvis." In an address to the Atlantic County Medical Society, delivered in Atlantic City, New Jersey, on December 10, 1897, Dr. Leonard explained that "by filling the hollow organs with opaque liquids, as emulsions of bismuth in the stomach . . . their exact area can be readily determined."

Many other radiologists must have had the opportunity to discover accidentally the value of bismuth as a contrast medium, for during the 1890's and early 1900's bismuth compounds were often prescribed as a gastric ulcer remedy, in doses so large that 60 grams of bismuth might well have been found in the stomach at one time. An X-ray taken at such a time would have astonished the radiologist. Dr. Pfahler, indeed, may as a result of just such an accident have been among the first to visualize the details of a human stomach on an X-ray plate.

In 1897, Dr. Pfahler recalled much later, he was examining some plates that he had made of a patient's abdomen, and discovered a "beautiful demonstration" of eventration of the diaphragm—that is, a bulging of the diaphragm upward due to pressure of the abdominal organs. "Incidentally," Dr. Pfahler added, "the photographic plate showed bismuth in the stomach which had been taken therapeutically." Thus, Dr. Pfahler was almost in the position of his Philadelphia colleague Dr. Goodspeed, who had made an X-ray plate in 1890 without knowing it. But, "like Goodspeed," Dr. Pfahler added regretfully, "I did not follow through and failed to show the value of bismuth meals in the study of the gastrointestinal tract. . . ." [9]

Another American who early made persistent efforts to visualize the alimentary tract by means of a contrast medium was Dr. A. L. Benedict of Buffalo, New York. His initial results were published in *Medicine* for February 1898. Dr. Benedict later recalled:

> After considerable preliminary work along both radiographic and fluoroscopic lines, most of it naturally being mainly negative, a definite attempt was made to locate capsules containing tablets of iron, by X rays and the fluoroscope on February 9, 1897. The tablets could be seen when held in the closed hand, or while in the mouth, but not after being swallowed—undoubtedly owing to lack of power of the apparatus used. March 13, 1897, at the Dental Department of the University of Buffalo, at a demonstration of X-rays by Prof. Van Woert, he kindly allowed me to make some further experiments, using radiography. A cent was strapped over the umbilicus and a 12-minute exposure was made. A circle probably corresponding to the coin was seen but not the [swallowed] capsule. About July 1, 1897, further experiments were made by the courtesy of Dr. Detweiler of Philadelphia, who was then demonstrating X-ray apparatus in Buffalo. In three cases, iron tablets enclosed in capsules were observed by the fluoroscope, the peristaltic movements being plainly visible. The movements explained the failure of the previous attempt at radiography by time exposure. As the apparatus available at that time was not considered powerful enough for instantaneous radiography—this term, of course, not being used at the time—no further efforts were made in this direction. Instead of "skiagraphic" attempts, the fluoroscope was used, both iron tablets and bismuth powder being administered in capsule. In two or three instances, a few minutes after giving capsules containing bismuth powder, the whole gastric area became visible as a faint shadow, the inference being made at the time that this was due to the distribution of the bismuth over the mucous membrane, after the melting of the cap-

sule. The shadow corresponded with the area determined by auscultatory percussion. "In the remainder of the patients" (about ten in all) "the test either failed entirely or was too faint to be relied upon." "In general, the thinner the patient, the clearer the shadow." A verbal report was made of these experiments to the Buffalo Academy of Medicine, in the fall of 1897.

Dr. Benedict went on, however, to call attention to a series of French experiments which preceded his own. "Roux of Paris ... seems to have antedated my work by a few months, as I understand from conversation with him in 1908 that his experiments, reported in 1897, were actually begun in 1896 and were carried to a relatively successful issue in the winter of 1896–7."

Despite these anticipations of his work, Rieder of Munich deserves credit for alerting both German and American radiologists in 1904 to the virtues of using this X-ray technique routinely for gastrointestinal diagnosis. The bismuth meal became known as the "Rieder meal," and the method as "Rieder's method." Dr. Pfahler and Dr. Henry Hulst of Grand Rapids, Michigan, promptly adopted Rieder's approach and in 1905 presented papers on their own use of the bismuth meal. At the August 1906 meeting of the American Roentgen Ray Society, the "President's Address" given by Dr. Hulst opened with "grateful recognition of the work done by Professor H. Rieder," and continued, "... No gastroenterologist, I dare say, ever looked for the first time at good roentgenographs of [the stomach and intestines] without being profoundly impressed by their diagnostic value, if not positively shocked by the striking inadequacy of the older methods which the pictures serve to reveal." [10]

Bismuth meals were increasingly used through 1910, then gradually gave place to meals mixed with barium sulfate. Dr. James T. Case of Battle Creek, Michigan, one of the outstanding gas-tube radiologists, explained why. His explanation of November 1912, incidentally, reveals the close ties between American and German radiologists during the gas-tube era.

> As the opaque medium in intestinal work the writer has used various compounds of bismuth and lately barium sulphate. Bismuth subcarbonate was first used but later the oxychloride, as being perhaps less likely to alter the chemical reaction of the gastric contents and less likely to interfere with the influences controlling the pylorus.
>
> A number of European Roentgen workers have introduced the use of barium sulphate, not only for bowel injection but also as a substitute for bismuth in the ordinary Rieder test meal. Schwartz, of Vienna, has given the barium by mouth for over a year without any untoward effects. [Alban] Koehler, of Wiesbaden, has used the barium sulphate without any untoward results; and was able to report

only two cases in which the use of the barium has proved harmful. In each of these cases, a soluble salt of barium was used in place of the insoluble barium sulphate by physicians not accustomed to routine X-ray examinations. . . . Barium is many times cheaper than bismuth which makes its use certainly desirable.[11]

Cannon of Harvard, however, rather than Schwartz of Vienna or Koehler of Wiesbaden, actually deserved credit for pioneering the barium sulfate meal. In his earliest 1896 experiments with Moser, Cannon subsequently reported, "barium and bismuth were selected from among the heavy metals, and barium sulphate and bismuth subnitrate were chosen as salts which, because practically insoluble, would serve our purposes. Since bismuth subnitrate was a pharmacopeial preparation we determined first to use that." Later Cannon also tried barium sulfate mixed with food, and showed that it "was quite as satisfactory as bismuth subnitrate." He reported on the virtues of the barium sulfate meal in the *American Journal of Physiology* for 1904, 6 years before it was introduced in Europe.

The onset of World War I in 1914 no doubt hastened the conversion from bismuth to barium by cutting American radiologists off from European bismuth sources, and barium sulfate remains today one of the many contrast media in general use by radiologists.

Many other physicians contributed to the development of gastrointestinal radiology during the gas-tube era, but, by common consent of radiologists who practiced the specialty in that era, the contributions of two were outstanding. One was Dr. Lewis Gregory Cole (1874–1954), professor of roentgenology at the Cornell University Medical College in New York City; the other was Dr. Russell D. Carman (1875–1926) of the Mayo Clinic in Rochester, Minnesota.

Lewis Gregory Cole

Dr. Cole was both a perfectionist and a maverick, not only willing but delighted to buck the opinions of his peers. His colleagues marvelled at the clarity and richness of his X-ray plates and films. Dr. George C. Johnston of Pittsburgh gave one explanation of their superior quality. "I learned my first lesson . . . from Dr. Cole," Dr. Johnston remarked at a medical meeting in 1910, "and I thought he was a perfect old woman in the way he went about to get a good picture. I thought it was absolutely unnecessary to do all the things he did, and yet I realized that his pictures were superior to anything I was getting out. The great secret of it all was that he was a crank on the subject of immobility. Then it occurred to me that there might be something in it. . . . I saw that to make such pictures as he made, there must be absolute immobility of all the tissues...and I now have things so arranged that I can keep my patients quite still." [12]

Immobility, however, was only one feature of the shrewdly integrated Cole technique. Another important feature was mastery of the finicky gas tubes. Radiologists of the era kept a rack of tubes at hand, knew the history of each, and selected with care the right tube for each purpose. "Nature seems capricious to the savage mind; tubes do to the X-ray worker," Dr. Henry Hulst of Grand Rapids, Michigan, had written in 1902. "He rests, pets, punishes, smashes tubes as the fetishist his idols. He learns to know them all by name, their temper and their capabilities. He has a number of them—the more the better. He has trained tubes, trick tubes, high-spirited, high-bred tubes as well as gentle steady tubes. . . . A flashy tube is worse than a hysterical woman, it is incurably useless." [13] Many radiologists gave their tubes women's names; "I think I'll try Isobel this morning" was a typical remark of the gas-tube era.

The condition of each tube could be gauged by turning on the current and watching what happened. When a new tube was turned on for the first time, Dr. Cole reported, "the anterior hemisphere lights up with a bright, yellowish-green fluorescence; this color gradually changes as the seasoning process advances into a purplish-yellow of less brilliancy [called] the 'sunflower' light, because of its rich, mellow color. Eventually, in a very old tube, there is scarcely any fluorescence whatever, and Roentgen spoke of this as a dead tube. . . .

"After a tube has been in daily use for three or four months...it will be found on some particular day that the vacuum is very high, and refuses to gradually respond to the usual methods employed." Even a voltage sufficiently high to produce a spark 12 inches long would not activate such a tube. Dr. Cole called this "the crisis of the tube," and he declared that it only lasted a few days. Thereafter, the tube could be activated at a moderate voltage again, and became even more effective than before, remaining "a most useful tube for six or eight months, or even a year or two." [14] In his practice, Dr. Cole was alert to each clue each tube provided.

Another feature of the Cole X-ray technique, and one in which he disagreed with the judgment of his gas-tube era contemporaries, concerned voltage and "hardness." Radiologists had learned that the X rays emitted by different tubes varied widely in their ability to penetrate human tissues. "Hard" tubes—that is, tubes which contained relatively little residual gas—required high voltages for their activation, and the combination of high voltage and hard tube produced a more penetrating ray. With such a ray, an acceptable plate could be secured with a shorter exposure, and therefore with less likelihood that the patient would move and spoil the plate. Higher amperage also shortened the exposure. Throughout the gas-tube era, accordingly, most radiologists strove toward higher voltage, higher amperage, harder tubes, and shorter exposure times.

Dr. Cole strongly dissented. He was dissatisfied with merely "acceptable" plates and sought for the very best. "It is my opinion," he told the December 1908 meeting of the American Roentgen Ray Society, "that with a high-vacuum tube, the rays penetrate the soft tissues, which are just the tissues we are most anxious to show. The first principle of radiography is that the higher the vacuum of the tube, the greater the penetration of the ray. If your tube is low enough you can show almost any tissue in the body, even the blood circulating in the veins. Therefore, I use as low a vacuum tube as I can and still throw the rays through the body." [15] Using such a tube, Dr. Cole would turn on the current and then slowly advance the rheostat until the rays, as seen through the fluoroscope, were barely able to penetrate a test object. Then he exposed his plate. This combination of low voltage and low amperage with a soft tube made a longer exposure necessary, but achieved plates replete with the most exquisite detail. In these plates Dr. Cole was able to spot many features which others had missed in their plates.

Cole was a master of "retrospectoscopy," and in collaboration with Dr. Arial W. George of the Tufts College Medical School in Boston, he extended the concept of retrospectoscopy in two directions. First, the two men pooled their plates, and each examined in the light of hindsight the plates of the other radiologist as well as his own. Second, hundreds or even thousands of plates, made over a period of years, were reviewed at one time in the search for consistent signs of disease which had been missed initially. Cole and George reported in 1915 two successful examples of this improvement on orthodox retrospectoscopy:

> Of late a re-examination has been made of those Roentgen plates taken during the last four or five years in which direct evidence of gall-stones was insufficient or undetected, but which showed enough evidence . . . to justify surgical procedure. In the re-examination, our increased knowledge of the Roentgenologic appearance of soft gall-stones has enabled us to detect direct evidence of the [gall-stone] on the Roentgen plate in a large number of cases where [a stone] was found at operation.
>
> The same results have been obtained from a re-study of those cases where the gall-bladder only was examined, and a negative diagnosis was made. The gall-stones found at operation in these patients can now be identified in the original Roentgen plates. *The evidence was there before, but we were then unable to recognize it.*[16] †

---

† Italics added.

After this experiment in retrospectoscopy, it was unlikely that either man would miss such cases thereafter.

Another Cole trademark was the vast number of plates that he made of each patient. When a patient came in for stomach radiography, for example, Cole in 1913 or 1914 routinely exposed 12 plates in very rapid succession with the patient in the prone posture, four to six exposures from the side, two from the rear, and 12 with the patient standing erect—but that was only the beginning. The patient next ate a full meal mixed with bismuth, and 2 hours later six to 12 additional plates were made, two of them stereoscopic views of the entire gastrointestinal tract. (Later he increased the number of exposures made at this stage in the procedure.) Often another series of plates was made 4 hours after the meal, and an additional pair was always made 6 hours after. If bismuth remained in the stomach at 6 hours, five or six more plates were made subsequently. Thus, 40 plates per stomach examination were a minimum in Dr. Cole's practice, and 50 or 60 were common. If other abdominal regions were also of interest, many more exposures might be made.[17]

To facilitate this multiple-plate technique, which he dubbed "serial roentgenography," Dr. Cole used Celluloid film instead of the glass plates used by most of his colleagues, although the films were still called "plates." He bought the film in long rolls, and he designed a special examining table which contained (in addition to many other complex and ingenious features) a semiautomatic mechanism to advance the film each time a lever was pressed, much as in the modern roll-film camera. Fifty exposures in succession could thus be made in a very short time without reloading. The films could also be projected in rapid succession to achieve a rough impression of actual motion—a primitive attempt at what is now known as cineradiography.[17]

Typical of Dr. Cole's successes was his diagnosis of a gastric ulcer in Mrs. X, described as "the wife of a well-known surgeon." [18] Mrs. X had been under observation for obscure gastrointestinal complaints for 3 years before she was brought to Dr. Cole. During this period many outstanding clinicians had examined her, at her surgeon-husband's request, and they could not agree on a diagnosis. Dr. Cole made his usual series of plates and reported, "From a study of these roentgenograms I believe we are justified in making a positive diagnosis of an ulcer of the lesser curvature of the stomach, about three inches from the pyloric sphincter, which requires immediate surgical procedure. This ulcer shows a tendency to perforation which to my mind would not justify any material delay."

Additional X-ray studies of Mrs. X had been scheduled for a subsequent day, but, to underline the need for haste, Dr. Cole cancelled the second appointment on the ground that he "did not consider the delay justifiable." He reassured Dr. X, however, that in his opinion the lesion was benign rather than malignant.

Dr. X could not believe the diagnosis. "Mrs. X's history contraindicated ulcer in every particular," he declared, "so much so that the very best men in town [New York City] refused to believe that an ulcer was present...." Despite Dr. Cole's warning that the ulcer might perforate at any moment, the operation was delayed for more than a month.

Then a surgeon, Dr. Deaver, operated on Mrs. X. When the outer surface of the stomach was exposed, Dr. Deaver examined it closely; he could not see the slightest sign of any lesion, and was no doubt tempted to sew Mrs. X up again. When he palpated the area indicated in Dr. Cole's report, however, he did seem to feel some irregularity. It was "very slight," he reported, yet, in view of all the facts, "I felt warranted in opening the stomach." There, on the lesser curvature, precisely as shown on Dr. Cole's plates, was the ulcer. "It was about the size of a five-cent piece," Dr. X wrote Dr. Cole, "and had penetrated through the mucosa and muscularis to the peritoneum." Thus, perforation was imminent, as Dr. Cole's report had stressed. "It [was] non-malignant," Dr. X added, "another confirmation of your diagnosis." [18]

"I excised the ulcer and took out the appendix," Dr. Deaver reported to Dr. Cole. "My heartiest congratulations on your skillful X-ray work." Dr. Cole himself added a postscript to the story in the *American Journal of Roentgenology* for November 1915: "The patient made an uneventful recovery and at the present time is perfectly well."

Dr. Cole was acutely aware of the distinction between functional disturbances of the stomach, for which surgery was not warranted, and organic pathology requiring surgical intervention. He did not hesitate to advise against surgery when he thought that the symptoms, however distressing, had a functional origin. Occasionally, however, despite Dr. Cole's recommendation, a surgeon went ahead and operated anyway, and in such cases Dr. Cole was delighted to engage in retrospectoscopy. As his experience thus expanded, his diagnostic skill improved.

In one typical case of this kind, Dr. Cole's report to the surgeon read as follows: "The irregularly shaped cap, the hazy edges of the sphincter, and the lack of normal expansion and contraction of the [pylorus] indicate that there is some lesion involving this portion of the stomach. The six-hour long stasis [retention of the bismuth meal beyond the normal six hours] would indicate an organic obstruction at the pylorus, *but I believe the stasis is due to some functional disturbance of the stomach and cap rather than to an organic obstruction.*" [19] ‡

Despite Dr. Cole's opinion that the condition was functional, and that an operation was therefore not warranted, the surgeon decided to go ahead with one. Dr. Cole accordingly wrote the surgeon again: "This case is typical of a group of about 20 cases in which there has been evidence of a definite lesion involving the [pylorus] and cap. I have not felt that I could advocate surgical interference in any of these cases, although I am exceedingly anxious to know what pathological condition causes these Roentgenologic findings. Therefore if the clinical history is sufficiently severe to indicate surgery, I should like if possible to be present at the operation."

The operation was in fact performed, and, as Dr. Cole had predicted, neither ulcer nor cancer was found. Indeed, it was necessary for the surgeon to make a second incision over the appendix—and through it a chronically diseased appendix was removed.

Such bold yet precise diagnoses earned Dr. Cole widespread recognition among physicians and surgeons, but there remained many doubters. At the 1914 meetings of both the Gastrointestinal Society and the Medical Section of the American Medical Association, for example, it was repeatedly asserted that the early diagnosis of gastric ulcer by X rays was impossible. Even surgeons who agreed that a *positive* X ray diagnosis of gastric ulcer could be relied on doubted the reliability of a *negative* diagnosis; they went right on operating, despite the negative X-ray findings, if clinical symptoms suggesting ulcer were present. Dr. Cole, bluntly although without arrogance, insisted that his negative as well as positive diagnoses were reliable. If he saw no ulcer on his plates, none was present.

To test Dr. Cole's claims, an objective study was arranged. A New York City surgeon, Dr. George Emerson Brewer—one of the doubters—sent Dr. Cole 27 patients.[20] In each case, Dr. Brewer told Dr. Cole nothing except that "an organic lesion of the stomach or duodenum was suspected; no history or data obtained by physical examination or gastric analysis being furnished." Dr. Cole then made his serial plates, and sent Dr. Brewer a typewritten report "giving the exact findings and an opinion regarding the presence or absence of a gastric or duodenal lesion, its location, extent, and probable cause." Regardless of Dr. Cole's X-ray findings, Dr. Brewer then operated—and reported back to Dr. Cole the physical findings at operation.

The results were conclusive. "In eleven cases, or 40 percent of the

---

‡ Italics added.

number investigated, examination by serial Roentgenography resulted in negative diagnosis of ulcer or cancer—or of any surgical lesion of the stomach or cap." [21] In all of these cases, the clinical findings seemed to Dr. Brewer strong enough to warrant an operation. *In not a single one of the eleven cases, when the operation was performed, did Dr. Brewer find any surgical lesion of the stomach or cap!* Dr. Cole's negative diagnoses were thus 100 per cent correct.

In another 11 cases, Dr. Cole made a positive diagnosis, and in nine of these he was correct.

In the remaining five cases, Dr. Cole was able to give Dr. Brewer only an opinion rather than a firm diagnosis, "owing to incomplete observation, or unusual findings which could not be definitely interpreted." [20] In these five cases, Dr. Cole's opinion was right four times and wrong only once. Thus, his over-all "batting average" for the series was 89 per cent—20 correct diagnoses, four correct opinions, and only three errors in 27 cases.

Dr. Brewer, who had long been known as a doubter, was wholly convinced of the value of gastrointestinal radiography long before the test series was completed. He and Dr. Cole jointly prepared the report which concluded the trials, and Dr. Brewer himself—no doubt as a penance—read it at the April 1914 meeting of the American Surgical Society.

The report began by summing up the current status of X-ray diagnosis from the surgeon's point of view. "While roentgenology has proved of great assistance in the solution of many diagnostic problems, such as joint and bone diseases, pulmonary tuberculosis, aneurysms, sinus infections, etc., the surgeon accepts the roentgenographic evidence of fractures and renal and ureteral calculi [stones] as final, and of greater value than the clinical history or the results of a most painstaking physical examination, or both methods combined. As a result of the accuracy with which these lesions are recognized by skilled roentgenologists, few if any experienced surgeons of the present day will accept the responsibility of treating a complicated fracture or of advising surgical intervention in a case of urinary calculi without the aid of a roentgenologic examination, if it is possible or practical to obtain one."

Gastrointestinal radiography, the report continued, was now on an equally sound footing as a result of Cole's serial roentgenography. "The objections to the method are obvious. It requires considerable time and is moderately expensive. If it could be shown that a simpler method would give equally good results, that method would undoubtedly become the popular one. In the opinion of the writers, however, serial roentgenography will give more accurate information concerning lesions of the stomach and duodenum than any other method now employed." [20]

At the beginning of the gas-tube era, radiologists often reported on a single case or pair of cases. Later they might report on a dozen or a score. By the end of the era, radiological results were on a far more solid statistical foundation. In 1914, for example, Dr. Cole reported on 566 cases in which he had made a negative diagnosis of gastric ulcer or carcinoma. Of these cases, he declared, 33 "presented sufficiently severe symptoms to justify surgical exploration; and it is upon the results in these 33 cases, operated upon by 23 different surgeons, that the present communication is based. The negative diagnosis ... was made in each case solely on the Roentgenographic findings, and *in not a single instance was a lesion of the stomach or cap demonstrated by surgical exploration.*" [21]

The fact that in 533 out of 566 cases the surgeons accepted Dr. Cole's negative diagnoses and did not operate indicates how much confidence they placed in Dr. Cole—and how much unnecessary surgery was thus avoided. Also significant was the fact that the 33 operations performed following a negative Cole diagnosis were performed by 23 different surgeons. A surgeon might operate once, or even twice, against Dr. Cole's advice, but it was a rare surgeon indeed who remained unconvinced after a few such distressing experiences. The reliance on Dr. Cole is even more striking when it is recalled that he was still a young diagnostician in his 30's when he was making these 566 negative diagnoses.

Russell D. Carman

Dr. Russell D. Carman, the other leader of gastrointestinal radiology during the gas-tube era, was 1 year younger than Dr. Cole and differed from him in many respects. Born in Ontario, Canada, Dr. Carman began his radiological career in St. Louis in 1902, and joined the Mayo Clinic as head of the Section on Roentgenology in 1913. There he and his associates had abundant opportunity to examine not just thousands but tens of thousands of patients who flocked to the clinic each year from all over the Middle West, attracted by the reputations of the celebrated Mayo brothers. Dr. Carman published a series of articles on X-ray diagnosis beginning in 1907, and in 1917 he and his Mayo Clinic associate, Dr. Albert Miller, published their influential textbook, *The Roentgen Diagnosis of Disease of the Alimentary Canal.* Although it appeared after the close of the gas-tube era, this 558-page classic was based primarily on work done with gas tubes.

Lewis Gregory Cole had used the fluoroscope primarily to line up his tube and plate with the patient, to check the hardness of the rays, and to make a preliminary survey; he relied on the plates for diagnosis. Carman used almost precisely the opposite procedure. He relied primarily on the fluoroscope for diagnosis, and exposed a few plates per patient to clear up a doubtful point or to record some unusual feature which he might later want to show students or other physicians.

"We believe that the advantages of the [fluoroscopic] screen in the examination of the digestive tract can hardly be too strongly emphasized," Drs. Carman and Miller wrote in their textbook. "Only by its use can exact information be obtained as to mobility and flexibility, the phenomena of peristalsis and antiperistalsis, the nature and permanence of irregularities of contour, and the effects of palpation, respiratory movement and varying positions. All changes can be seen at every instant, in the order of their succession, at any desired angle, and in these respects *a few minutes of screening is equivalent to hundreds of plates.*" § Thus, the issue between Dr. Carman and Dr. Cole was squarely joined.

The great value of the Carman-Miller textbook was that it brought together not only their own vast experience with patients at the Mayo Clinic, but also the published literature from the world's other leading clinical centers, and organized the whole in terms of specific techniques which other radiologists could adopt. The book included a review of the "normal" stomach, and noted that, in determining whether a stomach is normal, "account must be taken of its length, breadth, capacity, contour, position, form, tonus, mobility, peristalsis, and motility." Carman stressed that "stomachs which are markedly dissimilar in their roentgenologic characteristics may each be appropriate for its possessor and functionate in a normal manner," but he added that "these variations have limits, even though wide, which can be determined in a general way."

Next, Carman and Miller went on to describe and to illustrate specific abnormalities: the "hourglass stomach," the "niche" or protruding pocket indicating an ulcer, the "accessory pocket" seen near a penetrating ulcer, the "filling defect" seen when something in the stomach prevented the barium meal from filling a portion of its interior, the "incisura" or notch which results from spastic contraction of the muscle fibers near an ulcer, and many more. Carman was even willing on occasion to adopt techniques quite inconsistent with his general views, such as Cole's technique for diagnosing ulcer of the duodenum.

"Deformity of the duodenal contour," Carman wrote, ". . . was first established as a practicable sign of duodenal ulcer by Lewis

---

§ Italics added.

Gregory Cole of New York, who developed the plan of 'serial roent-genography.' ... On theoretical grounds, the method did not seem to be either convenient or wholly trustworthy, and was regarded skeptically by many roentgen workers, including ourselves.... However, more careful investigation has proved that bulbar deformity is feasible of demonstration and stands first among the roentgenologic signs in diagnostic value." This, from Carman, was praise indeed for his leading rival.

Each of the roentgenological signs was related by Carman and Miller to the appropriate diagnosis—cancer, ulcer, gallstones, syphilis, fibromatosis, chronic appendicitis, and many more. Their textbook was replete with illustrative case histories, and with references to the surgical wisdom of Carman's hero, Will Mayo. "Dr. W. J. Mayo says...," "According to Dr. W. J. Mayo...," and similar references dot the pages. But the confidence of readers was chiefly elicited by the vast numbers of Mayo Clinic cases reported—1000 examples of one condition, 2000 of another. Carman could refer as casually to "Case 107,944" as earlier radiologists might refer to "Case XLIII." In a single year (1919), he and his staff performed 50,668 X-ray examinations.

Dr. Carman's most celebrated diagnosis was made long after the close of the gas-tube era. The occasion was a tragic one, and was recorded by Carman's closest associate, Dr. Albert Miller, soon after the event.

In the fall of 1925, Dr. Miller recalled,[22] Dr. Carman was returning from Europe with his wife, happy and relaxed. He had just been elected president of the American Roentgen Ray Society. "In all his 50 years no bitter grief, no blasting ill, had been his lot. Fame had come to him, and fortune had been kind." As his train neared Rochester, however, he suffered a gastric upset.

On the assumption that the upset was a recurrence of an earlier gallbladder attack, a duodenal drainage tube was inserted; it brought a show of blood. Clearly an X-ray examination was required.

On October 8, 1925, Dr. Miller recorded, Carman "stood gaily before the screen where thousands of patients had confronted him. In the darkness the X-ray tube gave out its steady drone. No other sound was heard, for his associates were dumb as they gazed at a distorted gastric shadow." The image on the fluoroscopic screen left no doubt in their minds that this was gastric cancer. "Finally they found voice. Spasm, they told [Dr. Carman] evasively. They would make some films.

"Carman returned to his office. It was a gray afternoon. On his desk was a rough draft of a new paper on cancer of the stomach. It had been the theme of the first paper he had published from Rochester. When the films were ready his assistants could not withhold them. Gravely they were laid before the Chief."

Holding the films toward the window, Dr. Carman announced his diagnosis, as he had done so many tens of thousands of times before: "Cancer of the stomach, and inoperable."

Carman's staff now assembled. "To them he pointed out the tell-tale marks he knew so well. He was flushed, but only with animation." The others left, but Dr. Miller remained a bit longer. "If I could have lived only ten years longer," Dr. Carman commented.[22] A few minutes later he was back in the film room, dictating other diagnoses. He died 8 months later, in June 1926.

Did Carman get better results with his primary emphasis on fluoroscopy, or Dr. Cole with his serial roentgenography? A radiological tournament at which the two might pit their skills against each other was often discussed by other radiologists, and it has been said that Dr. Cole was actually invited to the Mayo Clinic to match his technique against Carman's, but no such confrontation actually occurred. Radiologists today, of course, draw upon both techniques; a complete gastrointestinal workup now includes both a series of films and a thorough fluoroscopic examination.

Hardly a region or organ of the body escaped careful diagnostic study during the gas-tube era. Behind each advance in diagnostic prowess lay a story—and a radiologist. Many more of these stories merit retelling, and many more radiologists of the gas-tube era deserve a place in this history. However, enough has perhaps been presented to suggest the flavor of the era, the ingenuity of the radiologists who expanded the boundaries of diagnosis, and the revolutionary influence of X-ray advances on surgery, on internal medicine, and on the lives and health of patients.

REFERENCES

1. *Amer. J. Roentgen., 75:* 14–22, 1956.
2. *Philadelphia Med. J., 9:* 268–273, 1902.
3. *Trans. Amer. Roentgen Ray Soc.,* 175–181, 1905.
4. *Trans. Amer. Roentgen Ray Soc.,* 45–83, 1908.
5. *J.A.M.A., 61:* 321, 1913.
6. *J.A.M.A., 62:* 1–3, 1914.
7. *Amer. J. Physiol., 1:* 435–444, 1898.
8. WILLIAMS, F. H., *The Roentgen Rays in Medicine and Surgery,* Ed. 3, pp. 360–372. The Macmillan Company, New York, 1903.
9. ANON., *American Roentgen Ray Society 1900–1950,* p. 18. Charles C Thomas, Publisher, Springfield, Illinois, 1950.
10. *Amer. Quart. Roentgen., 1:* 1, 1907.
11. *Amer. Quart. Roentgen., 4:* 78, 1912.
12. *Amer. Quart. Roentgen., 2:* 133, 1910.
13. *Physician and Surgeon (Detroit), 24:* 492–498, 1902.
14. *Amer. Quart. Roentgen., 1:* 35, 1907.

15. *Trans. Amer. Roentgen Ray Soc., 229,* 1908.
16. *Boston Med. Surg. J., 172: 326–330,* 1915.
17. *Amer. J. Med. Sci., 142: 92–118,* 1914.
18. *Amer. J. Roentgen., 2: 793–810,* 1915.
19. *Amer. J. Roentgen., 2: 497–506,* 1914.
20. *Ann. Surg., 61: 55–72,* 1915.
21. *Amer. J. Roentgen., 2: 497–506,* 1914.
22. *Amer. J. Roentgen., 16: 53–55,* 1926.

11   The X Rays in Therapy

While the usefulness of Roentgen's rays for diagnosis was implicit in Roentgen's own initial discovery, their value in the *treatment* of disease had to be laboriously discovered, confirmed, and explored.

No doubt many arrows pointed toward the discovery of X-ray therapy. One was simple, empirical curiosity: "Let's try it out and see what happens." This seems to have been the attitude of mind which led Dr. J. William White (1850–1916), professor of clinical surgery at the University of Pennsylvania, to launch in the fall of 1896 what must have been one of the earliest clinical trials of the X rays in the United States—perhaps the very earliest.

"I must confess that, as with every new discovery, my thoughts turn to its possible application to a subject which has an invincible attraction for me—the cure of cancer," Dr. White told a meeting of the American Surgical Association in May 1897. "I was led in a purely speculative and empirical manner to direct the use of X rays in a number of inoperable cases of cancer in various regions. . . .

"I have no results to report. Indeed, as yet, I have no results at all, but . . . I intend to continue my own experiments until I am convinced that they are useless. . . . I feel reasonably sure . . . of doing my patients no harm, even if the experiment is an entire failure." [1]

Dr. White claimed no priority, it should be added, for his early use of the X rays in cancer therapy; he claimed only that the idea had occurred to him independently. "I was surprised to find," he told his fellow surgeons in May 1897, "that what last fall seemed to me an entirely original thought had first occurred to V. Despeignes, who in July and August, 1896, had reported in the *Lyon Médical* [France] a case of gastric carcinoma which had appeared to be greatly benefited by the transmission of the rays through the seat of disease." News of the Despeignes case had been brought to American physicians in the *Medical Record* for August 29, 1896. Others, of course, may have preceded Despeignes.

Another arrow pointing toward the therapeutic use of X rays was the report in April 1896 that an excessive dose caused human hair to fall out (see above, page 81). Before the end of the year, several investigators were using the rays, both in Europe and in the United States, for the treatment of hypertrichosis (excessive growth of hair), especially on the faces of women.

This work, in turn, led by simple coincidence to the accidental discovery of other uses. An eminent Chicago specialist, Dr. William Allen Pusey, professor of dermatology at the College of Physicians and Surgeons of Chicago and a member of the Medical Department of the University of Illinois, reported an example from his own practice: "Miss ——, aged 22, brunette, was put under X-ray exposures in July 1900 for hypertrichosis," Dr. Pusey stated. In addition to the excessive hair for which she was being treated, Dr. Pusey noted that "on the chin and around the mouth she had an *acne simplex* of moderate severity." To his surprise, "the acne disappeared" following the use of X rays, "and she has had no recurrence in two years." [2] That accidental success with the X rays in acne led Dr. Pusey during the next 1½ years to treat 13 more cases. Other clinicians no doubt made similar accidental discoveries even earlier. European investigators, for example, had reported before 1900 on the successful use of the rays for tinea capitis (ringworm of the scalp), favus (a parasitic skin infection), sycosis (inflammation of the hair follicles), and chronic eczema.

A third arrow pointing toward the discovery of the therapeutic usefulness of the X rays deserves mention. During the late 1890's, Dr. Niels Finsen of Copenhagen was reporting good results from the use of ultraviolet light in the treatment of several skin conditions. His "Finsen light," as it was then known, produced a reddening of the skin like a sunburn. "Finsen therapy" became quite popular, and, since a sufficient dose of X rays also produced an erythema or reddening of the skin much like sunburn, the thought must naturally have occurred to many clinicians that the X rays might similarly have therapeutic effects.

These and no doubt other preliminary trials of the X rays as a form of medical treatment, however, fell far short of establishing X-ray therapy as an accepted medical procedure either in the United States or in Europe. The "great leap forward" occurred in 1900 and 1901, when dramatic reports were published of the successful treatment and even cure of two loathsome and devastating skin diseases far more prevalent then than now: skin tuberculosis, also known as lupus vulgaris; and carcinoma of the skin, a form of cancer then also known as epithelioma.

Skin Tuberculosis

The treatment of skin tuberculosis—lupus vulgaris—was reported from Vienna as early as 1898 by Eduard Schiff and Leopold Freund; an American physician, Philip Mills Jones (1870–1916) of San Francisco, soon followed in their footsteps. Dr. Jones treated his first lupus patient with the X rays in January 1899. He reported that the patient, a man of about 55, had had "a troublesome lesion on the right forehead, just above the outer angle of the orbit, for some 12 years. One spot after another would become involved, break down, ulcerate, be treated, and for a time heal. Invariably, however, it would subsequently reappear, involving a little more fresh tissue with each recurrence. He had been treated by a number of men in many ways. The actual cautery, curetting, creosote, silver nitrate, hydrogen dioxide, and many other modes of treatment had been employed."

Dr. Jones selected a "soft" tube and began X-ray exposures. "There were present three ulcerating points and one large, hard nodule which had not yet broken down. A sheet of lead was arranged so as to protect the whole of the head save the lupus area; a hole cut in the lead sheet allowed the X rays to reach all the diseased area, with the exception of one of the ulcerating points. This one small point was protected as a sort of control upon the treatment.

"The patient was exposed about four to six inches from the tube, two or three times a week, the exposures lasting from two to five minutes. At the end of four weeks the whole area, with the exception of the one ulcer protected, was healed and the nodule had disappeared."

The protected ulceration had meanwhile increased in size. "I then exposed the ulcerated area that had been previously protected by the lead plate. In three weeks this had quite healed."

Dr. Jones, despite this salutary result, did not rush into print. Instead, he cautiously waited 9 months or so. The lesions remained "healed"—Dr. Jones was careful not to claim that they were "cured," although he did note that "previously the longest time the lesion had remained healed was four months."

During his 9-month wait, Dr. Jones also treated a second lupus case with X rays, and secured excellent results again. With this patient, too, he shielded a part of the lesion from the rays initially to make sure there was no "spontaneous remission," and began treatment of the shielded portion only after the main lesion had healed. Thus, despite the fact that he had treated only two patients, Dr. Jones had in effect proved the effectiveness of the X rays four times in succession. He published an account of this work in the *Philadelphia Medical Journal* for January 6, 1900.

"So far as I am aware," he declared of his initial patient, "this was the first case of lupus treated by X-ray exposure in this country, though the method had been used in Germany and several cases reported as cured."

Dr. Jones was also careful not to tout the new method as the treatment of choice for lupus. "I believe," he wrote, "... that the method of treatment by ultraviolet light (Finsen) will be found to be quicker and better than the treatment by X rays."

Two other investigators, one in Cincinnati and one in Chicago, followed up Dr. Jones's case by trying the X rays on lupus cases themselves. The Cincinnati case was reported by Dr. J. T. Knox in the *Journal of the American Medical Association* for November 10, 1900.

His patient, Dr. Knox explained, was a young woman of 20, Miss C, with a tragically disfiguring lupus of the nose and facial skin, referred to him by Dr. W. L. Taylor. "Recognizing his inability to cure the disease by any of the ordinary methods," Dr. Knox continued, "the X-ray treatment suggested itself to [Dr. Taylor]; but not being equipped with the necessary apparatus, he consulted me. I informed him that I had never treated a case of lupus by this method, and it was with some hesitancy that I assumed charge of the case."

The patient's disfigurement was severe indeed. It had begun as a lesion of the eyelids, and had progressively eaten into the nose and upper lip. Thereafter it grew still larger, "and had so far progressed as to cause perforation of the nose septum."

For 2 years Miss C had been "treated by some of our most capable dermatologists, and was an inmate of St. Mary's Hospital for seven months of the time, under the care of the staff physicians. The disease steadily progressed, never at any time exhibiting symptoms of improvement." Then Dr. Knox began his X-ray treatments.

"I was very conservative in the beginning," Dr. Knox stated. ". . . The treatment consisted of the application of the rays for from six to ten minutes each sitting, every other day, placing the affected parts from four to eight inches from the tube, according to the density of the rays. The whole number of applications made during the treatment was 74. . . .The unaffected parts of the face and head were shielded by means of a mask, thus preventing the possibility of producing dermatitis and loss of hair. . . ."

The results, to the dermatologists who had struggled unsuccessfully for more than 2 years with this stubborn infection, must have seemed little short of miraculous. "Improvement was apparent very soon after beginning treatment." Thereafter Miss C's face continued to improve until the lesion had completely disappeared. As evidence, Dr. Knox published pictures of Miss C, taken before and after completion of therapy. The second photography, he noted, ". . . shows almost entire absence of scars, or any condition of the tissues that would indicate that the disease had ever existed."

It was hardly surprising that following such an experience Dr. Knox should feel exuberant. "Although this is the first case of lupus I have treated by this method," he affirmed, "I have no hesitancy in stating that I regard it as an infallible one, if properly applied and continued a sufficient length of time." He concluded on an euphoric note: "In closing this paper I cannot refrain from adding a word in favor of this wonderful and mysterious . . . therapeutic agent, and it is my opinion that there are possibilities within its range that as yet have not been dreamed of. . . ."

While Dr. Knox was treating his young woman patient in Cincinnati, Dr. Pusey in Chicago was similarly treating a 38-year-old married woman for severely disfiguring lupus of the face and neck. His results were equally impressive. A lesion so large and so foul that it could hardly be viewed without repugnance first shrank and then disappeared altogether, leaving only a few modest, healthy-looking scars. But Dr. Pusey, a scientist as well as a clinician, was more cautious than Dr. Knox in summarizing his results. "It is at once admitted," he wrote in the *Journal of the American Medical Association* for December 8, 1900, "that whether it is a complete cure or not can only be determined by the lapse of time." He correctly stated the basic problem of X-ray therapy, today as in 1900: "The object to be obtained by the exposures is, of course, to get the required effects of the rays without overstepping the bounds of safety."

Skin Cancer

The discovery that the X rays were effective against skin cancer—epithelioma—followed very promptly after the discovery that they were effective against skin tuberculosis. Credit for initiating the X-ray treatment of skin cancer is often given to two Swedes, Thor Stenbeck and Tage Sjögren, each of whom independently demonstrated a case of epithelioma treated with X rays at a meeting of the Swedish Medical Society on December 19, 1899. But, as has been noted, others had tried earlier.

In the United States, Dr. Charles Lester Leonard of Philadelphia began treating two patients with inoperable cancer of the breast on March 18, 1899, but the results were negative. Two investigators in Washington, D.C., however, began treating a patient with X rays for skin cancer on September 6, 1899, and completed their treatment on October 9, with startlingly favorable results.[3] They were Dr. Wallace Johnson, demonstrator of pathology at the Georgetown University Medical School and pathologist at Washington's Central Dispensary and Emergency Hospital, and Walter H. Merrill, a medical student who had been placed in charge of the X-Ray and Photographic Department at the Dispensary. Both men deserve more recognition than they have received.

Dr. Johnson's and Mr. Merrill's first patient, known as Mr. G, was a 45-year-old professional man who had noticed a small pimple on his left cheek 8 or 10 years earlier. When the pimple failed to heal, "his friends became alarmed and insisted that he see a surgeon. In 1894 the diseased area was removed and the actual cautery applied. A year later the ulcer had returned, larger than before; a second operation was performed with apparent success, but in three years the disease had returned in full force and a second center had developed on the right side of his nose. The several surgeons who had had charge of the case pronounced it epithelioma"—that is, cancer of the skin.

Dr. Johnson knew very well what that diagnosis meant. "There is no disease that physicians like less to encounter than carcinoma in any of its forms," he wrote, "especially when it has progressed to the stage where the probabilities of its complete removal are slight." Mr. G's was such a case.

The physician and his student selected a "soft" tube and administered a series of X-ray treatments on an every-other-day schedule—10 treatments aimed at the nose and five at the spot on the cheek. "A marked reduction in the quantity of the discharge was the first result noted. This appeared in about three days. Then the scab of dried secretion which formed over these surfaces would form more slowly and remain adherent longer each time." [3]

At the 15th treatment in the series, on October 9, 1899, the two men met with an occurrence quite common throughout the "gas-tube era." This treatment was no longer than usual, lasting only 5 minutes, yet quite unexpectedly it "set up a severe dermatitis. ... The surface became inflamed, the discharge profuse and watery; a typical X-ray burn was produced. Treatment was suspended for 6 weeks. At the end of that time, a healthy cicatrix [scar] had formed over both areas." Six months later, "smooth white scars...invisible at a distance from the patient, had replaced the original ulcers." After 2½ years, "the original scar...has remained smooth and soft, and is not noticeable at a distance." [4]

Dr. Johnson and Mr. Merrill, encouraged by this first success, went on to treat with quite favorable results five more epithelioma patients in 1900. They reported their initial findings in the *Philadelphia Medical Journal* for December 8 and 15, 1900:

> Few surgeons today doubt that carcinoma can be cured [by surgery] when it is localized and in a location favorable to operation. More often than not, however, cases are concealed until glandular involvement or widespread dissemination has occurred and the hope of a cure from operation is practically gone. This common and dangerous delay is due to popular dread of the knife. If, then, we have at hand an agent that will effect the cure without the use of the knife or of painful caustics, one of the most frequent causes for neglect of the disease has been removed. *We are firmly convinced that, by means of the proper application of X rays under conditions of no practical*

discomfort to the patient, we can bring about the painless removal of the slow-growing epitheliomas.

These growths, especially when they occur on the face, are very disfiguring; if allowed to progress they produce a condition loathsome in the extreme. Treatment of such cases by the X rays leaves a remaining defect that is incomparably better in cosmetic results than that which must accompany extirpation by knife or caustic. Furthermore, our experiments lead us to believe that even in inoperable cases of carcinoma attacking superficial parts, we may give great relief from pain and can even slightly prolong life. If we can dispense with the use of opiates in this class of cases and free the patients from pain while leaving the intellect clear, . . . we have made a great improvement in the therapeutics of this condition.*

Dr. Francis H. Williams of Harvard soon added the weight of his authority to the earlier reports. He confirmed the Jones, Knox, and Pusey findings with respect to skin tuberculosis in the influential *Boston Medical and Surgical Journal* late in 1900, and he confirmed the Johnson-Merrill findings with respect to skin cancer in the same journal for January 17, 1901. There was a saying abroad in those days, "Boston physicians won't believe something can be done until it has been done in Boston"; now Bostonians, too, were assured that skin tuberculosis and skin cancers could indeed be healed, and perhaps even cured, by the X rays.

Later in 1901, Dr. Williams presented his therapeutic work, as well as his outstanding contributions to X-ray diagnosis, in his textbook, *The Roentgen Rays in Medicine and Surgery,* which Dr. James T. Case three decades later called "perhaps the most important publication in English during the first decade of roentgenology."

A veritable boom in X-ray therapy was touched off by these and other detailed and convincing reports of successful healing, and by "before-and-after" photographs showing astonishing results. Just as everyone with an induction coil and a Crookes tube had begun making diagnostic X-ray plates in 1896, so everyone similarly equipped began treating skin diseases and cancers 4 or 5 years later. Perhaps the most celebrated of the early cures came to be known as "Skinner's case."

"Skinner's Case"

Dr. Clarence E. Skinner of New Haven began X-ray treatment of this patient in January 1902. He reported his case in full to the Electrotherapeutic Section of the International Electrical Congress in St. Louis in September 1904, and to the Connecticut Medical Society in May 1906; he published histories of the case in the *Archives of Electrology and*

---

* Italics added.

Radiology for October 1904, and in the *Journal of the American Medical Association* for November 10, 1906; and the case was further discussed at the October 1907 meeting of the American Roentgen Ray Society.[5] It may well have been the first reported *cure* of a deep-lying internal cancer by the X rays—a cure in the modern sense that the patient survived for more than 5 years with no detectable evidence of recurrence.

Dr. Skinner's patient was a 39-year-old Massachusetts school teacher who had been operated on in 1898 for what was presumably a benign fibroid tumor of the uterus. The surgeon who performed the operation, a Dr. Boothby, may have found more than a fibroid, however, for he removed the entire uterus, the tubes, and the ovaries.

"About 2½ years after this operation," Dr. Skinner reported, the schoolteacher "noticed a hard tumor in the lower abdominal wall" near the scar of the previous operation. There was a rapid growth, and the tumor soon reached the size of a coconut.

The schoolteacher thereupon consulted Dr. Maurice H. Richardson of Boston, who could do nothing for her himself but referred her to Dr. W. B. Coley at Memorial Hospital in New York City for treatment by the "Coley method"—the injection of erysipelas toxins. Dr. Coley excised a portion of the growth, found it to be a malignant fibrosarcoma, and gave her his injections for 10 months. The growth decreased in size during the first months of this treatment, but the toxins "then lost their power," and at the end of the treatment, in January 1902, the schoolteacher's fibrosarcoma measured 10 inches from side to side, 8 inches vertically, and about 5 inches from front to back, giving her "the appearance of a woman seven months pregnant." At this point she was referred to Dr. Skinner in New Haven, "losing flesh, markedly cachetic, very weak, and complained bitterly of pressure symptoms." Dr. Coley considered her case "entirely hopeless."

Dr. Skinner began X-ray exposures on January 28, 1902, "and during the next four months she received 46 applications. Her general condition commenced to improve at once." The tumor continued to grow, however, and the patient left New Haven for a visit to her home in Massachusetts.

When she returned a little later, Dr. Skinner was delighted to note that during the interim the tumor had shrunk in volume by about 20 per cent, making it necessary for the school teacher "to shorten her waist bands and the fronts of her skirts to keep them from dragging on the ground."

During the next 2½ months, Dr. Skinner gave his patient 31 more X-ray treatments. "Her general health continued to improve and the tumor steadily decreased in size." In September 1902, she resumed her teaching position for the first time in 1½ years. In October 1903, Dr. Skinner could proudly report to Dr. Coley that his "entirely hopeless" patient was feeling well and teaching school.

"To make a long story short," Dr. Skinner concluded 1 year later, "the whole treatment of the case extended over a total period of two years and three months, during which time she received 136 applications of the Roentgen ray.... She received her last roentgenization May 20, 1904, at which time no trace of the tumor was discoverable."

In October 1907, Dr. Pfahler of Philadelphia addressed the American Roentgen Ray Society on "The Treatment of Sarcoma by Means of the Roentgen Rays." In preparing his address, he checked the prior medical literature, and was naturally curious to know what had happened to the Massachusetts school teacher after May 1904. So he wrote to Dr. Skinner—and he led off his address to the radiologists with a summary of the reply.

"A letter from Dr. Skinner," Dr. Pfahler announced, "states that she is living and entirely well" three years and four months after the cessation of treatment, "and that she has never been so well as during the past two years. She has continued her occupation five years after she was pronounced incurable by all other means."

A final report on Dr. Skinner's patient came from Dr. Charles Allen Porter of Boston, who examined her and reported his findings in an April 1, 1909, addendum to his 1908 paper. At that time she was suffering from X-ray burns (see below, page 170), but Dr. Porter affirmed that her fibrosarcoma was still, after more than 7 years, "entirely cured." [6]

Treatment of Other Diseases

The welter of such reports pouring from the medical presses during the years after 1900 produced scientific chaos, for some of the reports were regrettably lacking in verisimilitudinous detail, and some were dubious on their face. How much should a prudent physician believe? Among the first efforts to bring order out of this chaos was a textbook prepared by Dr. Pusey of Chicago. Published in June 1903, this textbook was entitled *The Practical Application of the Roentgen Rays in Therapeutics and Diagnosis*, and it was so immediately successful that a second, revised edition appeared in July 1904. In addition to nearly 475 pages on therapeutics by Dr. Pusey, it contained shorter sections on X-ray equipment and X-ray diagnosis by Eugene Wilson Caldwell, then a young electrical engineer in New York City, but soon to become a physician and one of the leading radiologists of the gas-tube era. The 1904 edition reviewed the literature, and reported Dr. Pusey's own experience with the use of the X rays, in no fewer than 52 diseases:

Acne rosacea
Acne vulgaris
Actinomycosis
Alopecia areata
Blastomycosis
Callous
Carcinoma of the breast, head, neck, mouth, larynx, orbit, abdomen, pelvis, anus, and rectum
Clavus
Comedos
Eczema
Elephantiasis
Favus
Glioma
Goitre
Granuloma
Hyperhidrosis
Hypertrichosis
Ichthyosis
Keratosis palmaris and senile keratosis
Leprosy
Leucoma
Leukemia
Leukoplakia buccalis
Lichen planus
Lupus erythematosis

Lupus vulgaris
Mycosis fungoides
Naevi
Neuralgia
Paget's disease of the nipple
Prurigo
Pruritis
Pseudo-leukemia
Psoriasis
Rheumatism
Rhinoscleroma
Sarcoma
Scars
Scrofuloderma
Seborrhea
Sycosis
Syphilis
Tinea tonsurans
Trachoma
Tuberculosis of the bones, joints, glands, and larynx
Tuberculosis arthritis
Tuberculous rhinitis
Urticaria pigmentosa
Vernal conjunctivitis
Warts
Xeroderma pigmentosum

Even this impressive list was hardly an exhaustive roster of diseases treated by the X rays during the early 1900's. At most it was a list of conditions for which X-ray therapy was being recommended by at least a few medical authorities. As early as November 1902, Dr. Heber Robarts, editor of the *American X-Ray Journal*, had estimated that "there are about 100 named diseases that yield favorably to X-ray treatment." If diseases were added which physicians here and there exposed to the X rays "just to see what might happen," the list would no doubt be longer. A few physicians, for example, were using the X rays to produce infertility; a few others were using them to cure infertility; and there were also efforts to treat X-ray burns and X-ray-induced skin ulcers by means of additional X rays.

Almost all the early published reports, regardless of the patient's disease or of the technique used, were enthusiastic. After the first 2 or 3 years, however, more cautious statements began to appear here and there.

At Memorial Hospital in New York City, for example, Dr. Coley—who had treated the Massachusetts school teacher with erysipelas toxins in 1901—soon thereafter added X rays to his anti-cancer armamentarium. This was made possible when Mrs. Collis P. Huntington gave Memorial two X-ray machines and a $100,000 fund for cancer research—said to be the first such fund in the United States—in memory of her husband, who had recently died of cancer. In a report late in 1902, Dr. Coley discussed 84 cases of tumor treated with these machines. The results:

> *Twenty-eight cases of inoperable or recurrent sarcoma:* "Of these the tumors have entirely disappeared in three cases; yet in all of them there was a recurrence within the year. All are still under treatment, and in one the growth has again disappeared under X-ray and toxin treatment. In the remaining two there is steady improvement."
>
> *Twenty cases of recurrent inoperable cancer of the breast:* "In one there has been entire disappearance. In one the growth has nearly disappeared and the patient is much improved in health. In a large proportion of the remaining cases there has been alleviation of pain and temporary improvement. . . ."
>
> *Ten cases of cancer of the abdomen, including rectum, uterus, and intestine:* "Entire disappearance in one case of cancer of the cervix. Marked improvement in three other uterine cases. More or less temporary improvement in most of the remainder."
>
> *Twenty cases of cancer of the head, face, and neck:* "In two cases . . . the tumors have entirely disappeared, one the size of a silver dollar on the forehead, one three-fourths of an inch in diameter on the face. . . . In the tongue cases there have been no good results, nor in the epitheliomata of the larynx or glands of the neck."
>
> *Six miscellaneous cases:* "One case of extensive lupus of the entire nose has disappeared; one of tuberculosis of the pectoral region has disappeared entirely; and one case of advanced Hodgkin's disease, a practically hopeless condition, has shown the most remarkable improvement that has yet been reported. The large tumors of the neck, axilla, and groin have disappeared; the spleen, which nearly filled the abdomen, has decreased three-quarters in size, and the man has resumed his usual occupation. He was given the X-ray and toxin treatment together." [7]

One year later, Dr. Coley reported again. "The results of the second year's work, while not so encouraging as the first year's still are of much interest. Of a total of 129 cases, the tumor disappeared entirely in nine; eleven patients were discharged improved; the remainder were unimproved, or are still under treatment. . . .

"In three cases of sarcoma a recurrence took place within less than six months after the disappearance of the primary tumor. In one case of deep-seated cancer of the breast, in which the tumor disappeared, the patient has had a recurrence. . . ."

Dr. Coley concluded, "The amount of success that has been obtained, while less than we had hoped, is sufficient, we feel, to make it strongly advisable to continue the work in selected cases. . . ." [8]

Suppression of Pain

One reason for the excessive enthusiasm of many very early reports, it seems likely in retrospect, was the favorable *psychological* effect of the X-ray treatment on patients. A visit to the "X-ray doctor" was an impressive occasion indeed. Patients were awed by the hiss or the roar of the equipment, by the tingle of ozone in the air. An aura of something akin to magic surrounded the very word "X ray" in the public mind. Thus, a patient was almost sure to leave an X-ray séance (as some of the electrotherapeutists called their treatments) psychologically encouraged even though not physically benefited.

The early reports were also in all probability over-enthusiastic because of the impressive success of the rays in suppressing pain. This is still a salient effect of X-ray therapy today. Dr. Seabury W. Allen was among the early clinicians who studied the pain effect.

"Not infrequently," Dr. Allen wrote in *American Medicine* for March 22, 1902, "patients whom I have subjected to X rays for one cause or another have spoken of the relief of the pain or discomfort which previously existed in the part exposed. Only lately, when a patient with varicose ulcers of the leg emphasized the fact, was the subject thought worth looking into." Dr. Allen accordingly reviewed his case records and came up with eight striking examples.

The first concerned Mrs. S, a pianist, aged 36. "Two skiagraphs of [her] hands were taken for diagnosis of chronic rheumatic arthritis. On her next appearance, 5 days later, she said that since the exposure was made her hands had been comfortable, and that she had been able to resume practice on the piano, which she had previously had to abandon."

Another case was that of J. L., a man of 32, exposed to the X rays for the purpose of diagnosing a fracture of the ankle. "His wife, who came for the negatives 48 hours later, was skeptical about the existence of the fracture because 'the ankle felt so much better since he was here.' "

The last of Dr. Allen's eight cases was a woman of 85, treated therapeutically with the X rays for a chronic ulcer on her foot. The ulcer had been there for more than 50 years. "Three days after the first exposure," Dr. Allen reported, "she said that she 'knew it would heal, for it had stopped burning and paining.' No effort at healing could be seen, however, until a week later."

To what extent did the X rays actually cure diseases? Which diseases? Would relapses follow the enthusiastic preliminary reports—and if they did, could the recurrence be again successfully treated by the rays? Were doctors and patients alike misled by the psychological effects of treatment as distinct from the specific effect of the rays on diseased tissues?

And what of those dimly understood X-ray burns and other hazards; did the benefits outweigh the risks?

These were questions to which only very tentative answers could be secured during the gas-tube era. Many years of hard work, and the accumulated clinical experiences of many radiologists, would be needed to thresh the wheat (which proved to be abundant) from the chaff (which was also abundant). Chapter 20 in Part III of this history and Chapter 24 in Part IV are concerned with the threshing process.

REFERENCES

1. *Trans. Amer. Surg. Ass., 15:* 59–88, 1897.
2. PUSEY, W. A. AND CALDWELL, E. W., *The Practical Application of the Roentgen Rays in Therapeutics and Diagnosis,* Ed. 2, p. 368. W. B. Saunders, Philadelphia, 1904.
3. *Philadelphia Med. J., 6:* 1089–1091, 1900.
4. *Amer. Med., 4:* 217–218, 1902.
5. *Trans. Amer. Roentgen Ray Soc.,* 66–70, 1907.
6. *Trans. Amer. Roentgen Ray Soc.,* 123, 1908.
7. *Gen. Mem. Hosp. Rep. (New York),* 41–42, 1902.
8. *Gen. Mem. Hosp. Rep. (New York),* 46–47, 1903.

12 Rays from Radium Too

Radium was also introduced as a source of radiation for medical therapy during the "gas-tube era."

The story of the discovery by Henri Becquerel in 1896 that some substances emit radiation—that is, are radioactive—and the story of the subsequent discovery of radium and other radioactive substances by Marie and Pierre Curie are too well-known to require retelling in a history of American radiology. The first significant North American work with radioactive substances was undertaken at McGill University in Montreal by a young New Zealand-born, English-trained physicist, Ernest Rutherford (1871–1937), and his English-born associate, Frederick Soddy (1877–1956).

Rutherford, Soddy, and others, in a series of experiments undertaken soon after the discovery of radium was announced, were able to show that the Becquerel rays emitted by radioactive substances are actually composed of three quite distinct types of radiation[1] : *alpha rays* (the nuclei of helium atoms), which account for more than four-fifths of the energy radiated, but which are so "soft" that a single sheet of paper will block their progress; *beta rays* (electrons), which can pass through thin filters of aluminum but not through sheets of lead or other heavy metals, and which account for most of the remainder of the radiation; and *gamma rays* (X rays of very high energy, short wavelength and great penetrating power), which account for only about 1 per cent of the radiation.

One major contribution of Rutherford and Soddy to the rapidly advancing study of radioactivity was the theory of atomic transformation. Physicists and chemists previously had agreed that the atoms of each element are indestructible and unchangeable, that an atom of oxygen remains an atom of oxygen forever. Rutherford and Soddy showed that this was not true of radioactive atoms. An atom of uranium, for example, emits an alpha particle (helium nucleus) and is thereby transformed into an atom of a "daughter" element, uranium X_1 . This atom in turn disintegrates, emits radiation, and is transformed into an atom of uranium X_2 . After several more transformations, what was initially a uranium atom becomes a radium atom. A disintegrating radium atom in turn gives rise to a further series of radioactive daughter elements. These discoveries revolutionized the sciences of physics and chemistry. In addition, practical uses were soon found for the newly discovered radioactive elements.

In the United States, the first medical experiments with radium were undertaken by the Boston dentist, Dr. William Herbert Rollins (1852–1929; see above, page 67), and his associate, Dr. Francis H. Williams (see above, pages 70–80). Dr. Rollins had secured an M.D. degree from Harvard in 1879 to supplement his 1873 Harvard D.D.S. degree, but he continued to practice dentistry. He published his X-ray contributions in both engineering and medical journals, and he reprinted nearly 200 of them, dealing with both the X rays and radium, in his *Notes on X-Light,* privately published in 1904.

"In these notes," he explained in the preface, "are recorded some impressions derived from experiments made after the day's work, as a recreation, yet with hope of learning to design and construct apparatus for my friend, Dr. F. H. Williams, who has done most to show the importance of X-light in medical diagnosis."

Rollins was an almost compulsive experimenter and deviser of ingenious equipment; indeed, much of Williams's X-ray as well as radium work was performed with apparatus and accessories designed and built for him by Rollins. Rollins even made with his own hands the gold wedding rings used in the ceremony when he married Dr. Williams's sister, Marian. Many of the important later developments in radiological equipment, some not introduced into common use until the 1950's, are traceable to Rollins's work from 1897 to 1904 (see below, pages 180–188 and 425–427). That he accomplished so much is remarkable in any event, and particularly so when it is recalled that most of his work was done alone, in a basement laboratory in his home, during whatever hours he could spare from his successful dental practice.

Rollins's first radium experiment was suggested to him by Professor George F. Barker of Philadelphia, sometime before the summer of 1900. It was based on the hypothesis that Becquerel rays were identical with the cathode rays in the Crookes tube. If Professor Barker were right, Rollins wrote, "we could produce X-light from a vacuum tube with a radioactive cathode, without an electric generator. It would only be necessary to exhaust the tube to the usual X-light vacuum. The particles in the cathode stream from the radioactive cathode would then meet with no more obstruction on their way to the target to produce X-light than would be encountered by those of a cathode stream formed in the ordinary way."

This suggestion of Professor Barker's was a temptation to experiment

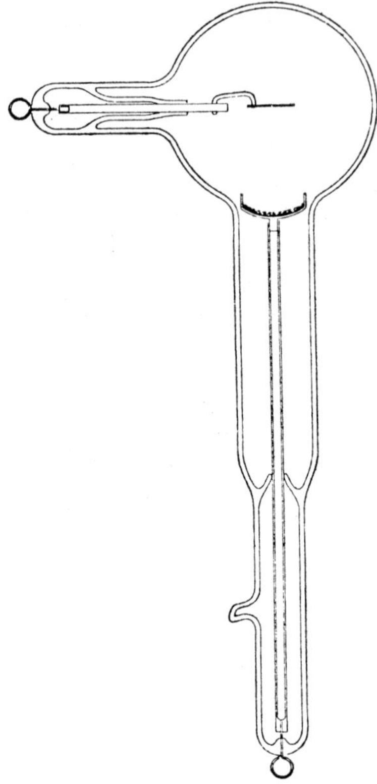

Fig. 26. From *Electrical Review, 38:* 169, February 2, 1901.

which a man of Rollins's temperament could not resist. Abandoning for the time being his research on X rays, he secured a supply of a compound containing radium chloride and constructed a vacuum tube with a conventional target plus a cup-shaped cathode in which the radium compound could be lodged (Fig. 26). During the summer of 1900, experiments with this equipment were performed for Dr. Rollins by Mr. J. O. Heinze, Jr. The results, reported in the *Electrical Review* for February 2, 1901, seemed promising at first, but nothing came of them.

Rollins now went on to evolve an idea of his own, more ingenious than Barker's original suggestion. Rollins knew from his work with Williams that the instability of the Crookes tube was the bane of the radiologist's existence. The functioning of the tube depended on the amount of gas remaining in it after it was evacuated, and this gas varied from moment to moment, depending on the potential applied to the tube, the heating of the cathode and target, and other factors which caused gas molecules to adhere to or detach themselves from the glass and the electrodes. Rollins correctly predicted that a stable tube might be achieved if all or almost all of the gas molecules were evacuated from the tube, but in that event, Rollins knew, the tube would not work at all, since without gas in the tube no "cathode particles"—in modern terms, electrons—would be emitted from the cathode to strike the target and generate the rays. "This problem should be solved," Rollins wrote in the *Electrical Review* for March 9, 1901, "for few discoveries could aid more in the relief of human suffering than this, as it would enable a physician always to have an abundance of X-light of proper wavelength without more trouble than the turning on of an incandescent lamp."

The problem with which Rollins was contending was not actually solved until 1913, when W. D. Coolidge of General Electric developed a tube with a "hot cathode" as a source of electrons in a gas-free tube (see below, page 196). But Rollins's 1901 suggestion came curiously close to anticipating Coolidge. He, too, proposed a "hot cathode"—one which would radiate cathode particles in a completely evacuated tube by virtue of a radioactive substance alloyed with the cathode metal. With such a radioactive cathode, Rollins suggested, the electrical "stress" or potential applied to the tube might cause the charged particles emitted by the radium "to be driven against the target with sufficient force to produce X-light."

Again nothing came of it. Yet it vividly illustrates the way in which Rollins's mind created fresh patterns out of such familiar concepts as charged particle, potential, vacuum, cathode, target, and radioactivity, and then devised new theories and new equipment for testing them.

The same point is illustrated by a third Rollins radium proposal. After a few months or a year of use, the gas tubes available to radiologists during the 1890's and 1900's became so hard that they could no longer be used at all, since too much of the gas adhered to the glass and electrodes. Rollins hoped that such a tube could be "regenerated" by means of particles emitted by radium entering the tube through the glass.

"As it seemed possible," he wrote in his 1904 *Notes on X-Light,* "that one cause for the deterioration of X-light tubes by use might be that some of the charged particles formed during the action of the tube passed out through the glass wall, the tubes were kept in an enclosure with radium salts to see if the charged particles shot off from the radioactive material might not by passing into the tube supply the loss." Nothing came of this experiment, either, but Rollins as late as 1904 was still hopeful. He thought that the relative weakness of his early radium compounds might be the cause of his failure. "The experiment should be repeated now with pure radium bromide," he wrote, "which can be purchased by any rich person."

Rollins did not record the source of his original radium chloride supply, but he did note that he had at least 1 gram of it, and that it had "an activity of 1,000"—meaning that its radioactivity was 1000 times as great as the radiations from pure uranium metal. Pure radium, in contrast, would have shown an "activity" of more than 2,000,000. In effect, Rollins therefore had the equivalent of only about ½ milligram of pure radium—a trivial amount. It is hardly surprising that his initial experiments came to so little. With more time and more radium, the kind of ingenuity he was bringing to bear on radiation problems might well have borne more fruit.

Dr. Rollins next conceived an idea which was indeed to bear fruit. Late in 1900, it will be recalled, his brother-in-law, Dr. Williams, had confirmed in Boston the findings, reported elsewhere a little earlier, that the X rays can heal the lesions of lupus. This seems to have suggested to Rollins that radium, too, might cure lupus. He accordingly placed 500 milligrams of his radium chloride compound in a sealed capsule, "to protect it from moisture," and gave the capsule to Dr. Williams "with the request that it should be tried on lupus, a disease which at that time was interesting to him." This occurred in 1900, probably late 1900, and was quite probably the first suggestion that radium might have therapeutic value.

It is astounding that at so early a date Rollins was already concerned to provide protection against the possible harmful effects of the radium. "The capsule was disk-shaped," he reported, "with the front of aluminum, a back of comparatively non-radiable metal." Thus, both the beta and the gamma rays could pass through the front of the disk to the lupus lesion, while stray radiation through the back of the disk would be minimized.

In a paper at the beginning of 1902 Rollins went on to describe his high hopes for radiation therapy. "It is believed to be important," he wrote, "to test these substances in the treatment of lupus, superficial cancer, and diseases of the skin in which X-light has been found useful. . . . Radioactive substances can be used in sealed capsules held against the body by adhesive plaster, or they can be made to cover larger areas by mixing them with rubber or celluloid to form moisture-proof plasters. These plasters may be still further protected by being coated on the sides nearest the body by aluminum foil and on the opposite sides by lead foil. They could be kept in stock by the yard by druggists and given to patients by prescription with proper directions as to the length of application. They could be worn at night. Their use would prevent the poor from making such frequent visits to a physician as are now required when X-light obtained from a vacuum tube is used. This is a matter of some importance, as the present treatment takes many sittings, which require time and cost money."

Although radium therapy did not take precisely the form which Rollins predicted, his suggestions in some respects came remarkably close to the mark.

The 500 milligrams of radium compound—equivalent to $\frac{1}{4}$ milligram of pure radium—which Dr. Rollins gave his brother-in-law in 1900 were only part of his supply. "Another [radium] capsule will be sent to any Boston physician who will give the matter a fair trial," Dr. Rollins offered in his January 1902 paper. But this offer came 1 or 2 years too early. "Considering the present interest in radium," Rollins commented wryly in his 1904 book, "it may be worth while to say that no application was received for this capsule."

Dr. Williams later confirmed Dr. Rollins's account of his radium gift and therapeutic suggestion. "In 1900," he told the June 1908 meeting of the Surgical Section of the Massachusetts Medical Society, "Dr. William Rollins of Boston suggested the use of the radiations from radium salts as a therapeutic agent, and put capsules containing radium into my hands.... To Dr. Rollins..., so far as I am aware, is due the credit of being the first to realize the probable value of these radiations as a therapeutic agent." [2]

Dr. Williams himself was quite probably the first physician to use radium therapeutically, late in 1900 or early in 1901. The first recorded European trial of radium was the treatment of a lupus patient by Dr. Henri Danlos in Paris later in 1901. However, Dr. Williams never made such a claim. He reported only that his initial clinical trials led to no "definite results," [3] and he explained that "The salts then obtainable were not powerful enough to be efficient."

Meanwhile, in Europe, a different chain of events was leading to the same suggestion that Becquerel rays from radium might prove of therapeutic value.

In 1900 two Germans, Friedrich Walkhoff and Friedrich Giesel, reported that the rays from radium have a destructive effect on human skin. "In order to test the results that had just been announced by Giesel," Mme. Curie subsequently recalled, "Pierre Curie voluntarily exposed his arm to the action of radium during several hours. This resulted in a lesion resembling a burn, that developed progressively and required several months to heal." [4]

Henri Becquerel made the same discovery by accident a little later. On a trip to London and back, April 3 and 4, 1901, to address the Royal

Society, he carried in his waistcoat pocket a sealed tube containing $\frac{1}{10}$ gram of a radium compound "of high activity." The tube was in his pocket for 6 hours. On April 13, 10 days later, he noticed a burn on his skin under the pocket where the radium was carried. The skin peeled off on April 24, and the burn healed very slowly. Mme. Curie recalled that Becquerel "came to tell us of this evil effect of radium, exclaiming in a manner at once delighted and annoyed, 'I love it, but I owe it a grudge!' " [5]

Becquerel's burn was sufficiently serious that he consulted a dermatologist, Dr. Besnier of the Hôpital St. Louis in Paris, who immediately noticed that Becquerel's radium burn resembled an X-ray burn and therefore suggested that radium might also have a therapeutic effect similar to that of the X rays. Dr. Besnier's colleague, Dr. Henri Danlos, tried using radium—said to have been supplied to him by the Curies— for the treatment of lupus and reported his promising results in the *Proceedings of the Society of Dermatology and Syphilology* for November 7, 1901. The view that radium therapy dates from Becquerel's burn, Besnier's suggestion, and Danlos's clinical trials has thus come to be generally accepted. It reveals, however, a regrettable ignorance of Dr. Rollins's and Dr. Williams's work the year before.

By the summer of 1903, radium was being used in a number of European hospitals, and Dr. Williams observed the good results on a trip abroad. "During the past summer," he told the Boston Society of Medical Sciences on December 15, 1903, "I have seen the successful work being done in London with radium by Mackenzie Davidson, who most kindly showed me all his patients; and also the work begun in Vienna by [Guido] Holzknecht." [6]

Impressed by what he had seen, Williams secured and brought back with him 120 milligrams of what was said to be *pure* radium bromide— more than 1000 times more active, milligram for milligram, than the sample given him by Rollins 2 or 3 years before. He also secured 6 grams of "impure" radium salts. At the end of 1903 Dr. Williams reported the effects of these stronger radium compounds on 42 cases he had treated at Boston City Hospital:

Epidermoid carcinoma	23
Rodent ulcer	5
Lupus vulgaris	4
Breast cancer	4
Eczema	2
Psoriasis	2
Keloid	1
Acne	1

His results were on the whole most promising, as may be judged from these excerpts from his paper: "In the two cases of psoriasis, the radium was used for small areas only, to test its efficiency. Healing took place in each of these areas a few days after one exposure. In the four cases of lupus, the results have been very satisfactory. In one of these cases I selected the area in which the disease was most severe for the employ-ment of the radium, and treated the other parts with the X rays. The portion to which the radium was applied improved much more rapidly than those for which the X rays were used. Two of the patients are now apparently well, and the two others, for whom treatment was begun later, are improving. The action of the radium in all these four cases was far more prompt than that of the X rays.... Of the 23 patients with epidermoid carcinoma ... 11 have healed and 12 are improving. Among the latter there is present promise that most of them will heal. One is a carcinoma of the lip that had been steadily treated with the X rays, but did not yield to them." Dr. Williams used a phrase which many others were to use subsequently: in certain cases, he wrote, a lesion treated by radium "seems to melt away."

Dr. Williams went on to compare in detail his recent radium experi-ence with his years of X-ray experience, and concluded that "the com-parison at the present time is greatly to the advantage of the radium. ... In the first place, when radium is employed for healing purposes no cumbersome apparatus is necessary; radium is portable and always ready for use. Further, the dose from radium is uniform; the strength of the output does not vary, so that the dose depends entirely on the length of exposure and the distance of the radium from the part to be treated. Radium may be applied to parts which are not readily accessible to the X rays, as the mouth or vagina. Furthermore, the healing action of the radium is more prompt. The treatment, therefore, extends over a shorter period, and fewer exposures are required than when the X rays are used. Radium has the further advantage of bringing about healing in some cases where the X rays have failed after careful and long-continued treatment." He conceded, however, that "it is yet too early to give a final and definite opinion as to the value of radium salts as a therapeutic agent." [6]

One feature of Dr. Williams's December 1903 report on his radium trials was his emphasis on radiation *protection*. "As with the X rays," he wrote, "caution must be observed when treating patients, for the sake both of the patient and of the practitioner; for radium, if not properly protected, causes severe burns, which do not manifest themselves for a week or more. These burns are painful and heal slowly. Already a number of cases of injury to persons working with radium have been reported.

"Radium, therefore, should be kept in a metal box or capsule with a thin mica front or other suitable covering, so that the radiations may be cut off in all directions except that in which the practitioner desires the rays to proceed. To such a capsule I have attached a long, flexible handle, in order to hold the radium at a distance when applying it. This handle is a protection to the practitioner. When not in use, the capsule should be placed in a thick lead box or tube, so that the radiations may be absorbed." And he noted that when he treated a small skin lesion, he exposed it to the radium "through an opening in a sheet of lead foil" to protect the healthy skin nearby.

A few weeks later, at the January 18, 1904, meeting of the Boston Society for Medical Improvement, Dr. Williams reported on eight additional cases, and renewed his warning that "the burns caused by radium, like those produced by the X rays, are, it is said, very difficult to heal." But, he added proudly, "*I have had no experience with them.*" [7] *

Dr. Williams also went on, in 1903 and 1904, to describe two further uses of radium. One was as a "fluorometer," or device for gauging the quantity of radiation from an X-ray tube. The principle was simple. Dr. Williams darkened the room, placed a fluoroscope screen in the X-ray beam from the tube, and then moved the screen away from the tube until the fluorescence on the screen precisely matched in brightness the fluorescence from a radium sample used as a standard of comparison. The greater the distance from tube to screen at the point where the screen fluorescence matched the comparison standard, the greater the emanation from the tube. Two tubes whose output matched the radium standard at the same distance were emitting the same quantity of rays. This use of radium as a fluorometer Dr. Williams described in the third (1903) edition of his classic textbook, *The Roentgen Rays in Medicine and Surgery.*

Finally, Dr. Williams used radium in an interesting procedure to assure a minimum of X-ray exposure to the patient during a fluoroscopic examination. Physicians then as now were accustomed to blindfold their eyes or sit in a dark room prior to fluoroscopy in order to adapt their eyes to the darkness, so as to see the image on the screen clearly with only a moderate current to the tube and thus a moderate X-ray dose to the patient. But how could the physician know when his eyes were sufficiently dark-adapted? Dr. Williams secured or made a *spinthariscope,* a device invented by Sir William Crookes in 1903. In this device, the charged particles emitted by radium cause tiny scintillations to appear on a calcium tungstate screen, each scintillation representing the

____
* Italics added.

effect of a single particle. "If the scintillations appear bright to the practitioner," Dr. Williams wrote in the *Boston Medical and Surgical Journal* for May 26, 1904, "his eyes are ready for use; if dull, he must wait for a while longer in the dark room before attempting to make a fluoroscopic examination."

The interest in radium generally, and particularly in radium therapy, expanded notably throughout Europe and the United States during 1903 and early 1904. The award of a 1903 Nobel Prize to Becquerel and the Curies, and the appealing pictures of Mme. Curie published in the newspapers at the time, no doubt contributed to this interest, as well as the reports of therapeutic successes from Paris, London, Vienna, and other cities appearing in the medical journals or brought back by travelers like Dr. Williams. Among the American physicians who either secured radium compounds or borrowed them from friendly physicists, and who launched therapeutic trials of their own in 1903 or early 1904, were the following:

> Dr. Robert Abbé, New York City
> Dr. Truman Abbé, Washington, D.C.
> Dr. Joseph Beck, Chicago
> Dr. L. Duncan Bulkley, New York City
> Dr. Walter B. Chase and his son,
>   Dr. Carroll Chase, Brooklyn
> Dr. Margaret A. Cleaves, New York City
> Dr. Max Einhorn, New York City
> Dr. Howard A. Kelly, Baltimore
> Dr. Myron Metzenbaum, Cleveland
> Dr. William J. Morton, New York City
> Dr. William Allen Pusey, Chicago
> Dr. Jay F. Schamberg, Philadelphia
> Dr. George H. Stover, Denver
> Dr. Samuel G. Tracy

No doubt there were other American pioneers as well. Indeed, by August 1904 Dr. Beck was reporting that "scarcely a number of any journal appears which does not contain an article or a report" on radium, "and most of them are extremely encouraging in their results." [8]

During the following decade (1904–1913), the use of radium for therapy continued to expand in Europe, but most American radiologists used X rays exclusively. Only a few of the radium pioneers—notably Dr. Robert Abbé, Dr. Kelly, and Dr. Williams—continued to treat patients with radium. Thus, of 48 books and papers on radium therapy listed in *Index Medicus* for 1913, only six were North American publications. The other 42 came from Germany (18), France (eight), and six other European countries. Of the six North American publications on radium therapy, moreover, four were concerned primarily with reporting European developments. Only one during the entire year—a paper by Dr. Robert Abbé—described work in the United States; the other described work done in Canada. At the end of the gas-tube era, North America was lagging far behind Europe in the use of radium for therapy.

The main reason for this lag was an inadequate radium supply within the United States. After 1913, fresh supplies became available, and progress thereafter was rapid (see pages 271–299).

REFERENCES

1. RUTHERFORD, E., *Radioactive Transformations.* Yale University Press, New Haven, 1906.
2. *J.A.M.A., 51:* 894–897, 1908.
3. *Boston Med. Surg. J., 150:* 207, 1904.
4. CURIE, M., *Pierre Curie,* p. 117. The Macmillan Company, New York, 1923.
5. *Ibid.,* p. 118.
6. *Med. News, 84:* 241–246, 1904.
7. *Boston Med. Surg. J., 150:* 206–209, 1904.
8. *Laryngoscope, 14:* 901, 1904.

13　With Death in Their Fingertips

As experience with the X rays accumulated during 1896, it will be recalled, quite serious X-ray "burns" were occasionally reported (see pages 81–90). During the years following 1896, additional X-ray injuries were occasionally described in the medical literature, but the outlook for the safe use of the rays seemed on the whole quite reassuring. In 1902, for example, a surgeon—Dr. E. A. Codman of the Harvard Medical School and the Massachusetts General Hospital—conscientiously reviewed all the papers on X-ray injuries that he could find, European as well as American, and unearthed fewer than 200 cases. There was a widespread impression that injuries had been more numerous, but Dr. Codman attributed this to the fact that individual cases were being reported repeatedly in one publication after another. "It was a matter of great surprise," Dr. Codman commented, "to find the number of recorded cases so small, and that each was so often copied in other journals." [1]

Moreover, injuries seemed to be getting rarer as the years rolled by. Of the 88 X-ray injuries which Dr. Codman could definitely date from published accounts,

55 had occurred in 1896
12 had occurred in 1897
6 had occurred in 1898
9 had occurred in 1899
3 had occurred in 1900
1 had occurred in 1901

This decline might be attributable in part, of course, to the fact that X-ray injuries were no longer news and therefore went unreported unless they exhibited unusual features. Dr. Codman preferred to believe, however, that the record was actually improving. Some of the later cases that he described could be attributed less to the hazards of radiation, properly used, than to the wanton folly of those who abused their apparatus.

One such case reported by Dr. Codman concerned a physician in Willimantic, Connecticut, who purchased an X-ray machine from Otis Clapp & Son of Boston early in 1899. Soon after installing the machine, he tested it by exposing himself to the rays for 45 minutes, with the tube only 5 inches from his groin.

A 45-minute groin exposure at 5 inches would have been risky even in 1896. With the far more powerful apparatus supplied by the Clapps in 1899, so prolonged an exposure came close to being self-mutilation, and if attempted on a patient it would almost certainly have been malpractice. "A most intractable burn followed," Dr. Codman reported, "necessitating a severe operation, and producing disability for a year and a half."

The physician thereupon sued the Clapp firm for $20,000 in damages, alleging that the company had warranted that its apparatus would not burn. Half a dozen of the country's foremost X-ray authorities testified on behalf of the manufacturer—Dr. Codman himself, Dr. Charles A. Porter of Boston, Dr. Walter H. Merrill of Washington, D.C., Dr. Louis A. Weigel of Rochester, New York, and Major W. C. Borden and Dr. W. M. Gray of the U.S. Army Medical Corps. Yet the physician was awarded $6750 in damages by a U.S. District Court on November 8, 1901.[1] Only such outrageous overexposures, it was quite generally believed as late as 1902 or 1903, rendered the X-rays unsafe, and, even after severe burns, patients seemed to recover.

Then a series of disasters, beginning in 1904, shook the infant specialty of radiology to its foundations.

Clarence Madison Dally (1865–1904), so far as is known, was the first American X-ray worker to die as a result of X-ray exposure.[2] Like his father and his three brothers, Dally was a glassblower in Edison's employ, and, as noted above (page 41), he had blown countless Crookes tubes for X-ray experimentation in Edison's laboratory back in 1896. He had tested the output of these tubes in the usual way—by placing one of his hands directly into the beam. (A photograph showing Edison examining a hand with his fluoroscope appears as Plate VIII; the man whose hand is being X-rayed may have been Dally.)

Later, Edison assigned Dally to work on a new "fluorescent lamp" which, it was hoped, would replace the ordinary electric lamp as a source of illumination. This lamp was an X-ray tube with a thin inner coating of calcium tungstate. X-rays caused the calcium tungstate to fluoresce and thus brighten a room.

Damage to Dally's hands must have occurred quite early. Elihu Thomson, it will be recalled, had noted on December 1, 1896, that two of Edison's assistants—one of them probably Dally—had been severely burned by X-rays, and that one of them "was told by his physician that if he continued to work it would be necessary to amputate his hands." [3]

Yet Dally did continue to work with the rays. Indeed, when one of his hands became too badly injured to be used for testing tubes, he began to use the other. Edison blamed the fluorescent lamps that Dally had been manufacturing for the injury, and subsequently wrote, "I started in to make a number of these lamps, but I soon found that the X-ray had affected poisonously my assistant, Mr. Dally, so that his hair came out and his flesh commenced to ulcerate. I then concluded it would not do, and that it would not be a very popular kind of lamp, so I dropped it." [4]

Dally continued, however, to work with X-rays through 1897 and 1898. When he later consulted Dr. Charles Warren Allen, professor of dermatology at the New York Post-Graduate Medical School, Dr. Allen recorded Dally's history: "Patient states that for three years he had worked continually, making and testing X-ray tubes. A year after beginning this work he noticed a sunburned condition of the hands. He stopped work for two or three days until the pain and swelling had subsided and then resumed his occupation." [5]

Dally "was treated at many different hospitals," one of his physicians later reported. "Skin grafting was tried without result, until finally epithelioma [skin cancer] developed on the right hand and on the base of the little finger of the left hand." [6] Thus, Dally's case was among the earliest in which skin cancer was diagnosed following radiation injury.

During 1900 and 1901, as noted above, the use of X-rays for the *cure* of skin cancer was being reported. Indeed, the medical literature of the period contains a number of cases in which patients suffering from X-ray burns, and from skin cancer following such burns, were treated with additional X-rays in an effort to cure the cancers. Dally was among them. Dally's New Jersey physician, Dr. Allen recorded in 1902, had been "applying the X-ray with the hope of undoing what the ray itself had done." Deciding after a while that "this was a futile course," the physician brought Dally to Dr. Allen at New York Post-Graduate on June 2, 1902. [5]

Dr. Allen found "purpura-like spots . . . scattered over the skin upon the arms and wrists and over the backs of the hands. On the right hand the tendons were exposed in an ulcer." An ugly ulcer measuring $3\frac{1}{2}$ by $3\frac{1}{2}$ inches also covered his right wrist; 144 skin grafts from Dally's leg applied to the surface of this ulcer had failed to produce healing.

Dr. Allen accordingly referred Dally to his associate, Dr. Samuel Lloyd, a surgeon at Post-Graduate, and on August 8, 1902, Lloyd amputated Dally's right arm at the shoulder joint and excised the neighboring glands. He also urged the amputation of Dally's left hand, but Dally refused consent until March 16, 1904, when amputation above the elbow was performed by Dr. W. B. Graves of East Orange, New Jersey.

"Death followed from mediastinal recurrence in October 1904," Dr. Graves subsequently reported. [6]

The next death to be reported was that of Elizabeth Fleischman Ascheim (1859–1905) of San Francisco. [6, 7]

Miss Fleischman had become interested in X-ray diagnosis in 1897 and had installed an X-ray machine in the office of her brother-in-law, a San Francisco physician. There she X-rayed patients for several years, exposing her hands repeatedly to the direct rays, as did other physicians, both to test the condition of the tube and to demonstrate to her patients that the rays were really quite harmless. She continued her X-ray work after her marriage in 1900, and was one of the few nonphysicians admitted to membership in the American Roentgen Ray Society. Her subsequent medical history was reported to Dr. Porter by her personal physician, Dr. Childs Macdonald of San Francisco, and was published by Dr. Porter in the *Transactions of the American Roentgen Ray Society* for 1908.

> Patient was a pioneer in X-ray work. In 1903, her hands commenced to show signs of X-ray dermatitis, the nature of which was not understood, and attributed to chemicals used in developing the plates. Patient worked 12 hours a day without protection. In the early part of 1904, she came for the first time under treatment.
>
> The fingers of both hands were badly ulcerated, chiefly the tissues over the middle phalanges and the middle joints; all the nails were affected, the surfaces presenting ulcerated, warty condition, the warts assuming the form of necrogenica, healing alternating with ulceration. All the secreting glands and hair follicles were destroyed, so that the skin was hard and dry and cracked easily. All sorts of treatment of ointments and washes was apparently without permanent benefit. In November, 1904, a wart appeared on the index finger, near the terminal phalanx, which was very raw and grew with great rapidity. A portion was removed, under cocaine, and submitted to Dr. Rifkogel, who reported a branching papilloma, with a tendency to downward growth, and advised amputation. This the patient refused, so the growth was freely excised and healed healthily.
>
> A few weeks afterwards, however, a nodule appeared near the scar, which pushed up through the epithelium, broke through it and appeared exactly the same as growth No. 1. The glands in the axilla were found somewhat enlarged. Radical operation was again refused, until after Christmas, when axilla was freely opened and the whole space cleared of glands. Pathological examination of these showed undoubted involvement with epidermoid carcinoma. In the course of a week more nodules appeared.... It was decided that the only chance of recovery lay in amputation at the shoulder.
>
> Accordingly, on January 27, 1905, ... the arm and scapula with the clavicle were removed. The patient rallied well from the operation and the wound healed rapidly, but about the end of April 1905, a recurrence took place at a point representing the position of the inferior angle of the removed scapula. This was excised and found to be carcinoma. Slowly and then rapidly other nodules appeared, until ultimately the whole of the vertical scar ... became involved. Metastases took place in the pleura and lungs and the patient died on August 3, 1905. On reading this history, it is obvious that the patient,

by refusing early radical surgical treatment, jeopardized her life, though it is, of course, possible that metastases had occurred early.

The death of Dr. Louis Andrew Weigel (1854–1906) was next reported.[6, 8] He was an orthopedic surgeon in Rochester, New York, who had used X-rays in diagnosis for 5 years. As noted above (page 87), some manufacturers of X-ray equipment insisted that it was not the X-rays themselves but the associated induction coils which cause the burns; Dr. Weigel had believed this dogma and therefore used a static machine instead of a coil, remarking on one occasion that he "considered it safer," and referring to the static machine's "greater safety" as compared with the induction coil.

Dr. W. B. Coley of Memorial Hospital in New York reported Dr. Weigel's medical history to Dr. Porter: "Ulcerations present for six months on the backs of both hands, specimens from which were examined by Professor [William H.] Welch of Johns Hopkins Hospital, and found to be undoubted epithelioma. The carcinoma had deeply involved the metacarpal bones of the index and middle fingers. Amputation of right hand above wrist, and thorough excision of ulceration on the left hand, October 10, 1904. Subsequent recurrence in axilla and liver."

Dr. Weigel died on May 31, 1906.

Deaths reported thereafter included those of Wolfram Conrad Fuchs (1865–1908), who had opened an X-ray laboratory in Chicago in 1896 (see page 64) and had made the first X-ray negative of a brain tumor in 1899 (see page 113), and Dr. William Carl Egelhoff (1872–1907) of Chicago.[6, 9]

Dr. Porter of Boston delivered his classic 65-page report on these and other cases at the December 1908 meeting of the American Roentgen Ray Society. Dr. Porter had had what he called "a unique experience," having personally operated on 13 of these X-ray victims, who had come to him from all over the East and Middle West for skin grafting and other surgery following his apparent success with his first few cases. In his 1908 paper, Dr. Porter reported in precise detail on his own 13 cases plus 34 others, and alluded to many more. He quoted Dr. William A. Pusey of Chicago, for example, as having stated: "I have seen many cases of this kind, certainly more than a score."[6]

Dr. Porter commented particularly on the pain associated with chronic X-ray burns and their precancerous or cancerous sequelae. "The amount of pain which these patients suffer is variable," he noted, "though usually extreme. From my experience, and personal communications from patients, I believe that the agony of inflamed X-ray lesions is almost unequaled by any other disease. . . . While morphia has been used in some of the cases, it is really surprising to find how many have borne their pain without resorting to its habitual use."

Among the cases Dr. Porter presented at the 1908 meeting was that of Dr. Charles Lester Leonard (1861–1913) of Philadelphia, one of the greatest of early American radiologists.[6, 10] Dr. Leonard had begun work with the X-rays early in 1896. At first he had denied the harmfulness of the rays, engaging in a controversy on this point with Elihu Thomson. By 1903, however, Dr. Leonard had changed his mind. "I have been suffering from X-ray burns for some time," he told a medical meeting in that year, "and I have been putting in some time in the endeavor to find some way of preventing these accidents, and also to make it possible for me to recover."[11] An ulcer on his left hand he described as "extremely painful, keeping me awake for hours, night after night." Among the remedies that he tried was further X-ray treatment of the lesion. At the 1908 meeting addressed by Dr. Porter, Dr. Leonard had the unusual experience of hearing his own case presented.

"Case Thirteen," Dr. Porter intoned. "Dr. C. L. L. Several years ago developed an epithelioma of his forefinger, and fearing excision or even amputation, lest metastases result, applied the X-ray very vigorously, with the intention of destroying all malignant cells before operation. He produced a slough that extended to the bone, after which the finger was amputated and healed by primary union. There are a few suspicious areas over the fingers of the same hand; no glandular involvement."

When Dr. Porter had concluded, Dr. Leonard joined in the discussion. "I suppose that as one of the sufferers from X-ray dermatitis I am well qualified to discuss this subject," he began. "I was educated as a surgeon, and I practiced surgery until my dermatitis prevented me from doing so any longer." He then went on, in disagreement with Dr. Porter and other speakers, to deny the importance of early surgical excision for X-ray-induced cancers. "Look at the cases in which operation has been resorted to," he suggested. "I have yet to find in the whole category of those who have died as a result of X-ray dermatitis one who was not subjected to repeated operations. That they are not living now shows that the operation did not cut short the disease."[6]

Nor was Dr. Leonard's disease cut short. Following the amputation of his finger, his left hand and forearm were amputated, and then his upper arm at the shoulder. He died of metastatic cancer in 1913. "He was active in scientific work up until the very end, however," Dr. Richard H. Chamberlain of the University of Pennsylvania Medical School reports, "and Dr. Pancoast gave a paper for him at the International [Radiological] Congress in London when his terminal illness prevented his own personal attendance."[12]

Among the victims who suffered most was Dr. Walter James Dodd (1869–1916) of Boston.[6, 13, 14]

Born in London, Walter Dodd came to Boston at the age of 10, and at 18 became assistant janitor at Harvard's Boylston Chemical Laboratory. In addition to sweeping the floors, Dodd studied, and in 1892, at age 23, he was appointed assistant apothecary at Massachusetts General Hospital. He was chief apothecary and official photographer there in 1896, when news came of Roentgen's discovery. He added an X-ray machine to his pharmaceutical and photographic equipment in March 1896, and by November he had incurred a severe dermatitis. Dr. Porter was his physician, and reported Dodd's subsequent tribulations in his 1908 paper.

The initial irritation had subsided, Dr. Porter declared,

but was followed in April 1897 by an extremely severe general dermatitis, with pain beyond description. All kinds of washes, ointments and powders were used with orthoform to relieve the pain. My first graft was applied to an ulcer on the tip of the left forefinger, on July 10, 1897. On August 13, 1897, fourteen different grafts were applied, after excision of as many ulcerated areas. The extreme pain ceased at once, and the great majority of the grafts healed soundly. Between this date and 1902, there were seven other similar operations under ether. Most of the grafts were successful, but, in spite of several attempts, failure was constant over ulcerations on the ends of the ring finger of both hands. In July 1902 another attempt at excision and grafting was made; it failed. In October, extremely painful, angry looking ulcers with indurated edges had formed upon the ends of both ring fingers; these were amputated. The report from the pathologist was unmistakable carcinoma. In consequence, on October 31, 1902, both of the ring fingers were amputated at the knuckles. From October, 1902, until June, 1905, a dozen or more operations, consisting of partial amputations, excision of growing ulcerations and keratoses, were performed.

In May, 1905, for the first time in eight years, the patient was free from pain and no dressings had to be worn. In June the left hand was practically well, but keratoses broke down on the base of the middle finger of the right hand, and ... numerous other ulcerations were skin grafted; some of these showed a precancerous stage. By April 25, 1907, after ten years of treatment, and *twenty-five operations under ether*, the condition of the hands was as follows.

Left hand: amputation of little finger through the interphalangeal joint; amputation of ring and middle fingers at knuckles; fourth finger shows slight ulceration at its base and a small ulcer in the middle of the back of the hand; there are numerous keratoses, but no ulcerations.

Right hand: the thumb is useful, but its ulnar side is covered with thickened epithelium, at the base of which is a small ulceration. For two months there has been ulceration over the joint between the

> first and second phalanx of the forefinger, with flexion of this joint; this ulceration strongly suggests malignant disease. The middle finger is stiff; the fourth is lacking, as is also the end of the fifth. The hand shows the presence of numerous grafts, which have taken, and a few keratoses.
>
> The patient was at work at a medical school and did not submit to an operation until July 5, 1907, at which time it was evident that the forefinger must be amputated.... Several suspicious areas were excised in other parts of both hands, and skin grafted. Microscopic examination of the amputated forefinger showed five different areas of carcinoma....
>
> As a result of this examination, it was decided on July 15 [1908] to amputate higher up. The head of the first metacarpal bone was removed and a large flap reflected on to the dorsum of the hand, thus forming a sound stump for approximation of the thumb. In September, 1908, after eating lobsters, there occurred a general urticaria and both hands became much swollen, and the serous discharge was extreme. The patient was confined to bed for ten days, then very gradually the exudate dried up and there followed desquamation. This, however, did *not affect* the *keratotic areas*. There have been one or two injuries to the base of the forefinger of the left hand, and to the base of the middle finger of the right hand, which set up extremely painful and obstinate excoriations. For several months there has been an inflamed warty growth over the stump of the little finger of the left hand.

Despite these tribulations, Dodd had enrolled as a student at the Harvard Medical School in 1900, at the age of 31. After 1 year there, he had transferred to the University of Vermont Medical School, where he received his M.D. degree in 1908. "I have operated on this patient under ether *thirty-two* times," Dr. Porter noted the year that Dodd was graduated, "the operations varying in duration from one hour and a half to three hours.... The number of different carcinomata in this one case has been *over a score*. I can have no reasonable doubt that general metastases would have taken place long ago had it not been for timely excisions and amputations."

The newly graduated Dr. Dodd, aged 39, now began the practice of radiology in Boston. He served as radiologist at his old hospital, Massachusetts General, and the next year was appointed "instructor in the use of the Roentgen ray" at the Harvard Medical School. In June 1915 he went to France as radiologist with the Harvard Medical Unit of the British Expeditionary Force. Before departing, he underwent one more severe operation at the hands of Dr. Porter. "The vehicle that took him from his house to the train for New York," says his friend and biographer, John Macy, "was an ambulance. The operation had left a deep wound, still unhealed, in his arm and breast." Dr. Dodd served in France with distinction, returned in 1915, and died of metastatic cancer of the lung on December 18, 1916.[6, 13, 14]

Elderly radiologists who had trained at Massachusetts General during the 1910's still remembered Dr. Dodd with affection in the 1960's, both for his interest in their careers when they were young and for the quiet way in which he used his own misfortune to impress upon them the need for precautions against a similar fate.[15]

Almost all the early victims of the X-ray were men in the prime of life; the two oldest of those noted above were both 52 when they died, and the average age at death was 45. Several were tube manufacturers, including Rome Vernon Wagner (1869–1908) and his brother Thurman Lester Wagner (1876–1912), Burton Eugene Baker (1871–1913), Henry Green (1860–1914), John Bauer (?–1908), and Robert Herman Machlett (1872–1926). Dr. Rome Wagner ruefully described the problems of a tube manufacturer in trying to protect himself.

"One of the most difficult things about this work," he told the October 1907 meeting of the American Roentgen Ray Society, "is to determine what absolute protection is. I meet many X-ray workers in my work, and I used to find, when I called on one of them, that the first thing he wanted was to show me some tube that was defective in some way, so that I could tell him what was the matter with it. He had no idea of protecting either me or himself. I found it a good plan to carry a little camera. Every operator knows how to protect the photographic plate, but he never stops to consider the protection of himself in the same way. The thing is to know whether you have exposed yourself during the day.... I concluded that I would not take chances with any ray that would affect a photographic plate, so I carry one in my pocket, and in the evening, after the day's work, I develop this film to see whether I have been exposed to the ray. Once in a while I find that I have, and then I try to figure out where I have been exposed. Now I often go for a week without any exposure; in fact, only seldom is the film affected. I believe that this plan is a good one because you need not worry about being exposed when you have not been exposed."[6]

Wagner's adoption of the "film badge"—a measure now common in hospitals and radiological offices—came too late, however. He already had cancer of the hands and cheek. A prominent radiologist of the "gastube era" who survived uninjured, Dr. Benjamin H. Orndoff of Chicago, described a visit to Rome Wagner and his brother Thurman at about this time.

"It was in 1906 or 7," Dr. Orndoff told a meeting of the Chicago Roentgen Society in February 1963, "that I paid my last visit to their factory. Sadness filled my heart to overflowing. Rome with multiple skin ulcers on his hands, body, and face, and skin showing early jaundice, and metastasis to the liver was evident. Thurman with back and chest ulcers, amputated fingers, and axillary glands. Here were two brothers, fine gentlemen, who had earned their medical degree the hard way of self-sacrifice and labor, attending colleges at night and working during the day. . . . Both pursued their duties intensely, and the path they followed to their useful position in life was steep and arduous. Both recognized the magnitude of the sacrifice they were soon to make, but with supreme fortitude and courage they carried on to the end." [16] Rome died of extensive metastatic cancer of the liver in the spring of 1908, less than 6 months after describing his film-badge method of gauging exposure. Thurman Wagner, after a series of amputations, died in May 1912.

During the 1930's, the biographical facts concerning these and other X-ray victims were patiently collected by an eminent Boston radiologist, Dr. Percy Brown. Dr. Brown published his collection of biographical essays, *American Martyrs to Science through the Roentgen Rays,* in 1936; a number of the facts in this account are drawn from his book. In addition to the cases noted above, he told the stories of Mihran Krikor Kassabian of Philadelphia (1870–1910), Eugene Wilson Caldwell of New York City (1870–1918), Heber Robarts of St. Louis (1852–1922), Frederick Henry Baetjer of Baltimore (1874–1933), and a number of others whose lives deserve to be remembered. However, one story—his own—was missing from his volume. Dr. Brown himself died of X-ray-induced cancer in 1950.

Although radiologists and others professionally engaged in X-ray work provided the bulk of the gas-tube era radiation-induced cancer cases and deaths, some patients, too were afflicted. One of them was Dr. Clarence E. Skinner's famed patient, the Massachusetts schoolteacher.

Back in January 1902, it will be recalled (see page 143), Dr. Skinner had begun to treat with X rays a schoolteacher dying of an incurable fibrosarcoma. By May 1904, "Skinner's case" had received 136 X-ray treatments, and her "incurable" cancer was cured. When Dr. Pfahler checked up on the teacher in 1907, he was informed that she was still living and entirely well three years and four months after the cessation of treatment, and "she has never been so well as during the past two years." [17]

But her medical history did not end there. In April 1909 Dr. Porter of Boston brought the story up to date, in an addendum to his 1908 paper.

The schoolteacher had remained "perfectly well" until August 1907, Dr. Porter then reported, "though she had noticed that the skin of the hypogastric region was irregularly mottled and much thicker than normal, especially on the right side. Pain, from which she had been free, began to be severe and ulceration commenced. No treatment seemed of avail, the ulcerative process gradually spreading, undermining the skin, which subsequently necrosed. She lost weight and strength, becoming anemic, and suffered severely from the pain. She was referred to me by

Dr. Dennett, of Winchester, and I first saw her at the Baptist Hospital on March 7, 1908. Examination at this time showed in the hypogastric region, more on the right than on the left, an irregular, undermined ulcer about the size of the palm of one's hand, roughly an equilateral triangle, extending to the right side of the pubis, then nearly to the right iliac spine, the other angle approaching the umbilicus. The base of this ulceration is sloughing in parts; in others presenting poorly vascularized granulation tissue, in which necrosis is advancing rapidly. Several areas in the surrounding skin show characteristic appearances. The irregular undermined ulceration, with a firmly adherent, fibrinous base, is surrounded by a very bright scarlet-red areola, which bled on the slightest touch. Certain points in the ulceration are exquisitely painful on pressure. There was slight fever. After attempting to cleanse wound with antiseptics for a few days, on March 6 the whole ulcerated area, with a margin of about an inch, was excised down to the underlying tissue. This excision left apparently normal fat, except over an area 2 × 3 in., to the right of the median line, where extremely firm scar tissue marked the site of the original growth. The skin at the periphery, however, was very tough and three times the normal thickness."

The tissue removed was sent to the Harvard Medical School; the pathological diagnosis was epidermoid carcinoma. Although cured of her fibrosarcoma, Skinner's patient now suffered from "characteristic X-ray lesions" and skin cancer in the area where she had been irradiated.

Following a series of further operations and many months of suffering, Dr. Skinner's schoolteacher at length recovered again. "There is no tenderness in the scar and no pain," Dr. Porter noted on April 1, 1909. "Patient has been up and about for three weeks, having been in the hospital 13 months.... There is no evidence of recurrence of the sarcoma [seven years after X-ray treatment began]. Her general condition is excellent." [6]

A search of the medical literature has unearthed no subsequent report on "Skinner's case."

The medical profession, it need hardly be added, rallied to the care of the X-ray victims, and all possible measures were taken to alleviate their suffering and improve their condition. As one result, some of these patients were among the most thoroughly studied in the entire history of medicine, and much was learned about disease and its treatment in the course of their continuing care. The case of Dr. Walter B. Cannon of Harvard was in this respect outstanding. [18]

Dr. Cannon, it will be recalled, used the X rays beginning in 1896, when he was a freshman medical student at Harvard, to study the physiology of the gastrointestinal tract (see page 118). "An insatiable worker," his colleagues later declared, "his exposure to the X radiations must have been great as he hovered over the fluoroscopic screen above the X-ray table."

Dr. Cannon had adopted some safeguards. For example, he used a galvanized iron box which "completely surrounded the X-ray apparatus except for a small opening at the top. As a result, he was relatively well protected from X rays except for his hands, which were seriously burned repeatedly, and, to a less extent, his face and the upper part of his body."

In 1908 Cannon completed his experiments on digestion and moved to other research not requiring X-ray exposure. For 23 years he remained in good health. Then, early in 1931, when he was 59, a papilloma was removed from his bladder, and in the summer of that year, "There appeared itching of the skin and fiery red papular cutaneous lesions on his back, chest, thighs, knees, and elbows." The skin lesions grew worse during the year that followed, and a skin biopsy made in the fall of 1932 showed that Cannon was suffering from a rare malignant condition known as *mycosis fungoides*. Dr. Cannon knew, of course, what that diagnosis meant; patients generally survived, in discomfort, for only about 5 years on the average.

Specialists at three Boston hospitals—the Collis P. Huntington, the Massachusetts General, and the Peter Bent Brigham—contributed to Dr. Cannon's care and to the study of his condition during the years which followed; four of them—Drs. Joseph C. Aub, S. Burt Wolbach, B. J. Kennedy, and Orville T. Bailey—published the final report on his illness in the *A.M.A. Archives of Pathology* for 1955. Despite the medical tradition of withholding the names of patients in published reports, Dr. Cannon's name instead of merely his initials or case number was used; his physicians explained why.

"With the objectivity so well known to his friends and associates," they began their report, Dr. Cannon had "suggested that repeated biopsies be made whenever they would provide information on the development of this incompletely understood condition. The material thus obtained over a period of 14 years, and that from the necropsy, were carefully prepared for histologic study. They now afford an opportunity to trace the sequences involved in mycosis fungoides with development of lymphatic leukemia, to elucidate some controversial points concerning the cellular components involved, to review the hematologic data, and to consider the relation of the condition to exposure to unfiltered X radiation. Therefore, the record demands careful reporting, and it is coupled with Dr. Cannon's name because a great man who taught so many students so much should also be associated with the record of his instructive illness."

The four physicians then went on to review in detail the prolonged course of Dr. Cannon's group of related illnesses. "In October 1933," they noted, "the skin involved was irradiated weekly with small amounts of low-voltage X ray to give temporary relief from the severe and progressive itching." Many other palliatives were also tried, for, as his physicians noted, "Dr. Cannon was a man who expected continuous investigation" in his own case as well as in medical science generally.

During 1937, "a progressive rise in the white blood cell count occurred," and leukemia was diagnosed. In March 1940, an ulcerated lesion on the left wrist was excised and proved to be "a slowly growing epidermoid carcinoma." In 1941 "a basal-cell carcinoma beneath the right nares [nostril] was treated with 25 mg.-hr. of radium." This was the fourth type of malignancy to be diagnosed.

In April 1944, a recurrence of the basal-cell carcinoma below the right nostril was excised. In 1945 Dr. Cannon passed the 14th anniversary of the onset of his mycosis fungoides—an amazingly long survival. "Three enlarged lymph nodes could be felt in the left groin on September 5, 1945," his physicians noted, "but the liver and spleen were not palpable." There was marked anemia, however, and later in the month Dr. Cannon experienced difficulty in breathing, his weakness became severe, and his liver became enlarged. On October 1, 1945, he died of intercurrent pulmonary infection. He was just short of 74 years old.

On the basis of their 14-year study of his case, and of the autopsy findings, Dr. Cannon's physicians concluded: "It seems a legitimate speculation that mycosis fungoides should not be considered a neoplasm but a reaction (to agents unknown) which, like other known premalignant processes, leads to the development of neoplastic properties in responsive cells." [18]

Thus ended Dr. Cannon's contributions to the progress of the medical sciences.

REFERENCES

1. *Philadelphia Med. J., 9:* 438–442, 1902.
2. BROWN, P., *American Martyrs to Science through the Roentgen Rays,* p. 32. Charles C Thomas, Publisher, Springfield, Illinois, 1936.
3. *Boston Med. Surg. J., 135:* 610–611, 1896.
4. BROWN, *op. cit.,* p. 37.
5. ALLEN, C. W., *Radiotherapy and Phototherapy,* pp. 335–336. Lea Brothers and Company, New York, 1904.
6. *Trans. Amer. Roentgen Ray Soc.,* 101–170, 1908.
7. BROWN, *op. cit.,* pp. 43–49.
8. *Ibid.,* pp. 50–61.
9. *Ibid.,* pp. 62–71.

10. *Ibid.*, p. 11.
11. *Trans. Amer. Roentgen Ray Soc.,* 253, 1903.
12. CHAMBERLAIN, R. H., Personal communication.
13. BROWN, *op. cit.*, pp. 141–154.
14. MACY, J., *Walter James Dodd—A Biographical Sketch.* Houghton Mifflin Company, Boston, 1918.
15. GOLDEN, R., Personal communication.
16. *Illinois Med. J., 124:* 530–533, 1963.
17. *Trans. Amer. Roentgen Ray Soc.,* 67, 1907.
18. *Arch. Path. (Chicago), 60:* 535–547, 1955.

In his 1909 presidential address to the American Roentgen Ray Society, Dr. George C. Johnston of Pittsburgh sounded a worried note: "The insurance companies are beginning to look upon us as undesirable risks. There is no need to rehearse here the actual peril which is about every man who spends much time in a Roentgen laboratory." [1]

How did the radiologists of the "gas-tube era" react to this "actual peril"? They sincerely and earnestly sought, of course, to safeguard both their patients and themselves from the ray's deleterious effects, but almost all of them misjudged the extent of the effort needed.

Most early radiologists assumed that if the initial effect of the X rays— the "burn," or severe erythema—could be prevented, they and their patients would also be protected from the delayed effects—cancer and death. Since they had no method of measuring with any precision the dosages that they and their patients were receiving, they tended to rely on particular devices to prevent burns rather than on an over-all program of radiation protection. The safeguards that they adopted, therefore, fell seriously short of the safeguards deemed essential today.

FILTERS TO PROTECT THE PATIENT

One protective device was described by Dr. George E. Pfahler in 1903.[2] It was a large round metal disk or diaphragm, with a small round hole in the middle, suspended from a hatrack. By moving the diaphragm closer to or further from the patient, the diameter of the cone of rays reaching the patient, and hence the patient's exposure, could be decreased or increased. But unfortunately, this diaphragm did not cut off "stray" rays from Dr. Pfahler's open tube.

At the September 1905 meeting of the American Roentgen Ray Society, Dr. Pfahler introduced a more sophisticated protective device: the "Pfahler filter." [3] He was, of course, familiar with the fact that the rays from a Crookes tube are not homogeneous. Some are "soft," and are therefore mostly absorbed by the skin and other superficial tissues; the "hard" rays are more penetrating, and are absorbed deeper in the body or pass all the way through to strike the photographic plate beyond. Dr. Pfahler thus conceived the possibility of finding a filter that would "strain out" the soft, skin-burning rays while letting the others through—

much as window glass strains out of sunlight the ultraviolet rays which cause sunburn.

Dr. Pfahler also knew that when an X-ray beam passes through an aluminum filter, soft rays are absorbed. If a second aluminum filter is then placed in the beam, little further absorption takes place, for the first filter has already removed most of the rays absorbable by aluminum. Generalizing from such observations, earlier researchers had formulated what they called the "principle of selective absorption"—the principle that each material absorbs rays of a particular quality from the heterogeneous X-ray beam. Dr. Pfahler's new filter was ingeniously derived from this principle.

"In radiotherapy," he told his colleagues, "the rays which give us the most concern are those that affect the skin when we are treating deep-seated disease. If the law of selective absorption be correct, then the skin has a peculiar absorbing power. Now, I reasoned that in order to filter out these harmful rays we must select a substance that resembles the skin as closely as possible. The substance resembling the skin most closely is leather. In order to make assurance doubly sure, I have selected the thickest leather possible, namely, sole leather, which is about four times as thick as the human skin. Therefore the rays which pass through this leather should pass through the skin without affecting it in any way. . . ."

"Based upon this theory, during the past four months I have made use of this 'Roentgen ray filter' with the most gratifying results." The filter, he added, was a simple disk of sole leather five inches in diameter, soaked in water "in order to resemble the skin more closely."

Dr. Pfahler went on to cite the case of a woman whom he had been "treating for about a year for round-celled sarcoma . . . and whose face had been reddened many times, and who was so sensitive to the rays that she noticed a burning sensation each time the rays were applied." With the sole-leather filter in the X-ray beam, he reported, she no longer noticed this sensation, and, even when the X-ray dose delivered to the patient through the filter was substantially increased, "no redness [was] produced."

The Pfahler filter did provide considerable protection to the skin, but at least part of this protection was cancelled if a radiologist relying on the filter increased the dose too enthusiastically. Some radiologists did. Thus, Dr. Henry K. Pancoast of Philadelphia reported at the next meeting of the American Roentgen Ray Society, in August 1906, "I have made general use of Dr. Pfahler's filter . . . and have found that as a rule from two to three times as much dosage could be applied when the wet filter was used as could formerly be done without it. But still a dermatitis may follow, and a very severe one, too." [4]

Even when Dr. Pfahler used both his diaphragm and his filter, more-over, his patients might still suffer accidental burns, as he himself noted at the 1905 meeting of the Society. One such burn had occurred while he was treating a man with X rays for cancer of the bones of the hand. "Daily exposures were made. By mistake, the stray rays at times struck his face, as he was in a sitting position. A severe erythema developed upon his face." [3] The stray rays from the unshielded tube which burned this patient's face must also have spread through the room and struck Dr. Pfahler himself.

None of Dr. Pfahler's listeners—the leading radiologists of the time—commented on the burning of a patient's face while his hand was being treated, nor did Dr. Pfahler reveal any embarrassment in describing the incident. Indeed, the only moral that he drew was that his filter was effective. Despite the fact that the patient's hand was actually closer to the tube than his face, Dr. Pfahler reported proudly, his hand was not burned, "the rays having passed through this 'filter.' "

Shielding the Radiologist

At the 1907 meeting of the American Roentgen Ray Society, the as-sembled radiologists returned to the problem of radiation protection. By then the deaths of Clarence Dally, Elizabeth Fleischman Ascheim, Louis Weigel, Wolfram Fuchs, and a number of European X-rays workers were well known. Two papers on safeguards were scheduled for the meeting: "Protection of the Roentgenologist," by Dr. Charles Lester Leonard of Philadelphia, and "Protection of [the] Patient During Roentgen Expos-ure," by Dr. Russell H. Boggs of Pittsburgh.

Dr. Leonard, as noted above (page 166), was himself a victim of severe hand burns before 1907, but his talk began with a reassurance to his listen-ers. "The care essential to the protection of patients has been carefully studied," he declared, "and diagnosis and therapy have been rendered safe in the hands of experts. Accidents are now no more frequent, when this agent is employed by those fitted to use it, than those from any other thera-peutic agent of equal potency. Rules and limits of safety have been deter-mined which render accidents rare. . . ." [5]

Dr. Leonard was concerned, however, about the misuse of X rays by practitioners "with little theoretical and no practical knowledge or ex-perience. This is the grave danger of Roentgen therapy at the present time. Its mysterious and powerful action, its brilliant results, are leading many practitioners to attempt its employment in their own practices. The majority acquire no theoretical knowledge and their clinical ex-perience is limited. . . . Their results are necessarily poor and injure the name of Roentgen therapeutics. . . . The general medical public should be warned not to entrust their patients to those inexperienced in employing [X rays] safely and effectively."

A particular hazard of inexperienced use which Dr. Leonard pointed out was the risk of *too small* a dosage. "The novice is fearful of producing ill effects and hence produces none. He prefers to employ inefficient dosage protracted over long courses of treatment rather than court invisible dangers."

However, while trained and experienced radiologists could readily protect their patients, Dr. Leonard continued, they were still not doing enough to protect *themselves* from the ray. "A seeming disbelief renders . . . experienced operators careless. They [think that they] are immune to its action. It may be dangerous for others but not for them. Because they cannot see immediate effects they cannot appreciate that any injury is being done. The earlier operators had the excuse of an ignorance that was common to the whole scientific world. They exposed themselves freely for experiment and scientific research. The injuries they suffered were not manifested for four or more years. The operator of today who has had only four or five years' experience, and has in a measure protected himself, feels certain he will suffer no ill effects. His dose has been less powerful, it probably will not manifest its ill effects so speedily—*but if he continues to expose himself to repeated though minute doses, the injury though slow in appearing may be more chronic in course and more resistant to treatment.*

"The warning of past experience has not been heeded."

The protective measure which Dr. Leonard went on to stress in 1907 was an adequate enclosure around the tube to cut off stray or "vagabond" rays, such as the rays which had burned the face of Dr. Pfahler's patient while his hand was being treated in 1905. "The only safe protection," Dr. Leonard told his colleagues, "is metallic lead of at least a thickness known commercially as six pounds to the square foot over the active hemisphere of the tube." The remainder of the tube, except for the beam opening, should be encased in lead weighing at least 3 pounds per square foot. There should be a diaphragm to "cut off all secondary and vagrant rays and increase definition."

Some radiologists of the period left their tubes unshielded but retired behind a lead-sheathed partition before activating the tube. Dr. Leonard knew, perhaps from personal experience, that such a procedure—which requires affirmative action over and over again—leads to slips, and is therefore inferior to protection built into the apparatus itself. "The practice of some operators of working behind a lead screen with an open or semi-protected tube is unsafe," he emphasized, "because familiarity breeds carelessness, and while the occasional exposure may not result in *visible* injury, such exposures will certainly become more frequent, with results that are certain to be serious."

Equipment manufacturers came in for their share of the blame in this connection. Many alleged safety devices were being offered by the manufacturers, Dr. Leonard declared, "that are apparently safe, others are of questionable value, while others are totally valueless and by engendering a false sense of security lead the operator into grave danger." [5]

Dr. Boggs's paper, which followed Dr. Leonard's, covered such points as maintaining an adequate distance between the tube and the patient, and cited a table by Dr. Francis H. Williams of Harvard showing how distance should vary with duration of exposure and quantity of radiation emitted by the tube. Dr. Boggs also noted the importance of an adequate filter. However, during the discussion period which followed, several participants warned of the folly of *excessive* caution.[6]

"It seems to me that there is no such thing as absolute protection," Dr. W. S. Laurence of Memphis, Tennessee, remarked, "unless you go to an adjoining town and operate by telephone. Then the question is, how much protection is it wise to take? I believe that there is a point of tolerance in the human body to the X ray as there is to other injurious agents. We all know that tobacco in certain quantities will kill the individual, but if one will limit himself to a certain number of cigars a day he can smoke and still live to be old and die from some other cause than tobacco poisoning. . . . I am sure that the body will tolerate a certain amount of X-ray energy, either the direct or the secondary ray. For that reason I do not believe that it is necessary to clothe ourselves in armor or to leave the city and operate our apparatus from a distance. To work without protection is foolhardy and inexcusable, but I believe attempts at absolute protection have been carried to rather absurd extremes." [7]

Other participants added to the discussion out of their own experience. "I agree with Dr. Leonard that insufficient protection is a danger," Dr. H. W. Van Allen of Springfield, Massachusetts, stated. ". . . I also believe in the greater danger of the small, oft-repeated dose. Nearly two years ago I published a paper on the result of exposure of the genital region. I found that those men who had a long series of light exposures, some as many as thirty times, remained sterile much longer than the men who were exposed harder but a less number of times. It is the constant effect of the ray that is deleterious." [8]

Dr. Eugene W. Caldwell of New York City, who had had an operation for cancer of the hand a few months before, and who was destined to die of the effects of the rays 11 years later, was on the whole reassuring at the 1907 meeting, and argued against surrounding the tube with lead: "Undoubtedly we should avoid all unnecessary exposure, but I believe there has been undue alarm over the dangers of the secondary rays, and that we are not warranted in sacrificing facilities for observing and controlling our tubes in order to exclude the last vestige of secondary radiation. It is well known that overexposure to sunlight may produce very disastrous results, but it does not follow from this that we must live in darkness. . . . I think that a screen which will protect a photographic plate so well that only a little fog is shown on development after two or three weeks' exposure in the position occupied by the operator is practically safe, even if all the secondary rays are not excluded." [9]

That radiologists in 1907 were not in agreement on safeguards should hardly be surprising. They had only recently become familiar with the delayed effects of excessive exposure, and the very late effects—arising two decades or more after the exposure—had not yet had time to make their appearance. No prior experience in the entire history of medicine prepared radiologists in advance for cases like that of Dr. Walter B. Cannon (pages 171–173 above), who was exposed to the rays from 1896 to 1908 but did not develop late effects until 1931, nor could gas-tube era radiologists be expected to foresee the case reported by Dr. Robert S. Stone to the Radiological Society of North America in 1951:

> A radiologist acquired a new fluoroscopic table in 1915. The X-ray tube had no built-in protection, but was enclosed in a wooden box which was supposed to be lined with lead. Five years later, in 1920, when this radiologist moved his office, he found that part of the lead lining had been omitted, so that his right foot, which was frequently under the table, must have been exposed to radiation. He noticed no effect on the foot until 1946, 26 years later, when the skin began to crack and the nail of the big toe to break. When we saw him in 1947, a complicating epidermophytosis was present, but it was possible to recognize the thin, scaly skin with some telangiectasia and marked changes in the nails characteristic of radiation damage.[10]

WILLIAM ROLLINS MINIMIZES X-RAY EXPOSURE

The question which most of the radiologists of the gas-tube era sought to answer was, "How large a dose of radiation can be safely given to the patient or absorbed by the radiologist?" Since they lacked a crystal ball, they necessarily omitted from their calculations the as-yet-unobserved, long-delayed effects of relatively small doses. But one man did not wait for damage to become visible before taking precautions against it. He was the Boston dentist, Dr. William Rollins, and with almost prophetic foresight he pioneered the prophylactic approach to radiation damage which is generally accepted today.

Instead of seeking to determine how large a dose could be safely administered, Dr. Rollins almost from the beginning urged radiologists to use, especially in diagnostic work, *the smallest exposure that would accomplish the purpose.* Thus, Dr. Rollins's techniques, although they seemed overpunctilious at the time and were quite generally neglected, have assumed greater and greater importance as additional experience has accumulated. Looking backward, it is readily apparent that, in this as in other respects, Dr. Rollins—both in philosophy and in practical proposals for radiation protection—was decades ahead of his time.

Rollins early in his research was involved in the continuing debate between those who attributed X-ray damage to the X rays directly and those who alleged that the cause was the induction coil used as a power supply for the X-ray tube. Instead of arguing the matter, however, he resorted to experiment, and reported his findings in the *Boston Medical and Surgical Journal* for February 14, 1901. He used for his experiment a "Faraday chamber"—that is, a grounded metal box in which a second metal box was suspended by means of insulators, so that electrical energy could not penetrate the inner chamber.

"A strong male guinea pig," he reported, "was placed in a grounded Faraday chamber and exposed to X-light for two hours a day, the source of light being outside. He died on the eleventh day. The experiment was repeated, with death on the eighth day." These experiments, Rollins pointed out, "separated the effects of electricity from those of X-light and showed clearly what a powerful agent X-light was." He summarized for his physician readers the three radiological precautions which in 1901 he believed essential:

> A—The physician in using the fluoroscope should wear glasses of the most non-radiable material that is transparent.
> B—The X-light tube should be in a non-radiable box from which no X-light can escape except the smallest cone of rays which will cover the area to be examined, treated, or photographed.
> C—The patient should be covered with a non-radiable material, exposing only the necessary area.

Two weeks later, in the same journal, Dr. Rollins reported a further experiment: "A pregnant guinea pig was placed in a closed metallic chamber hung by silk cords within a closed metallic chamber connected with the ground. This is the same arrangement for excluding electricity as a factor in the results which was used in the other experiments. The source of X-light was outside. Exposure to X-light killed the foetus.... This note is published because pregnant women are being exposed to X-light to determine the size of the pelvis or to examine the condition of the foetus."

In these early papers Dr. Rollins reported an ominous observation which most radiologists during the following years ignored, to their own great peril. *The guinea pigs died even though no burns appeared on their skin.* Thus, the lack of a visible burn could not be cited as adequate evidence that a given X-ray exposure was safe. (No doubt the two metal walls of the Faraday chamber filtered out most of the soft "skin-burning" rays.)

Dr. Rollins's reports on these guinea-pig experiments aroused a furore of rebuttals. Perhaps the guinea pigs had suffocated in the Faraday chamber. Perhaps they had died of some infection. Rollins gleefully replied to his critics in the *Boston Medical and Surgical Journal* for March 28, 1901, "As the experiments have been doubted, the deaths being attributed to other causes, the condition of the control guinea pigs is reported. These were kept in the same pen as those exposed to X-light. All were given the same food and care. Some of the control guinea pigs gave birth to young that have now reached the adult stage. No death or visible sickness has occurred except in those exposed to X-light. If activity, appetite, fine coats and bright eyes are signs of health, these control animals are well."

The following year, in the *Electrical Review* for June 14, 1902, Rollins discussed the problems of radiation protection in more detail. "It seems hopeless," he wrote, "even at this late date, when so much is known about the possibilities of injury from X-light, to get others to use an X-light tube entirely enclosed in a non-radiable case, because of the supposed inconvenience of a box." Rollins therefore presented plans and pictures for an improved tube-enclosing box. It had a front made of "polished lead glass, three centimeters thick" through which the radiologist could examine the fluorescence of the tube without exposing himself to the direct rays. The lead glass "absorbs the X-light on account of the great number of sub-atoms crowded into the atoms of lead of which the glass is largely composed.

"The criticism was made," Rollins continued, "that these glass fronts would be too expensive. . . ." But the tube case with a lead-glass front "is so convenient as to outweigh the cost, about five dollars."

To render the rest of the box impervious to X rays, Rollins recommended that it be "coated on the inside with a non-radiable paint, white lead in japan, which dries so quickly six coats can be put on in a day." He also proposed a quantitative standard which such a tube case should meet. "The test . . . is to expose a photographic plate in contact with the outside of the case. *If the plate is not fogged in seven minutes, the coating is sufficient.*" *

Dr. Robert S. Stone, who made a search of the early medical literature on radiation safeguards for the Manhattan (atomic bomb) Project during

---

* Italics added.

World War II, reported that this Rollins recommendation was the earliest use of the concept of a "maximum permissible exposure" or "tolerance dose" that he had been able to find.

Rollins's standard has been superciliously criticized in later years as inferior to the standards now accepted.[11] But when it is recalled that at the time, and for years thereafter, many radiologists were exposing themselves and their patients to the stray radiation from tubes with no shielding at all, Rollins's 7-minute standard—measured at the face of the tube enclosure, not at the radiologist's position—represented an enormous initial stride toward the minimization of exposure.

One way to reduce the diagnostic X-ray exposure to a patient, of course, is to use a very sensitive plate which will capture the image with a minimum of radiation. The exposure can be further reduced by using an "intensifying screen," as described above (page 55). The fluorescing of such a screen multiplies many times the direct effect of the X rays on the photographic plate and thus permits a very great reduction in the X-ray dose to the patient. Early intensifying screens, however, were coarse-grained and lacked uniformity. As a result, Rollins noted, "a single screen makes the developed image blotchy." He accordingly recommended a procedure which simultaneously speeded up radiography, reduced the patient's exposure, and improved the quality of the plate. It is the procedure used in radiography today. "More than one [intensifying] screen is . . . better, because the time of exposure is shorter and the blotches are less apparent, for the bright places on one screen usually correspond to darker places on the other." [12]

Another source of unnecessary radiation to patients during the early 1900's was the common practice of "warming up" the tube with the patient in its beam. The radiologist waited until the fluorescence emitted by the tube indicated that conditions were right, and then he exposed his plate. Rollins deplored this custom and built an improved technique into his own tube enclosure. "A tube case needs an instantaneous shutter . . .; then by pressing and releasing a bulb the shutter is opened, the plate exposed to the most suitable radiation and the shutter closed." The shutter, of course, "should be lined with white lead in japan until non-radiable." And it should overlap the tube-case opening by about 15 millimeters "to prevent the escape of X-light" through the cracks.

Radiologists of the gas-tube era often placed their tubes quite close to the patient. Rollins very early recognized that it was safer as well as optically more satisfactory to station the tube farther away. The apparatus that he built had a protruding rod to keep the tube at least 1 meter away from the photographic plate, thus in effect requiring the user to maintain a safe separation. "Apparatus which requires a less dis-

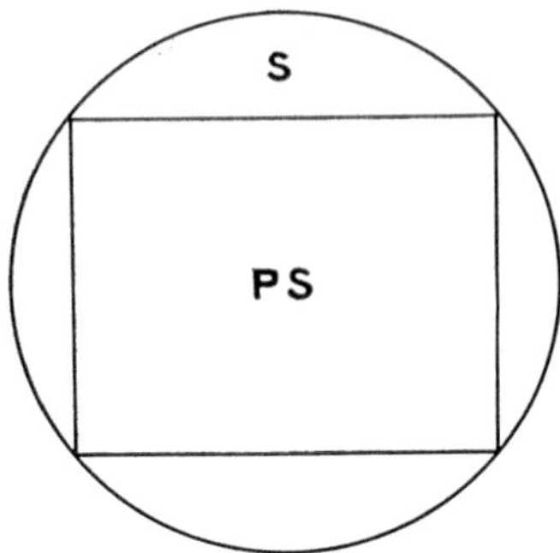

FIG. 27. From ROLLINS, WILLIAM, *Notes on X-Light*, Plate 116. Privately printed, Boston, 1904.

tance than one meter between the [tube] and the photographic plate is not satisfactory," he declared.

Over and over again, both in medical and in electrical journals, Rollins pleaded with his contemporaries to obey what he called the "first axiom" of radiological protection: *No X-light should strike a patient except the smallest beam which will cover the area to be examined, photographed, or treated.*" [13]†

In his early writings he spoke of the beam as a "cone." He soon came to realize, however, that this was in error, and in the *Electrical Review* for April 4, 1903, he enunciated the sound modern principle of rectangular collimation. "The opening in the diaphragm plate of the X-light tube box," Rollins now explained, "should be rectangular for diagnostic and photographic work, because this is the form of the fluorescent screen and photographic plate. If we use a round opening, the section of the cone of X-light escaping from the tube box is a circle.... While the patient will be illuminated by the whole cone, it is evident that the only part of the illumination which will be useful will be that included in the rectangular area."

To illustrate, Dr. Rollins drew a simple sketch (Fig. 27). "All the X-light which strikes the patient outside the rectangular area PS is objectionable," he went on, "for it is unwise to expose a patient unnecessarily...." To interest those unimpressed by his safety arguments, Rollins also called attention to a further argument for a rectangular diaphragm opening: "Besides, the excessive illumination fogs the photographic plate and blurs the image on the screen...." [13] Thus, concern for the welfare of the patient and for the quality of the work alike dictated rectangular exposure fields instead of round fields.

---

† Italics added.

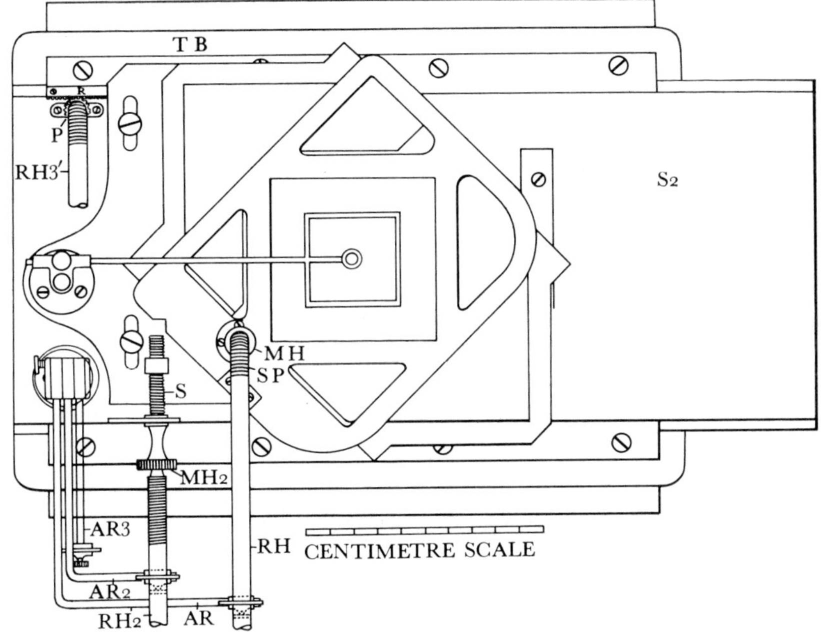

FIG. 28. From ROLLINS, WILLIAM, *Notes on X-Light,* Plate 101. Privately printed, Boston, 1904.

Lewis Gregory Cole used rectangular as well as round "blendes" to cut off stray rays in 1908, and rectangular as well as round devices were offered in the Kelly-Koett Manufacturing Company catalogue for November 1916. But for the most part, radiologists continued to use round fields for decades after Rollins had called attention to their inferiority.

How could the size of a rectangular opening be adjusted to the size of the area of interest in the patient? Rollins offered several solutions to this crucial problem. "Means have been devised," he wrote in his April 4, 1903, paper in the *Electrical Review,* "of making this and all other adjustments of the tube and light by electric motors controlled by switches on a console within reach of the hand . . . but they are too refined to be accepted at present, therefore all the methods which will be illustrated will be mechanical."

The equipment for one such method Rollins illustrated with a drawing (Fig. 28). "The opening of the diaphragm plate when fully expanded, as shown in the figure," Rollins noted, "has an area of 49 square centimeters. By turning the milled head MH, the size of the opening can be reduced or the X-light entirely cut off."

Rollins's next drawing (Fig. 29) revealed how this was accomplished.

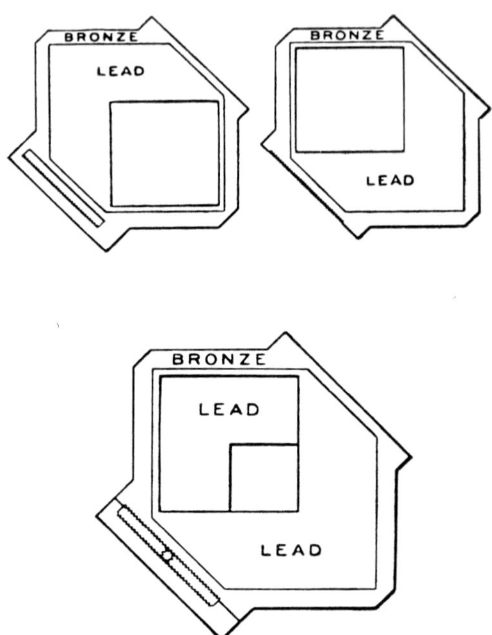

FIG. 29. From ROLLINS, WILLIAM, *Notes on X-Light,* Plate 102. Privately printed, Boston, 1904.

"Each of the diaphragm leaves has a rack," he explained. "When the two leaves are superimposed . . . , a pinion passes through both, and when turned, moves one leaf in one direction, the other in the opposite an equal amount, making the opening and closing symmetrical about a center. The central portion of the leaves are made of lead plates two or more millimeters in thickness, that the surroundings of the diaphragm opening may be non-radiable." [13]

This device, of course, is the modern "rectangular collimator," not introduced into general use until the 1950's and early 1960's.

Rollins then went on to show how an arrangement of handles made it possible to control the size of the collimator opening by remote control, so that the radiologist could enlarge or reduce the size of the opening— and hence the area of the patient's body radiated—while watching the effect through the fluoroscope. And he described a centering device which would aid in aiming the collimator.[13]

The X-ray exposure of a patient while a diagnostic plate is being made is exceedingly small. Did Rollins really accomplish anything of significance by reducing so small a dose still further with his rectangular collimator? No one then knew, and there is still difference of opinion today. Rollins himself did not claim to know. Rather, he considered this very lack of knowledge adequate grounds for adopting such safeguards.

Rollins also realized that fluoroscopy necessitated a much greater exposure both to the radiologist and to the patient than the making of an X-ray plate. To reduce the fluoroscopic exposure of the radiologist, Rollins made numerous sound proposals.

He recommended in the *Boston Medical and Surgical Journal* for April 2, 1903, for example, that the fluoroscope—or, as he called it, the cryptoscope—"must have a plate of heavy lead glass to absorb the X-light which has passed unchanged through the fluorescent screen, to prevent injury to the observer's eyes. The walls of the cryptoscope must be made of nonradiable material. The patient should be covered during the photographic exposures with a non-radiable sheet, exposing only the necessary area. An experimenter who works much with X-light should use a non-radiable face mask, the eyeholes of which are glazed with thick plates of heavy lead glass."

To reduce the patient's exposure to the X rays during fluoroscopy, Rollins recommended in the *Boston Medical and Surgical Journal* for October 1, 1903, that a pulsating rather than a steady current should be fed into the X-ray tube. The image on the fluorescent screen, he explained, persists for a brief interval after the rays cease to excite it; the human eye, too, exhibits a brief persistence of vision. It is possible to take advantage of these two types of persistence "to reduce the total amount of X-light required to make the diagnosis. The best way to do this is [by] sending the electric current in surges, each of very short duration, producing pulses of X-light, that persist as fluorescent light on the screen and in the eyes, allowing intervals between the surges during which, though the light appears continuous to the eye, no [X] light is shining on the tissues." [14]

Rollins was aware, of course, of the extent to which his contemporaries used their own hands as test objects in the X-ray beam, and warned repeatedly against such negligence. "In using the cryptoscope, while testing the tube ... he should not take his hand for examination, but should attach to the cryptoscope a Roentgen gauge and a Williams fluorometer [see above, page 158] for determining the penetrating power of the X-light and its brightness. The hand that holds the cryptoscope should be protected with a non-radiable covering. During the pumping and tuning of X-light tubes, they should be kept in an oven with non-radiable walls.

"Most of these precautions are neglected even at the present time [April, 1903], as may be seen by examining the illustrations in the catalogues of the makers of apparatus and in the papers and books of those who are writing on the subject, where open tubes are almost invariably figured. If masks are used to protect patients during the therapeutic application of X-light, they are in many cases made of rubber cloth or other radiable material." [13]

Rollins also urged that in radiating patients "selective filters should be used to strain out undesirable radiations." This he published in the *Electrical Review* for December 12, 1903, 2 years before Dr. Pfahler's filter.

This review does not exhaust Rollins's contributions to the safety of radiologists and patients. It should be sufficient, however, to warrant the conclusion that, in philosophy as well as in technique, Dr. William Rollins of Boston was the founder of today's science of radiation protection (see pages 425–435).

Dr. Rollins's safeguards proved themselves in actual practice. His brother-in-law Dr. Williams adopted the same philosophy of minimum exposure and introduced many of Dr. Rollins's procedures for minimizing exposure at the Boston City Hospital. Thus, Dr. Williams was able to report that at the hospital, between 1896 and 1915, "more than 150,000 patients were examined by the Roentgen ray or had Roentgen-ray or radium treatment, and none of the patients was injured or burned." [15]

REFERENCES

1. *Amer. Quart. Roentgen., 2:* 52, 1909.
2. *Philadelphia Med. J., 11:* 305–306, 1903.
3. *Trans. Amer. Roentgen Ray Soc.,* 217–224, 1906.
4. *Amer. Quart. Roentgen., 1:* 67, 1906.
5. *Trans. Amer. Roentgen Ray Soc.,* 95–102, 1907.
6. *Ibid.,* pp. 103–109.
7. *Ibid.,* pp. 117–118.
8. *Ibid.,* pp. 109–110.
9. *Ibid.,* pp. 111–112.
10. *Radiology, 58:* 639–661, 1952.
11. GLASSER, O. (ED.), *The Science of Radiology,* p. 334. Charles C Thomas, Publisher, Springfield, Illinois, 1933.
12. *Electrical Rev., 40:* 795–799, 1902.
13. ROLLINS, W., *Notes on X-Light,* pp. 260–272. Privately published, Boston, 1904.
14. *Ibid.,* p. 327.
15. *Amer. J. Roentgen., 13:* 253–259, 1925.

PART III. RADIOLOGY COMES OF AGE

15   Enter the Coolidge Tube

The "gas-tube era" drew to a close, and the modern era in radiology was ushered in, at a banquet held at the Hotel St. Denis in New York City on the evening of December 27, 1913,[1] for it was at that banquet that Dr. Lewis Gregory Cole announced to the eminent radiologists assembled there for the purpose a new kind of X-ray tube—a tube vastly superior in a wide variety of respects to the best of the Crookes tubes theretofore available.

Radiologists equipped with the new tube could do new things. They could do the old things better. They could more readily teach their techniques to their colleagues and their successors. As one result of the simplicity and the vastly greater dependability of the new tube, many additional physicians were attracted to radiology. Thus, radiology was able to evolve as one of the major specialties in the practice of medicine.

Dr. William David Coolidge (born 1873), the inventor of the new tube, took his degree in electrical engineering at the Massachusetts Institute of Technology in 1896 and a graduate degree in physics, *summa cum laude,* at Leipzig in 1899. He then returned to M.I.T., where he was first an assistant in physics and later an assistant professor in chemistry.[2] His first experiments with X rays were at M.I.T. in 1896.

"Nothing was then known of the great danger from overexposure to X rays," he later wrote, "and [in 1896] I . . . became the second patient to be treated for an X-ray burn by Dr. Francis Williams, of Boston. . . . So it was with a wholesome respect for X rays, but with no diminution of interest in them, that I later turned back to them when our laboratory developments pointed that way." [3]

In September 1905, Coolidge moved from M.I.T. to the General Electric Research Laboratory in Schenectady, New York, and was put to work on the problem of improving the filaments in electric light bulbs.[4] Tungsten seemed the most promising metal for filaments, and tungsten filaments were being produced at about that time, but they were brittle and had other defects. In due course, Coolidge discovered that, by working tungsten at a lower temperature than usual, ductility was imparted to the metal. His process for producing ductile tungsten was announced in May 1910,[5] and, within 1 or 2 years, electric lamps with ductile tungsten filaments came into general use.

Having developed an important new metallurgical product, Coolidge next went on to find additional uses for it. Soon his ductile tungsten was adopted instead of platinum for contact points in automobile ignition systems.[4] Another possibility, which Dr. Coolidge discussed at a 1912 meeting of the American Institute of Electrical Engineers, was to use tungsten instead of platinum for the targets (anodes) in X-ray tubes.[6] Such targets, Dr. Coolidge pointed out, must fulfil several requirements.

The first was *high specific gravity* or density. "From the concave cathode, electrically charged particles, the electrons, are shot out at high velocity in a direction normal to the surface. The paths of these particles converge and the target is placed at or near the point of strongest convergence, the focus point. When the electron meets . . . the target, its velocity is reduced, and the denser the target the more rapid is the deceleration. The more rapid the deceleration the greater is the amplitude of the electromagnetic pulse, the Roentgen ray, sent out. Here, then, is a need for high specific gravity; that of forged tungsten is but little less than that of platinum."

The target in an X-ray tube, Dr. Coolidge continued, must also have a *high melting point.* "In modern Roentgen-ray practice, powerful apparatus, running sometimes to a capacity of ten or even fifteen kilowatts, is used to excite the tube. The greater part of the energy delivered to the tube is transferred into heat at the point where the cathode rays bombard the target. Where platinum is used it has been found necessary, to prevent melting, to place the target beyond the focus of the cathode so as to spread the bombardment over a larger area. As a radiograph is a shadow picture, and as the source of the Roentgen ray is the bombarded area of the target, this enlarging of that area is clearly an undesirable thing to do, as the larger area will mean more overlapping and less definition in the resulting picture. In this way, the melting point of platinum has been the limiting feature of the Roentgen tube. The capacity of the tube has been increased by water-cooling the platinum or by using as a target a large mass of copper having a very thin platinum face. But the limit, although raised by these artifices, has still been the melting point of the platinum.

"Tungsten has a much higher melting point (3000°C, as against 1755° for platinum) and so, even with sharp focussing of the cathode rays on the target, permits the use of much more energy than has hitherto been possible. . . ."

An ideal target metal should also have *high heat conductivity.* Tungsten, Dr. Coolidge reported, was superior to platinum in this respect as well; "its better heat conductivity permits a more rapid flow of heat from the focus spot to the surrounding metal."

Finally, Dr. Coolidge specified *low vapor pressure at high temperatures* as an important characteristic of a target material. Platinum vaporizes freely when too hot, and the vapor thus released "condenses on the glass in finely divided form and absorbs relatively large amounts of gas, thus changing the vacuum. At high temperatures tungsten vaporizes least of all the metals." [6]

For these reasons, Dr. Coolidge reported in June 1912, X-ray tubes with tungsten targets were being tried out at General Electric. The results, however, were disappointing. In a subsequent paper,[7] Dr. Coolidge explained why.

"In the development of this target," he reported, "many different designs were made and mounted in tubes, and these tubes were operated on what was then the most powerful Roentgen apparatus on the market, a 10-kilowatt transformer coupled to a mechanical rectifying device." But even with the improved tungsten target, the tubes turned out to have so many *other* limitations that their over-all performance was not much better than that of the conventional tubes of the gas-tube era. Dr. Coolidge listed these limitations, common to his tungsten-target tubes and to the earlier platinum-target tubes. Radiologists already knew them all too well.

"1. With low discharge currents the vacuum gradually improves, with a consequent increase in the penetrating power of the rays produced." This meant that the penetrating power varied from moment to moment, and that even an artist with the rays—a man like Lewis Gregory Cole—could never be sure from moment to moment how penetrating a beam his tube was emitting.

"2. With high discharge currents there are very rapid vacuum changes, sometimes in one direction and sometimes in the other." This was what early radiologists meant by a "cranky" tube; it also explained why the many regulating devices introduced to enable a radiologist to raise or lower the vacuum in his tube at will did not really solve the problem. The rapid changes in vacuum were too complex and too unforeseeable to be compensated for effectively in so crude a way.

"3. If a heavy discharge current is continued for more than a few seconds, the target is heated to redness and then gives off so much gas that the tube may have to be re-exhausted." This was truer of platinum-target tubes than of tungsten-target tubes, Dr. Coolidge added, but in gas tubes it happened with his tungsten targets as well.

Dr. Coolidge then went on to enumerate seven other limitations of the conventional gas tube, of which three may be noted here.

6. The focal spot on the target in many tubes wanders about very rapidly. (In radiographic work, movement of the focal spot during an exposure is of course detrimental to good definition.) In many cases

where it does not show a tendency to wander, it will be found after a heavy discharge to have permanently changed its location.

7. While it is relatively easy to lower the tube resistance by means of the various gas regulators, it is a relatively slow matter to raise it much. . . .

9. No two tubes are exactly alike in their electrical characteristics.

Coolidge next made efforts to improve his tungsten-target tubes by using his ductile tungsten for the cathode as well as the anode, but the resulting tube, he sooned learned, would be "absolutely hopeless from the standpoint of a practical radiographer." The use of tungsten, in short, had removed the gas tube's most obvious limitation, but in the process it had unmasked a whole series of other limitations which would also have to be corrected before a significant improvement was achieved.

"A consideration of the above-mentioned limitations," Coolidge reported, "showed that they were for the most part incident to the use of gas and that they could therefore be made to disappear if a tube could be operated with a very much higher vacuum." But here another obstacle blocked his path.

The ordinary Crookes tube is activated when the electrical potential imposed between the cathode and anode causes positive ions of gas in the tube to bombard the cathode. This bombardment triggers the emission of electrons which in turn bombard the anode and generate X rays. As radiologists had known to their distress since the late 1890's, a tube without enough gas to produce the initial ion bombardment of the cathode would not work at all. Hence, the problem of producing a stable tube by raising the vacuum seemed insoluble—*unless,* as Coolidge noted, electrons for bombardment of the target could be "supplied in some other way." [7]

Here lay the crux of the problem: how to supply the tube with electrons without leaving in it a supply of the gas which made all the trouble. Dr. William Rollins, it will be recalled (page 153), had concerned himself with this same problem a decade earlier and had tried radium as a source of electrons, but had not succeeded in obtaining the effect he sought.

An Austrian working in Leipzig, Julius Edgar Lilienfeld, came remarkably close to a solution in 1911 or 1912. He viewed the problem in a somewhat different light. Crookes tubes, he agreed, were unstable because they contained gas, and were too resistant to generate X rays if too much of the gas were removed. He therefore built into an experimental tube an incandescent filament which, when heated, emitted electrons. These electrons, he reported, lowered the resistance of the tube and thus made possible X-ray production in a tube from which almost all the gas had been evacuated (Fig. 30). Lilienfeld applied for an Amer-

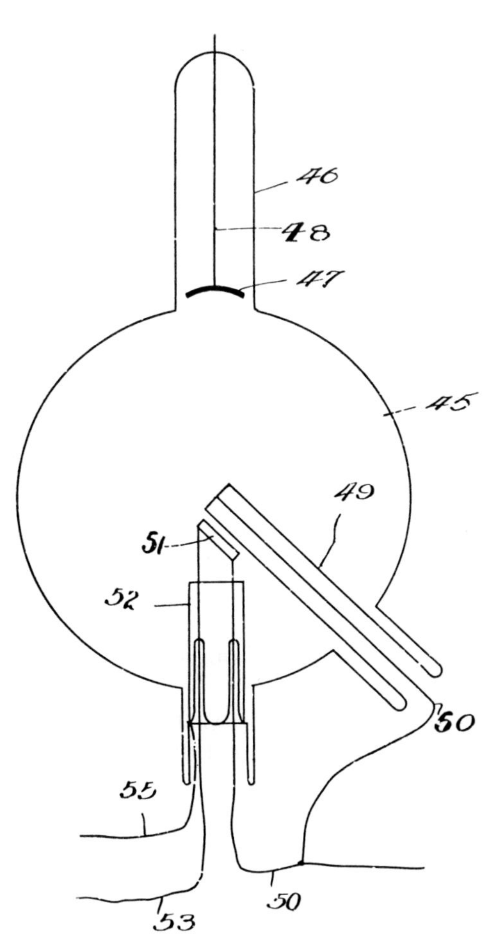

Witnesses:
F. M. Meyer
Floyd B. Cornwall.

Inventor.
Julius Edgar Lilienfeld
Attorney

FIG. 30. From Julius Lillienfeld's U.S. Patent Application No. 1,122,011, filed Oct. 21, 1912.

ican patent on such a tube, with a heated filament to supply electrons, on October 2, 1912.[8]

The Lilienfeld patent application raised an interesting theoretical problem. The emission of electrons from a hot filament in a tube had been discovered by Thomas A. Edison years before and was known as the "Edison effect." Earlier experimenters had reported, however, that the Edison effect, like the emission of X rays, depended upon a residue of gas inside the tube. Now the Lilienfeld patent alleged that electrons were emitted even in a highly evacuated tube.

Dr. Irving Langmuir of General Electric went to work on this problem and confirmed Lilienfeld's findings; electron emission was stable and very high in a tube with as nearly complete a vacuum as the available pumps could achieve.[7] Langmuir discussed these experiments with Coolidge on or shortly before December 12, 1912, for Coolidge wrote in his notebook on that day,[9] "I. L. tells me that in his study of the Edison Effect, current from hot cathode is greater with vacuum of .01 or .02 micron than at higher pressure (except in the case of argon). I will try this at once in an X-ray tube in which I can heat the cathode."

His experiments were soon successful, and on May 9, 1913, Coolidge applied for a patent on his new "hot cathode" tube. Unlike Lilienfeld's tube, which had a conventional cathode *plus* a hot filament to supply electrons, the cathode in Coolidge's tube was itself the electron-emitting tungsten filament. Also, whereas Lilienfeld's patent application specified that the electrons from the hot filament were to be used to lower the resistance of the tube, Coolidge's application specified that the electrons from the filament-cathode were to bombard the target and thus directly produce the X rays.

This was the heart of the new discovery. It appears in Coolidge's patent application of May 12, 1913, but not in Lilienfeld's application of October 2, 1912.

The new tube, instead of containing gas at a pressure of several microns, had a pressure "as low as it has been possible to make it, that is, not more than a few hundredths of a micron." It emitted far more X rays than Dr. Coolidge had anticipated. Human skin could be burned in a few seconds. "In our first experiments with this new type of X-ray tube," he later recalled, "I temporarily and unintentionally sacrificed my own back hair. So I didn't like to practice on other living subjects. For further experiments I was, through the kindness of a medical friend, provided with a human leg which had outlived its usefulness." [4]

After preliminary tests on this leg with his high-vacuum, hot-cathode, tungsten-target tube, Dr. Coolidge turned the tube over to a practicing radiologist for clinical trials on living patients. He wisely chose for this purpose a radiologist whose standards of quality were recognized as exceedingly high: Dr. Lewis Gregory Cole of New York City. Dr. Cole was ecstatic, and sponsored the introduction of the new tube to the medical profession at the banquet on December 27, 1913. He described the Coolidge tube as "undoubtedly the most important contribution to Roentgenology since the birth of that science," [10] and he listed a whole series of ways in which the new tube excelled the old gas tubes.

1. Accuracy of adjustment. "It is not until one uses the Coolidge tube," he noted in this connection, "that he realizes the limitations of the ordinary tube with regard to accuracy of adjustment." Any change in the current fed to a gas tube might change both the quantity of rays emitted and their hardness or penetrating power. With the Coolidge tube, in contrast, quantity and hardness could be independently controlled—the former by increasing or decreasing the current to the hot cathode and thus its temperature and electron emission, the latter by increasing or decreasing the voltage applied between the cathode and the target and thus the velocity of the electrons striking the target.

2. Stability. "During the short time that we have been privileged to test this tube the different degrees of penetration required for the various parts of the body were perfectly sustained during every exposure."

3. Exact duplication of previous results. "It is the experience of every operator that occasionally he obtains a roentgenogram of admirable brilliancy, but personally I have never been able to obtain such results with any degree of certainty. On a few occasions I have made roentgenograms showing really remarkable detail. My experience with the Coolidge tube leads me to believe that these exceedingly brilliant roentgenograms, hitherto obtained only occasionally, may be made quite uniformly with the new tube. . . . The apparatus can be set for a given penetration, and by using the same milliamperage through the tube, a hundred roentgenograms can be made so nearly alike that it is impossible to tell them apart."

4. Flexibility of the tube. "The tube may be operated one instant at a penetration so slight as to show the anastomosis of the blood vessels of the extremities and the next instant, without leaving his seat in the operating booth, one may operate the tube at a penetration far exceeding anything possible with the ordinary tube."

5. High output. "The tremendous output of Roentgen rays from the Coolidge tube, the concentration of which is accurately adjustable and absolutely stable for an unlimited time, and, moreover, can be exactly duplicated at any subsequent time, places in the hands of the roentgenologist a diagnostic and therapeutic agent of immeasurable value." [10]

Thus lauded by Dr. Cole, the radiologist who might be expected to be a new tube's severest critic, the Coolidge tube was promptly sought after by almost all radiologists. From all over the country they mailed, wired, or phoned in their orders to General Electric; some even journeyed to Schenectady in an effort to speed up delivery. Dr. Cole's acclaim for the tube was echoed by others, and the Coolidge tube became standard equipment.

Many radiologists, however, had nostalgic moments remembering their beautiful, cantankerous, individualistic gas tubes, high-strung as a stable of thoroughbred fillies who had to be coaxed and cajoled and called by name before they would perform at their best. Indeed, gas tubes were not altogether abandoned. Dr. Cole himself continued to use them for certain diagnostic procedures at least as late as 1923, and "soft" rays from an old gas tube were still being used for some types of superficial therapy by Dr. Traian Leucutia at the Harper Hospital in Detroit as late as 1964.

Following 1913, many improvements in and variations on the Coolidge tube were introduced by General Electric and by other American and European tube manufacturers. Only a few of these need be noted here. All the tube improvements in the list below, interestingly enough, had been foreshadowed by Dr. William Rollins, the Boston dentist, in his *Notes on X-Light* (1904) and in earlier papers.

> Water-cooled targets (described by Rollins in the *Electrical Review* for December 1, 1897)
> Line-focus tubes (explained and described by Rollins in the *Electrical Review* for December 29, 1897)
> Internal diaphragms near the target to block stray rays (described by Rollins in the *Electrical Review* for January 26, 1898)
> External vanes to carry off heat from the target (described by Rollins in the *Electrical Review* for August 17, 1898)
> Broad-focus tubes for therapy (described by Rollins in the *Electrical Review* for July 25 and August 1, 1903)

In reviving these old ideas after the introduction of the Coolidge tube, did later tube designers go back to Rollins's pre-1904 writings, or did they rediscover for themselves what he had described more than a decade before? The answer may never be known. Dr. Coolidge was familiar with Rollins's *Notes on X-Light* and referred to it on at least one occasion, in connection with the line-focus tube.[11] Beyond that we can only speculate—and wonder what other fruitful ideas may still lie buried, unexploited, in Dr. Rollin's prophetic volume.

REFERENCES

1. Amer. J. Roentgen., *1:* 90–91, 1913.
2. Coolidge, W. D., *Autobiographical Notes,* prepared for the "Project on the History of Recent Physics in the U.S." of the American Institute of Physics, Feb. 21, 1962.

3. General Electric Research Publication 141B, *William D. Coolidge Scientist*. No date.
4. General Electric Research Laboratory publication, *My Early Work in Tungsten—Coolidge Speech on Receiving I.R.E. Medal at Columbia University, May 20, 1952*. 1959.
5. Trans. Amer. Inst. Electrical Engineers, *29:* 961–965, 1910.
6. Trans. Amer. Inst. Electrical Engineers, *31:* 870–872, 1912.
7. Phys. Rev., 2nd series, *2:* 409–430, 1913.
8. U.S. Patent 1,122,011. Application filed Oct. 2, 1912.
9. Photocopy of Coolidge notebook. Supplied by the General Electric Company; patented Dec. 22, 1914.
10. Amer. J. Roentgen., *1:* 125–131, 1914.
11. GLASSER, O. (ED.), *The Science of Radiology*, pp. 85–95. Charles C Thomas, Publisher, Springfield, Illinois, 1933.

16   Other Advances in Equipment

While the Coolidge tube was the most prominent feature of the "Great Divide" separating the "gas-tube era" from modern radiology, three other technological advances should also be credited with substantial contributions. They were the improvement in power supplies, the conversion from glass plates to films, and the introduction of the Potter-Bucky grid.

POWER SUPPLIES

The very earliest X-ray experimenters, it will be recalled, used either static machines or induction coils as a source of electric power for their gas tubes. The induction coils, in turn, were at first powered by alternating current. A pulsating direct current, interrupted many hundreds of times a minute, was soon found to be preferable, and after 1900 the Wehnelt "electrolytic interrupter" was often used for this purpose. Then other types of interrupter, invented by the New York radiologist Eugene W. Caldwell and others, came into common use.

But even the best of these interrupters had a major defect. For a Crookes tube to function at its best, the current through it must always flow in one direction—from the cathode to the target. When an interrupter was used in the power supply, an "inverse current" flowed in the wrong direction through the tube during a part of each cycle; this reduced the efficiency and impaired the operating life of the tube.[1]

A Swiss-born instrument maker and inventor employed by General Electric, Hermann Lemp (1862–1954), invented in 1897 a device which came close to solving this problem.[2] He called his device an "alternating current selector" in his patent application; later it became known as a rotating rectifier switch.

Essentially Lemp's device was a switch which was rotated by a synchronous motor so that it completed exactly one revolution—or an exact multiple of one revolution—during each alternating current cycle (Fig. 31). When one terminal of the induction coil secondary was strongly negative, the rotating switch connected that terminal to the cathode of the Crookes tube; when the other terminal was strongly negative, the switch connected it to the cathode. Thus, the Crookes tube received, in theory, a high-voltage pulsating direct current from an induction coil which was operating on an alternating current. During low-voltage por-

H. LEMP.
ALTERNATING CURRENT SELECTOR.
APPLICATION FILED DEC. 1, 1897.

NO MODEL.

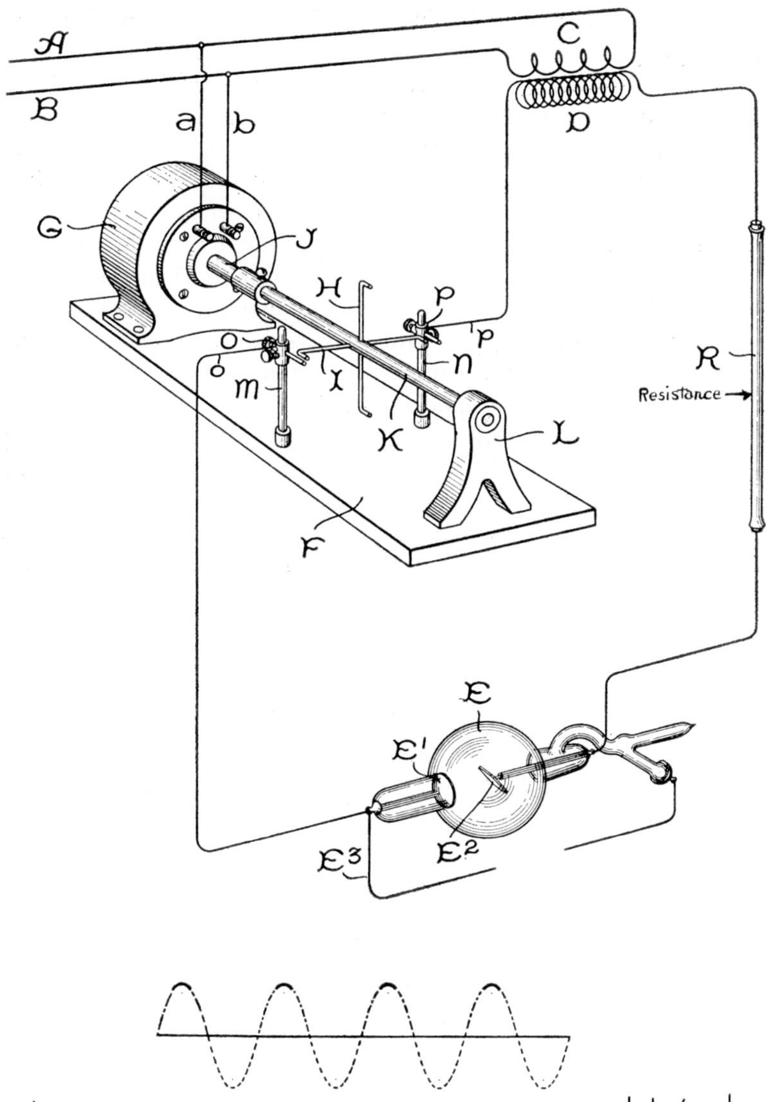

WITNESSES,
Arthur H. Abell.
A. F. Macdonald.

INVENTOR,
Hermann Lemp, by
Geo. R. Blodgett,
atty.

Fig. 31. From U.S. Patent No. 774,090. *Patent Gazette,* p. 251, Nov. 1, 1904.

tions of the cycle, no voltage was fed to the tube, thus reducing the quantity of heat generated in the tube without reducing the X-ray output.

Lemp's switch proved useful in supplying direct current for arc lights and other purposes, but for X-ray work the circuits based on it had at least two shortcomings. The alternating current supplies available at the time were poorly regulated, so that the switch fell "out of sync" with the current, and the induction coils in common use were inefficient when powered with alternating current. Hence, most radiologists continued to use direct current and very troublesome interrupters.

A Philadelphia physicist and X-ray equipment manufacturer, Homer Clyde Snook (1878–1942)—one of the few nonmedical members admitted to the American Roentgen Ray Society—made a thorough study of these and other power-supply problems faced by radiologists, and in July 1907 he applied for a patent[3] on a new "X-ray system" differing from Lemp's in two major respects (Fig. 32).

First, Snook recognized that the existing alternating-current supplies were too unstable to keep in step with Lemp's switch. So he started with direct current and used a rotary converter to change it to alternating current. The rectifying switch was then mounted on the converter shaft. This locked the switch to the alternating-current cycle and en-

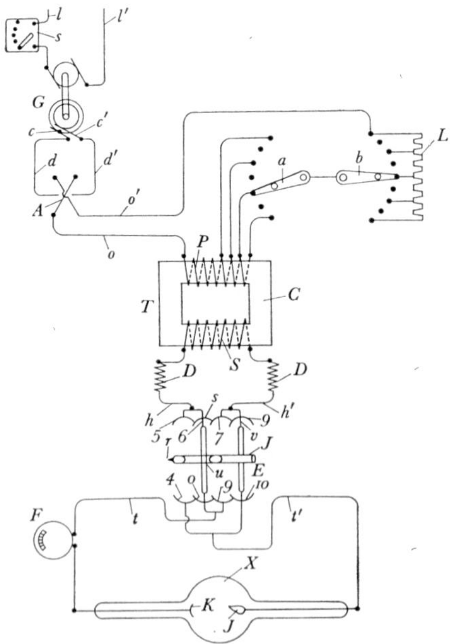

Fig. 32. From U.S. Patent No. 954,056. *Patent Gazette,* p. 131, April 5, 1910.

sured that only the negative phase of the current would be fed to the cathode of the Crookes tube.

For locations where no direct current was available, Snook used the alternating current supply to run a motor which drove a dynamo. This dynamo generated alternating current with a cycle independent of the cycle of the original supply; he then locked the cycle of the rectifying switch to the cycle of the dynamo by mounting the switch on the dynamo shaft. The rest of the circuit was the same as for direct-current installations.

The *mechanical* connection between the switch and the converter or dynamo supplying the alternating current, Snook stressed, "is an essential feature of the combination. Other attempts to rectify high-tension alternating currents for Roentgen work have failed partly because synchronous motors were used to drive the rectifying switches."

Snook's second step was to substitute for the conventional induction coil a much more efficient closed-magnetic-circuit transformer, with minimum magnetic leakage, sealed in an oil-filled tank.

His system also included a rheostat for varying the current continuously from a fraction of a milliampere to the full output of the transformer, and a switch for varying the voltage in steps from 70,000 to 120,000 volts. Thus, the voltage and amperage fed to the tube, and the quantity and hardness of the X rays generated, could be independently controlled.

"Two principal results have been the aim of all investigators who have attempted to improve the induction coil for Roentgen work," Snook noted. "The first of these is the complete suppression or effacement of the inverse discharge. The second is the ability to increase the usual secondary current without limit, and whilst so doing to introduce no new undesirable conditions.

"This new machine accomplishes both of these results, since it delivers *absolutely no inverse discharge;* and there is no practical limitation to the electrical energy output for which it may be constructed." [4] *

Snook's power supply soon became known as the "interrupterless transformer," although much more was involved than simply eliminating the troublesome interrupter. He made his first installation at Jefferson Hospital in Philadelphia in June 1907, and soon he was advertising: "The Snook Roentgen Apparatus Has Made Good ... used by over 30 members of the American Roentgen Ray Society." His power supplies were amazingly sturdy; a photo made at Jefferson Hospital in 1916 indicated that the first 1907 installation was still in use—and in May 1940 Dr. Robert R. Newell of Stanford University told the California

---

* Italics added.

Medical Association that he was "still using daily a large transformer that Clyde Snook built in 1909."

With the Snook apparatus available, the power supply was no longer the limiting factor in the generation of X rays. Indeed, the 10-kilowatt Snook installations were capable of producing more current at a higher voltage than any existing X-ray tubes could handle. Hence, when the Coolidge tube was introduced, the Snook apparatus remained the standard power supply. Dr. Coolidge himself used a Snook-type circuit in a 10-kilowatt apparatus for his first work with X-ray tubes.

The Lemp rotating switch in the Snook apparatus, however, was its Achilles' heel. A vacuum-tube rectifier—the "Fleming valve"—had been invented years before; this valve-tube permitted current to flow from its cathode to its anode but not in the reverse direction. Dr. Lewis Gregory Cole and perhaps other American radiologists used valve-tube rectification before 1907, but later abandoned it.[5] The problem was that the Fleming valve, like the Crookes tube itself, contained residual gas and was therefore inherently unstable. A radiologist catering to the vagaries of an unstable Crookes tube might be driven almost to distraction if in addition he had to manage a pair or a quartet of unstable Fleming valves in the same circuit.

This problem was solved in principle at General Electric by Saul Dushman, an associate of Langmuir's and Coolidge's, who announced in 1915 a new rectifier tube named the kenotron—essentially a hot-cathode Fleming valve from which almost all the gas had been evacuated.[6] Kenotrons for other purposes were soon put into production, but models suitable for use in X-ray power supplies were delayed for more than a decade. They are now in common use.

Dr. Coolidge himself made one further contribution to the power-supply problem. He developed "self-rectifying" models of the Coolidge tube, capable of operating with adequate efficiency even when unrectified alternating current was fed to their terminals.[7]

GLASS PLATES *vs.* FILM

Although photographic film as well as photographic paper was tried for X-ray negatives as early as 1896, glass plates were routinely used for the overwhelming majority of work during the gas-tube era, despite the fact that the plates were heavy, bulky, and fragile. Modern radiology, on the vast scale on which it is currently practiced, could hardly have developed if glass plates had remained in favor.

World War I no doubt accounted in part for the conversion from glass to film, for the United States was cut off from the European glass suppliers who had furnished most of the plates. Supplying glass plates to the farflung installations of the Army Medical Corps, moreover, was so difficult a logistic problem that many Army units had to "make do" with film. Thus, Army radiologists gained experience willy-nilly with film's greater convenience.[8]

The introduction of a new film-holder or cassette by Carl V. S. Patterson of the Patterson Screen Company also hastened the conversion to film. This cassette contained two intensifying screens, one in front of and the other behind the negative—an arrangement urged by Dr. William Rollins of Boston in 1902. The fullest advantage of this two-screen technique could be achieved if "duplitized" film were used—that is, film with a sensitive coating on both faces.[9] This made possible both shorter x-ray exposures and reduced X-ray dosage to the patient.

The film base used during the early 1920's, however, was made of cellulose nitrate and was therefore highly flammable. When it burned it emitted a poisonous gas in enormous quantities. A film fire in the office of Dr. Lewis Gregory Cole in New York City in 1924, another in Syracuse, New York, and a near miss at Columbia-Presbyterian Hospital in New York City alerted fire departments and radiologists to this hazard, and a nonflammable cellulose aetate film (invented in 1906 or earlier) was marketed in that year. But it was unsatisfactory; it wrinkled, grew mouldy, and was somewhat more expensive. Hence, flammable film continued in general use and continued to accumulate in enormous quantities in radiological offices and hospital radiology departments. Then, in 1929, disaster struck. A film fire at a clinic in Cleveland claimed 124 lives. Thereafter, improved cellulose acetate film became available, and remains in use today.[10]

The Potter-Bucky Grid

Equally as significant as the improvement in power supplies and the conversion from glass to film as factors in launching truly modern radiology was the introduction in 1921 of the Potter-Bucky grid, which "cleaned up" the blurred or fogged appearance from which X-ray negatives had long suffered.

Dr. Coolidge himself had assumed that his new tube, with its sharp, stable focus spot, would end any objectionable blurring, and the Coolidge tube did produce relatively "crisp" negatives. But there remained far more blurring than was desirable or readily explainable. With a General Electric associate, C. N. Moore, Coolidge undertook to investigate this phenomenon, which he assumed must be due to a shortcoming of his beloved tube.[11]

Negatives made of a lead sheet through which holes had been bored showed a shadowy penumbra trailing off from the image of the holes instead of a sharply outlined periphery. Dr. Coolidge and Mr. Moore concluded that the blurring must be caused by stray rays originating inside the tube from portions of the target outside the focal spot. To "clean up" the negatives, they accordingly constructed several new tube models. The best of these experimental models proved to be a tube with a molybdenum or tungsten diaphragm near the target, placed so that it would intercept the stray rays[12]—much as in a tube described by William Rollins in 1898. This tube proved completely successful in eliminating the penumbra around the image of the holes in a lead sheet.

But clinical trials on human patients instead of on lead sheets showed that the Coolidge-Moore hypothesis was incorrect. When plates made with the experimental tube and an ordinary Coolidge tube were compared, Coolidge and Moore confessed, "it proved very difficult to show beyond reasonable doubt that there was *any* perceptible difference.... Such a pair of plates has been submitted to quite a number of prominent roentgenologists, and some of these have chosen the right plate and some the wrong one as the work of the tube with the internal diaphragm."[11] The blurring of the negative occurred, it appeared, even when all the "stray" rays inside the tube were intercepted by the diaphragm.

The correct explanation of this blurring, or fogging, and the reason why no modification of the X-ray tube would cure it, had been discovered by Professor Arthur W. Wright of Yale back in January or February 1896. Professor Wright, it will be recalled, made his first X-ray negative—no doubt the first to be made in North America—on January 27, 1896, and in March 1896 he reported on his first weeks' work. "In some of the earlier experiments," he then noted, "the objects to be tested were separated from the sensitive plate by a screen of wood.... Strong effects were produced easily, but the pictures had a blurred appearance." This blurring Wright correctly attributed to the "diffusing or scattering effect of the wood."[13] The blurring which was troubling the radiologists in the 1910's was similarly due to the "diffusing or scattering effect" of the human body itself as it lay interposed between the tube and the photographic plate.

This scattering effect is a complex phenomenon resulting from the fact that when an X ray traverses a substance, it often triggers the ejection of an electron from an atom in its path, and the atom simultaneously emits a new "secondary" X ray as a part of the same event. The ejected electron and the secondary X ray, in their turn, may trigger the ejection of additional electrons and X rays from other atoms in their path, and the process may continue through a series of such ejections and X-ray emissions. It was these secondary rays, *generated within the human body itself* and proceeding outward from it in all directions, which had been blurring the negatives of radiologists all through the years. Dr. Coolidge's tube with an internal diaphragm could produce an unblurred negative through holes in a lead plate because the lead plate did not send secondary rays to the negative, but no tube could possibly produce an unblurred negative with a human body in the beam. Some device *outside* the tube was needed.

The magnitude of the blurring was very great. Studies reported in 1920 by Rex B. Wilsey of the Eastman Kodak Research Laboratory indicated that "under conditions similar to those in the radiography of thick parts, the scattered radiation reaching the film is roughly from four to ten times the intensity of the primary focal radiation." [14] In other words, from 80 to 90 per cent of all radiation reaching the films was blurring radiation; only 10 to 20 per cent was information-carrying radiation.

Wright's 1896 explanation of the blurring was also understood by a German-born physicist, Dr. Otto Pasche of the Insel Hospital Roentgen Institute in Bern, Switzerland; Pasche was perhaps the first to suggest (in 1903) that the solution lay in blocking the secondary rays by means of a device introduced *between the patient and the X-ray plate,* rather than inside the tube or between the tube and the patient. He designed a diaphragm with a slit-shaped aperture, and he proposed to have this slit travel across the plate, exposing each portion of it successively to a thin rectangular beam of rays. This system is used in some cameras. Pasche used a pair of synchronized traveling-slit apertures—one between the X-ray tube and the patient, the other between the patient and the X-ray plate. A device of this kind was fabricated for Dr. Pasche by German General Electric, and he described it in the *Deutsche Medizinische Wochenschrift* for April 9, 1903. Dr. Lewis Gregory Cole used a similar system of two travelling slits a decade or more later.[15]

A German radiologist, Dr. Gustav Bucky of Berlin, similarly realized that if the blurring rays were to be blocked out, the blocking would have to be accomplished between the patient and the X-ray plate; in a paper read to the German Roentgen Society, published in its *Proceedings* for 1913, Dr. Bucky described a new method for accomplishing this. Like Dr. Pasche, he used two diaphragms, one between the tube and the patient, the other between the patient and the plate. Each was a metal grid or lattice, oriented in such a way as to permit primary rays emerging directly from the focal spot of the tube to pass through, but blocking secondary rays emitted at other angles by atoms in the body of the patient.

His grid, Bucky explained in 1913, "consists of metal strips two to four centimeters wide, made into a grating, with each strip pointing edgewise at a single point, the focus of the tube." Bucky applied for a German patent on this kind of grid on February 6, 1913.[16]

Bucky's original grid, however, had a major defect. The shadow of the criss-cross grid was impressed on the X-ray plate. Thus, the price of eliminating the blurring was to superimpose an objectionable grid pattern upon the desired image. Could this handicap be overcome? Three researchers in rapid succession tried to solve the problem in much the same way, independently of one another.

The first was Dr. Bucky himself. On April 8, 1913, 2 months after his original patent application, he applied for an additional German patent on a *moving* grid, and on February 3, 1914, he applied for a United States patent.[17] His theory was simple. If the grid were moved uniformly through the X-ray beam, so that each point on the photographic plate would lie in the shadow of the grid for the same length of time, the grid movement would in effect erase the shadow, and no distracting lines would appear upon the plate.

The second researcher to conceive the same idea was the New York radiologist and engineer, Dr. Eugene W. Caldwell. Dr. Caldwell imported a nonmoving Bucky grid, manufactured by Siemens and Halske, in 1913.

"Immediately after the publication of the Bucky [stationary-grid] apparatus," Dr. Caldwell wrote in 1917, "I conceived the idea of moving the grid to get rid of the shadows of the grid, and did a little experimenting in this direction."[15] At the same time, however, Caldwell checked the patent applications and discovered that Bucky had already filed for a patent on a moving grid. Caldwell nevertheless continued work on the problem—no doubt realizing that Dr. Bucky had not really solved it—and on October 12, 1915, he applied for a United States patent on an improved method of controlling the motion of the grid.

Neither Bucky nor Caldwell presented a description of their moving grids in a medical publication, however, and so a third researcher—Dr. Hollis E. Potter, a brilliant Chicago radiologist—tackled the problem afresh without knowing about the patent applications. He soon discovered the same basic solution as Bucky and Caldwell. He reported on one model of a moving grid at a meeting of the Central Section of the American Roentgen Ray Society in February 1915,[18] and on a second model at the September 1916 meeting of the Society.[19]

None of the early grids designed by Bucky, Caldwell, and Potter was completely successful. Indeed, so long as criss-cross grids were used to block the indirect rays, the problem was insoluble. As Dr. Potter later wrote, "A long series of distressing experiments caused me to abandon entirely for roentgenography all grid constructions which involved the crossing of metallic strips. . . ." [15]

Instead, with a fresh burst of insight, Dr. Potter went on to simplify his approach and ask an altogether different question: if the pattern of a criss-cross grid could not be completely erased from the negative by motion, what kind of a pattern *could* be completely erased?

The simplest answer was a wire.[18] When a wire was moved back and forth uniformly in the X-ray beam, at right angles to its own axis, no shadow was recorded on the plate.

Next, Dr. Potter tried a lead strip, swung back and forth in the X-ray beam along an arc, in such a way that its flat sides always pointed directly to the focus area on the target. Such a strip also recorded no shadow when moved uniformly.

Finally, Dr. Potter tried a series of parallel strips similarly oriented and moved through an arc. Again no shadow was recorded on the negative. In theory such a device, because it lacked crosspieces, should intercept only a portion of the blurring rays, but Dr. Potter found to his surprise and delight that "the total amount of [blurring] rays suppressed by the parallel system was about the same as in the Bucky crossed grating, and it is far easier to build. . . ." [15]

Such a device—now known as the Potter-Bucky grid or diaphragm, though it is in fact neither a grid nor a diaphragm—Dr. Potter presented at the February 1917 meeting of the Central Section of the American Roentgen Ray Society. "The filter strips are mounted radially so as to form a portion of a cylindrical shell," Dr. Potter explained, "with the idea that the motion be along this same arc and across the strips. It is easily seen that with this construction there will result practically even illumination over a large area, that with a uniform motion the shadow of the strips will be neutralized and all requirements for invisibility satisfied in the simplest manner. . . .

"The results are highly gratifying for the demonstration of the lumbar spine, hip joints and pelvis and particularly for calculi. In several cases where small urinary calculi in portly individuals were difficult of demonstration the results obtained . . . were so far superior as to justify almost any statement. In one case of intra-cranial bone tumor it aided materially in showing the spongy network within the tumor. Although at this writing no positive gallstone cases have been encountered, the aid in this field cannot be doubted. With a suitably modified construction allowing a longer stroke and a higher speed, gastrointestinal work might be improved." [15]

Following another radiological meeting, Dr. Potter again displayed negatives made with his moving parallel-strip "grid." One radiologist, he later recalled, turned away from the sharp negatives in anger and announced accusingly, "You've touched those negatives up!" He could not be convinced that so blur-free a negative could be produced with an X-ray tube. (Dr. Bucky recounted a similar experience.)

An incidental effect of the Potter-Bucky diaphragm was to hasten the conversion from glass plate to film, described above. The blurring of a plate by secondary rays, in the absence of a Potter-Bucky grid, increases very rapidly with increase in size of plate. Hence, early radiologists were restricted to relatively small plate sizes (such as 4 by 5 inches) in order to hold blurring to a tolerable level. Following introduction of the Potter-Bucky grid, it became possible to secure images 14 by 17 inches or even larger with negligible blurring. But glass in these large sizes was so heavy, clumsy, and fragile that radiologists who wished to take advantage of the large size were forced to convert to film.

General Electric marketed the Potter-Bucky grid in 1921, and its acceptance was immediate. One General Electric representative, Glenn Files, started out on a tour of Oregon radiologists with a display sample, but one of the first radiologists to whom he demonstrated it, Dr. Frederick E. Diemer of Portland, "refused to let Mr. Files take it from his office; he paid for it on the spot and Mr. Files's triumphant tour was suspended until the factory could rush him a new demonstrator." [20]

REFERENCES

1. *Amer. Quart. Roentgen., 1:* 36–43, 1907.
2. U.S. Patent 774,090. Application filed Dec. 1, 1897; patented Nov. 1, 1904.
3. U.S. Patent 954,056. Application filed July 20, 1907; patented April 5, 1910.
4. *Arch. Roentgen. Ray (London), 13:* 186–188, 1908.
5. *Trans. Amer. Roentgen. Ray Soc.,* 110, 1907.
6. U.S. Patent 1,287,265. Application filed Feb. 20, 1915.
7. U.S. Patent 1,211,092. Application filed June 5, 1916.
8. FUCHS, A. W., in GLASSER, O. (ED.), *The Science of Radiology,* p. 97. Charles C Thomas, Publisher, Springfield, Illinois, 1933.
9. FUCHS, A. W., in BRUWER, A. J., *Classic Descriptions in Diagnostic Roentgenology,* p. 102. Charles C Thomas, Publisher, Springfield, Ill., 1964.
10. FUCHS, A. W., in GLASSER, *op. cit.,* p. 102.
11. *G. E. Review, 20:* 272–281, 1917.
12. *Amer. J. Roentgen., 2:* 881–892, 1915.
13. *Amer. J. Sci., 1:* 4th series, 235–244, 1896.
14. *Amer. J. Roentgen., 8:* 328–338, 1921.
15. *Amer. J. Roentgen., 25:* 396–402, 1931.
16. German Patent 287,652.
17. U.S. Patent 1,164,987. Application filed Feb. 3, 1914.
18. *Amer. J. Roentgen., 3:* 142–145, 1916.
19. *Amer. J. Roentgen., 4:* 47–50, 1917.
20. WOOLLEY, I. M., *Roentgenology in Oregon: The First Fifty Years,* p. 19. Privately printed, Portland, Ore., 1955.

   The Growth of Radiology

Equipped with the Coolidge tube, the Potter-Bucky diaphragm, stable and abundant power supplies, fast and convenient film, other technical aids, and an increasing supply of radium, radiology after 1920 entered a period of very rapid development.

As compared with only a few hundred radiologists in 1913—many of them also engaging in some other specialty or in general practice—the American Medical Association Directory for 1931 listed 1005 radiologists. During the next 7 years, this number more than doubled; 2191 radiologists were listed in 1938. The proportion of radiologists to the population was amplest in the Middle Atlantic states and least adequate in the East South Central states.

Distribution of Radiologists According to Geographic Divisions, 1938[1]

Geographic division	Number of radiologists in U. S.	Population per radiologist
New England	178	48,000
Middle Atlantic	704	39,000
East North Central	444	58,000
West North Central	172	80,000
South Atlantic	220	78,000
East South Central	86	124,000
West South Central	147	87,000
Mountain	48	79,000
Pacific	192	46,000
United States	2191	59,000

In 1938, the Bureau of Medical Economics of the American Medical Association sent questionnaires to 1434 of these radiologists—the members of the four national radiological societies. Replies were received from 876.[1] These questionnaire returns supply interesting data concerning the practice of radiology on the eve of World War II.

More than 75 per cent of the radiologists responding limited their practice to radiology. Fewer than 5 per cent engaged in general practice along with radiology. The remainder were surgeons, internists, pathologists, or dermatologists or were engaged in other specialties as well as radiology.

The split between diagnostic and therapeutic radiology, noted in the 1910 survey (above, page 109), had apparently healed by 1938. Only about 10 per cent of those replying to the 1938 questionnaire practiced diagnostic radiology exclusively, and only about 5 per cent practiced therapeutic radiology exclusively. The remaining 85 per cent practiced both, and a majority of them devoted less than one-third of their practice to radiation therapy.

The physicians who limited their practice to radiology were a seasoned cadre in 1938. They averaged 49 years of age and had specialized for a median period of 18 years. Teaching in medical schools was an important part of their work; 176 of the 874 replying to this question reported that they taught as well as practiced radiology.

During the "gas-tube era," it will be recalled, radiology was practiced both in hospitals and in private offices. This pattern continued in 1938. More than 800 of 840 radiologists answering the question stated they were members of hospital staffs, but 610 of them maintained in addition private offices outside of a hospital. Of these, 82 per cent practiced alone; the remaining 18 per cent reported partnership arrangements with one or more other radiologists.

Of the radiologists with hospital affiliations, 175 reported that they spent full time in one hospital, 322 that they spent part time in one hospital, 196 that they served two hospitals, 108 that they served three hospitals, nine that they served four hospitals, and five that they served five or more hospitals. These five must have been busy men indeed.[1]

After 1938, the specialty of radiology continued to take giant steps. Dr. S. W. Donaldson, then director of the Professional Bureau of the American College of Radiology, cited relevant data in the *American Journal of Roentgenology and Roentgen Therapy* for December 1951. There were about 3000 board-certified radiologists practicing full time in 1951, Dr. Donaldson reported, in addition to an undetermined number who were not board-certified or who practiced part-time. Thus, instead of one radiologist for every 122,000 residents (1931), or one for every 59,000 (1938), there was one radiologist for every 42,000 in 1951.

Dr. Donaldson estimated that, of the 2,500,000 Americans seen as patients each day by a physician, more than 83,000 daily were referred to radiologists. The average radiologist, he noted, received about 6000 patient visits per year. All general hospitals with more than 50 beds and more than three-quarters of all hospitals with fewer than 50 beds had X-ray equipment by 1951.

Further estimates were published in *Public Health Reports* for January 1953 by three members of the staff of the U.S. Public Health Service: Dade W. Moeller, James G. Terrill, and Dr. Samuel C. Ingraham II. They estimated that more than 125,000 X-ray units were then in use in the United States for diagnosis and therapy: 50,000 by general practitioners, radiologists, other medical specialists, and in hospitals and clinics; 65,000 by dentists; and 11,000 by doctors of osteopathy and chiropractors.

More than 215,000 medical-technical personnel, they indicated, were engaged in operating these units, including 40,000 X-ray technicians and perhaps 40,000 dental technicians and nurses. They noted that an estimated 15,000,000 persons received chest X rays in 1950, and that 84 million films were being used annually for dental X-ray examinations.

A further report by Dr. Donaldson and Dr. Carroll J. LaVielle for the American College of Radiology in 1958 noted that the number of board-certified radiologists in active practice had increased from 3000 in 1951 to 4500 at the beginning of 1958, bringing the ratio down to one radiologist for every 27,000 men, women and children.

Dr. Earl E. Barth, chairman of the department of radiology at Northwestern University Medical School, Chicago, published further striking estimates in *The New Physician* for December 1961. The number of physicians in the United States increased only 40 per cent from 1946 to 1961, Dr. Barth reported, while the number of radiologists increased by 170 per cent.

"A population of 25,000 or less," Dr. Barth continued, "will support the full-time services of a radiologist. On this basis we could now use 7,000 men in active practice in offices and community hospitals.... There are now about 6,000 actively practicing diplomates of the American Board of Radiology and a number of these are in full-time government service, research, and teaching." Thus, despite the rapid and continuing growth in the number of radiologists, the need still exceeded the supply.

Of all patients admitted to hospitals, Dr. Barth estimated, 42 per cent received one or more diagnostic radiology procedures in 1951, and 47 per cent in 1961. The average radiologist in 1961, Dr. Barth added, examined 5950 patients. Thus, the flow of patients to the nation's 6000 radiologists for diagnosis during the year had apparently exceeded 35,000,000.

Detailed data concerning American radiologists were assembled by Drs. Paul Q. Peterson and Maryland Y. Pennell and published in 1962 by the U.S. Public Health Service in its *Health Manpower Source Book*. It was noted that 7327 physicians had indicated to the American Medical Association in mid-1961 that they were engaged full time in radiology; an additional 230 were engaging in radiology part time. Two-thirds of the radiologists were certified by the American Board of Radiology.

Of the 7327 full-time radiologists, 638 were employed by the Federal government, 1458 were full-time members of hospital staffs, 1256 were residents in training, 107 were full-time members of medical school faculties, and 20 occupied miscellaneous posts—leaving 4486 in clinical practice. Sixty-three per cent of the radiologists were under 45—a much higher proportion of younger men than in 1938. All but 243 of the radiologists were men, and all but 75 were white. In addition to the 107 radiologists who reported full-time teaching posts in medical schools, 641 taught part time.

The radiological portion of the first National Health Survey, conducted by the U.S. Public Health Service in 1960–1961 and published in October 1962 as *Health Statistics, Series B, No. 38,* provides rich additional data on what the country's 4486 clinical radiologists were accomplishing.

During the period July 1960–June 1961, information for this survey was secured through interviews in 38,000 households comprising 125,000 persons. The sample of households was carefully drawn to be as typical as possible of the United States civilian, non-institutional population. Respondents were asked many questions about the recent X-ray experience of members of the household, as well as about other medical and dental experiences.

The most astonishing finding was the enormous volume of X-ray visits reported. Extrapolating the results to the civilian population of the United States as a whole, the Public Health Service estimated that 85 million visits were paid to medical facilities for X rays during the year, plus about 49 million visits for dental X rays—a total of 134 million X-ray visits.

Every 100 persons covered by the survey reported, on the average, 47.9 visits to a doctor or hospital for medical X rays during the year. The number of X-ray visits increased with age until 65 and then dropped.

Urban dwellers reported somewhat more medical X-ray visits (53.0 per 100) than rural non-farm dwellers (44.2) or farm dwellers (31.1). Residents of the West paid a higher proportion of visits (57.9 per 100) than residents of the North Central region (47.3), the South (46.4), or the Northeast (44.3).

The rate was almost as high among nonwhite respondents (47.0 visits per 100) as among white respondents (48.0 per 100). Surprisingly enough, respondents with a family income under $2000 reported a slightly *larger* number of medical X-ray visits (54.4 per 100) than respondents with a family income in excess of $7000 (52.4). The lowest rates were for respondents with an income of $4000 to $7000 (44.2 per 100) and for the few who did not report their income (38.9). On the whole, there was remarkably little variation from one income group to another in X-ray services received. The survey left little doubt that X-ray services were being made available in almost equal quantity to high- and low-income groups.

A surprising finding was the predominance of chest X rays (28.7 visits per 100 respondents) over X rays of all other parts of the body combined (23.4). This could be accounted for in large part by the nationwide anti-tuberculosis drive, using mobile X-ray units, sponsored by schools, employers, state and local health departments, local units of the National Tuberculosis Association, and other governmental and private agencies, and by the practice of many hospitals at the time of requiring chest X rays of all or almost all patients admitted. It is surely an astounding fact that more than one-quarter of the entire population surveyed received a chest X ray during the year.

Of the 93 million parts of the body X-rayed during the year, the overwhelming majority (95 per cent) were X-rayed for diagnosis. But 4,000,000 *parts of the body* received X-ray therapy during the year. All of the figures cited above, moreover, exclude visits for radium treatments and for the use of other radioisotopes either diagnostically or therapeutically.

Just half of all X-ray visits paid during the year were to hospitals. An additional 26.8 per cent were paid to doctors' offices. The remaining 23.2 per cent were visits to mobile chest X-ray units, to other places, or to places not reported. The vast bulk (87 per cent) of the X rays not made in hospitals or in doctors' offices were chest X rays.

X-ray therapeutic treatments were given to more parts of the body in doctors' offices (51.0 per cent) than in hospitals (44.5 per cent) and other places (4.6 per cent) combined. But this predominance of office practice was accounted for largely by X-ray treatments of the skin, 94.4 per cent of which were performed in doctors' offices. Hospitals were the site of most X-ray treatments of the chest (76.9 per cent) and abdomen (80.9 per cent).

Dental X rays were reported for 27.4 out of every 100 respondents covered by the survey; this was an average of about one X-ray procedure for every five visits to a dentist. The distribution of dental X rays was quite different from medical X-ray distribution, however. Thus, white respondents reported almost twice as many dental X-ray visits (29.0 per 100) as nonwhite persons (15.5 per 100). Also, the rate was more than three times as high for respondents with a family income in excess of $7000 per year (45.3 per 100) as for those with family incomes under $3000 per year (12.9 per 100). Dentists, clearly, had not succeeded in making their X-ray services as widely available to all races and income groups as had hospitals, radiologists, and other physicians.

This explosive growth of modern radiology can be accounted for in considerable part, of course, by the technological improvements in equipment. More physicians were attracted to radiology once stable apparatus was available—apparatus which a man could learn to use, and which would then behave in his office or hospital as it had in medical school, and which would behave tomorrow as it had yesterday. Neither hospitals nor doctors nor dentists, it seems likely, would have installed X-ray apparatus in such enormous quantities (an estimated 200,000 medical and dental X-ray machines were in use in 1964[2]) if the cranky old gas tubes, rotating rectifier switches, fragile glass plates, and other uncertainties of gas-tube era radiology had continued to be all that was available.

A second factor in the post-1913 radiological explosion was no doubt World War I. Immediately after the United States entered the war, many of the nation's leading radiologists joined the Roentgenological Division of the Army Medical Corps under Dr. (then Colonel) Arthur C. Christie. Army training schools for additional radiologists were established in New York City, Boston, Philadelphia, Pittsburgh, Baltimore, Richmond, Chicago, Kansas City, and Los Angeles; later these were superseded by Army schools of roentgenology at Camp Greenleaf in Georgia and Fort Riley in Kansas. An *Army X-Ray Manual* was issued which became the *vade mecum* for countless newly trained radiologists. The radiologists who had joined the Army and those newly trained by the Army went on duty in all theaters of action and at bases throughout the United States. Many received in Army service their first experience with the new Coolidge tubes and other improved apparatus. Their accomplishments on active duty awakened other physicians in the medical corps to the many uses of the X ray. Thus, at the end of the war, many physicians newly trained in radiology by the Army returned to civilian practice, many left the service resolved to take radiological training, and almost every demobilized physician returned home with a heightened respect for radiology.[3]

Yet another essential factor in the phenomenal growth of radiology emerged during the 1930's: Blue Cross, Blue Shield, and other hospital and medical prepayment plans and health insurance programs. Radiologists were not always happy with the details of the prepayment plans; they protested, for example, against plans which covered X-ray services in hospitals but not in their private offices, and they sought to retain the right to bill their patients individually rather than having their services blanketed into the hospital bill. However, despite friction at the periphery on these and other points, there can be little doubt that it was the prepayment and health insurance plans which made possible modern radiology on the vast scale revealed in the 1960–1961 Public Health Service survey, and which achieved the relatively uniform distribution of radiological services to all income groups.

Modern radiology prospered and expanded, moreover, because of the increasing confidence it earned among physicians and laymen alike. "I was going to take out that gallbladder," a surgeon might well report, "until I got the radiological report"; and a patient might well tell his neighbors, "They didn't know what was wrong with me until they took X rays." Remarks such as these, repeated in greater and greater volume each year during the period of rapid growth, established a high level of confidence which nourished even more rapid growth.

A final factor, perhaps the most important, in the explosive expansion of radiology is the theme of the remainder of this volume. This final factor was the development of an incredibly broad range of new radiological procedures, both diagnostic and therapeutic. More patients received radiological services from year to year in considerable part because the number of different kinds of service which radiologists were equipped to offer expanded from year to year.

This development of new procedures was stressed by Dr. Fred Jenner Hodges in *The New Physician* for December 1961: "To a phenomenal degree, X rays have been used to amplify older methods of physical examination as well as to supersede them with unique diagnostic procedures entirely dependent on the X-ray principle. By leaps and bounds X-ray examination has permeated practically every subdivision of medical practice, providing physicians with factual information about their patients which today seems indispensable."

The scope of diagnostic and therapeutic radiological procedures in 1963 can be roughly gauged from a list of them prepared for health insurance purposes by the American College of Radiology. This was far from a complete list; it was limited to those procedures used frequently enough in private and hospital practice to warrant coding for computer purposes. Despite this limitation the list included[4]:

    37 diagnostic procedures involving the head and neck
    16 diagnostic procedures involving the chest
    17 diagnostic procedures involving the spine and pelvis
    21 diagnostic procedures involving the arms and legs
    11 diagnostic procedures involving the gastrointestinal tract
     6 urological procedures
     8 gynecological and obstetrical procedures
    28 "special studies" not classifiable by body region

In addition, a wide variety of X-ray therapeutic procedures were listed, plus scores of both diagnostic and therapeutic procedures requir-

ing use of radium and other radioactive substances. The chapters which
follow are concerned with these new procedures.

REFERENCES

1. *JAMA, 113:* 943–948, 1939.
2. U.S. Public Health Service Press Release. Nov. 8, 1964.
3. GLASSER, O. (ED), *The Science of Radiology*, pp. 187–197. Charles C Thomas, Pub-
    lisher, Springfield, Ill., 1933.
4. American College of Radiology, *Relative Value Scale*. Chicago, February 1963.

   Progress in X-Ray Diagnosis

By far the most fruitful lines of investigation leading to broader diagnostic usefulness of the X rays during the years after 1913 were concerned with new contrast media and with new ways of using contrast media to make visible on the X-ray plate or fluoroscopic screen phenomena not otherwise visualizable. Bismuth and barium meals for the visualization of the gastrointestinal tract, described above, were an early example; the deliberate introduction of air into bodily organs to provide a contrast with the darker shadows cast by tissues was also begun quite early.

AIR AS A CONTRAST MEDIUM

Ventriculography

Dr. Francis H. Williams of Boston had noted as early as April 1896 the valuable radiological function served by the air naturally present in the lungs, making it possible to visualize the ribs, the heart, the diaphragm, and various lung lesions against the "negative shadow" cast by the air. From this observation Williams and others were naturally led to the possibility that air might be deliberately introduced. By 1901, in the first edition of his classic textbook *The Roentgen Rays in Medicine and Surgery*, Williams was able to describe a variety of radiological procedures based on air injection:

INTRODUCTION OF AIR OR GAS INTO ORGANS.—First, air or gas may be introduced into the hollow organs, and thus their position may be made clearer than before by the presence of the light areas thus produced on the screen. For instance, air may be pumped into the large bowel, and the outline of the sigmoid flexure and the descending colon may be easily followed. Not only does this procedure enable the practitioner to follow the position occupied by this portion of the large intestine, but he can thus more readily detect abnormal conditions in neighboring parts of the abdominal cavity; for example, some pathological conditions in or about the left kidney; or if the stomach, instead of the bowel, has been distended, some conditions about the pancreas, an organ which has been quite inaccessible to methods of physical examination.

INTRODUCTION OF AIR OR GAS TO DISPLACE ORGANS.—Second, air or gas may be used to displace the parts near the special organ we wish to examine; for example, the outline of the spleen may be followed more fully by filling the stomach and lower bowel with air or some gas; by this means the lower portion of the spleen is surrounded by a medium through which the X-rays pass easily, and light areas are brought near the denser spleen, and contrast is thus produced. Gas is also under certain conditions present naturally in the intestines, and under these conditions, of course, contrast obtains.

The injection of air into the ventricles of the brain might have followed immediately from these pre-1901 uses of air injection, but in fact it was delayed until 1918, for reasons which are hard to identify.

Certainly the medical need for improvements in cranial radiology was great and widely recognized. Interest in X-raying the brain, as has been noted, arose very early; Edison was attempting that feat in February 1896. Dr. Church in Chicago successfully localized a brain tumor in 1898, and Dr. Pfahler of Philadelphia achieved a similar coup in 1903 (see above, pages 111–116), but such successes were few and far between for a simple reason. Most brain tumors are composed of tissues differing in X-ray opacity only slightly, if at all, from normal brain tissues or from cerebrospinal fluid. Thus, the usual brain X-ray plate fails in many cases to distinguish a tumor or other lesion from the normal brain tissue and cerebrospinal fluid surrounding it.

One researcher who narrowly missed discovering the usefulness of air as a contrast medium for intracranial radiology was Dr. H. C. Jacobaeus, chief of the medical department of the Serafimerslasarett in Stockholm, Sweden. Several years after the discovery of ventriculography, Dr. Jacobaeus reported:

> It is hardly a new procedure to substitute air for the spinal fluid removed by lumbar [spinal] puncture. As early as 1909 or 1910, I did so myself in tuberculous meningitis, where I attempted influencing the process of the disease through replacing, to as large an extent as possible, the pathologically changed cerebrospinal fluid with air. It was not unusual that nearly 100 c.c. of cerebrospinal fluid were removed which were then replaced with a corresponding quantity of air. As no therapeutic effect, apart from a quite whimsical improvement during the first 24 or 48 hours, could be proved, these experiments of mine have not been published, nor have they been continued.[1]

Air thus substituted for fluid in the spinal canal, as investigators later discovered, bubbles up into the brain ventricles, outlining that organ on the X-ray film in revealing detail. Thus, if Dr. Jacobaeus had happened to expose the head of one of his patients to X rays after such an air injection, he would have been richly rewarded—but he did not.

The first patient in whom the brain was in fact visualized against the background of air-filled ventricles—or at least, the first patient in whom such a visualization was reported—was a 47-year-old machinist hit and thrown to the pavement by a trolley car in New York City on November 24, 1912.[2] The machinist was rushed to Harlem Hospital, obviously suffering from some kind of head injury. The hospital radiologist, Dr. William H. Stewart, made X-ray plates and discovered a fractured skull. The machinist's condition, after initial improvement, grew worse; on December 13, 1912, Dr. Stewart made a second series of plates.

"To my surprise," he reported, "I found we were dealing with a condition different than on the former examination." Indeed, the new series of plates revealed shadows neither Dr. Stewart nor anyone else (so far as the published record reveals) had ever seen before. "From the shape, location, and course of those shadows," Dr. Stewart declared, "their varying density and character simulating gas in the intestines, I was led to conclude that we were dealing with a case of fracture of the skull complicated by distended cerebral ventricles [inflated] with air or gas."

To check this unprecedented conclusion, Dr. Stewart showed the X-ray negatives to one of the country's most eminent radiologists, Dr. Eugene W. Caldwell, and Dr. Caldwell agreed that the shadows were caused by air-filled ventricles.

"The radiographic diagnosis . . . was received by the staff with some doubt," Dr. Stewart stated, but events proved that he and Dr. Caldwell were right. Dr. W. H. Luckett operated on the machinist on December 16, 1912, and reported "two or three quick spits of air and fluid" when he entered a ventricle; bubbles of air were also found in the spinal fluid. At autopsy a few days later, Dr. Otto H. Schultze submerged the brain in a tub of water; bubbles of air emerged from the ventricles when they were opened. The patient had had an attack of sneezing between the first and second series of X-ray plates, and Dr. Luckett surmised that "air was probably forced up through the fracture in the frontal sinus into the ventricles" by the sneezing.

So remarkable a case was naturally reported very widely. Dr. Luckett published an initial account in the *Journal of Nervous and Mental Diseases* for May 1913 and a second account, with the X-ray negatives reproduced to illustrate how clearly the ventricles were portrayed, in the *New York Medical Record* for August 1913. Dr. Stewart published his own account, again with illustrations, in the *American Journal of Roentgenology* for December 1913. Thus, radiologists, neurologists, and surgeons alike were challenged to take the next step: to introduce air into the ventricles deliberately for diagnostic purposes. But if this crucial idea—the idea of *ventriculography*—occurred to even one reader, there is no evidence that he acted on it.

During the next few years, a surprising number of the foremost American radiologists of the period similarly saw sharp outlines of the brain due to air accidentally introduced into the ventricles. Dr. E. H. Skinner of Kansas City recognized the telltale air shadows in the brain of a worker injured in a gas-well explosion in May 1914.[3] Drs. Stewart and Luckett at Harlem Hospital discovered a second case in October 1915— air in the ventricles of a plumber knocked down by a motorcycle.[4] Dr. George W. Holmes of Boston reported in August 1918 a similar case involving an Army aviation instructor hit on the head by a propeller blade, and Dr. Holmes further noted in his report: "Dr. Walter J. Dodd [of Boston] also had one case of air in the ventricles which followed a fracture of the skull." [5] Dr. Hollis E. Potter of Chicago reported air in the ventricles of a 40-year-old male patient who fractured his skull in a fall.[6] Dr. R. J. May of Cleveland reported air in the cranial cavity of a 55-year-old spinster knocked down by an automobile.[7] However, none of the six eminent radiologists who saw the cases—Stewart, Skinner, Holmes, Dodd, Potter, May—and none of the countless others who read the case reports and viewed the illustrations reproduced in the medical journals made the creative leap from accidental to deliberate ventriculography. In the entire history of radiology there can hardly have occurred a more startling series of failures to leap to a conclusion.

These failures are even more noteworthy, moreover, when the experience of neurosurgery is reviewed. On countless occasions through the years, surgeons had operated on the brains of patients and removed tumors of substantial size. Unless special precautions were taken, such as filling with salt water the space left by the removed tissue, air remained in the tumor cavity when the scalp was closed. Several days must elapse in such cases before the air is fully absorbed and replaced by fluid. Although no published reports have been found, it seems almost certain that this air remaining in the brain must have shown up from time to time on post-operative X-ray plates. The radiologists and neurosurgeons who viewed these plates were precisely the men most in need of an improved procedure for visualizing the brain. Thus, the scene was repeatedly but vainly set for a sudden flash of insight and a major radiological advance.

The investigator who, in 1918, did at long last inject air for the specific purpose of visualizing the brain was a 32-year-old surgical resident, Dr. Walter E. Dandy (1886–1946), working in Dr. William S. Halsted's Department of Surgery at the Johns Hopkins. Dr. Dandy, interestingly enough, reached his epochal discovery along a path altogether different from the paths described above which might have led to the goal.

Dandy's initial concern was with the diagnosis and localization of brain tumors. He knew that the only brain tumors which can be directly visualized on an X-ray negative are those whose opacity has been enhanced by an accumulation of calcium, and that this process of tumor calcification occurs only rarely. Indeed, when Dandy and a Johns Hopkins colleague, Dr. George Heuer, reviewed in 1916 the X-ray plates of 100 consecutive brain tumors proved at operation, they found only six cases in which the tumors had cast a shadow distinguishable from that of the surrounding tissue prior to operation. In an additional nine cases, the tumor could be noted because it encroached on the air spaces in the sinuses. In the remaining 85 cases, the X-ray negatives were silent, even when viewed with the "retrospectoscope." [8]

In an effort to improve the diagnostic box score, Dr. Dandy "considered the possibility of filling the cerebral ventricles with a medium that will produce a shadow in the radiogram. If this could be done, an accurate outline of the cerebral ventricles could be photographed with X rays, and since most neoplasms either directly or indirectly modify the size or shape of the ventricles, we should then possess an early and accurate aid to the localization of intracranial affections." [9]

Finding a suitable contrast medium to inject into the cerebrospinal system, however, proved no easy task. Such a contrast medium, as Dandy himself noted, "must satisfy two very rigid exactions: (1) it must be absolutely non-irritating and non-toxic; and (2) it must be readily absorbed and excreted."

Dr. Dandy thereupon tried "the various solutions and suspensions used in pyelography—thorium, potassium iodide, collargol, Argyrol, bismuth subnitrate and subcarbonate, all in various concentrations." Patiently he injected these substances, one at a time, into the ventricles of laboratory animals, "but always with fatal results, owing to the injurious effects on the brain." After numerous such experiments Dandy regretfully concluded: "It seems unlikely that any solution of radiographic value will be found which is sufficiently harmless to justify its injection into the central nervous system."

If, in this frustrating situation, Dr. Dandy or his associates had happened upon one of the published reports concerning air accidentally introduced into the ventricles, his problem might have been solved. Instead, Dr. Dandy was alerted to the possible usefulness of intracranial air by a humorous remark of his surgical chief, Dr. Halsted. Often, when Dr. Halsted and his staff viewed an X-ray plate, they could see on it the negative shadows cast by bubbles of gas in the intestinal tract—shadows clearly visible even though the gas was overlaid by a layer of bone. On such occasions, Dr. Halsted was accustomed to crack a little joke, referring to the way in which the gas seemed to bubble right up through the bone. "It is largely due to the frequent comment by Dr. Halsted on the remarkable power of intestinal gases 'to perforate bone,'" Dandy wrote when explaining his moment of discovery, "that my attention was drawn to [the] practical possibilities [of introducing gas] in the brain."

Once Dr. Dandy's attention was alerted by Dr. Halsted's mild witticism, numerous other analogies arose in his mind to buttress it. "Striking gas shadows are present," Dandy noted, "in all abdominal and thoracic radiograms. The stomach and intestines are often outlined by the contained air, even more sharply than when filled with bismuth. A small collection of gas in the intestines often obliterates the kidney outlines. A perforation of the intestines may be diagnosed by the shadow of the air that has accumulated under the diaphragm.... The paranasal sinuses and mastoid air cells show up in a thick skull by virtue of the air, and pathological conditions of the sinuses are evident because inflammatory or tumor tissue replaces the air. From these and many other normal and pathological clinical demonstrations of the radiographic properties of air it is but a step to the injection of gas into the cerebral ventricles—pneumoventriculography."

The usual procedure when so revolutionary a new approach is conceived is to try it out first on laboratory animals. Dr. Dandy, however, reported no animal experiments. Instead he published, in the *Annals of Surgery* for July 1918, an account of his first 20 human cases, most of them infants and young children. Two features of his account may explain why he felt warranted in proceeding without delay to human trials.

First of all, he—like other neurosurgeons—had already had experience with air in the ventricles following intracranial operations. "For a few days pending its absorption..." Dandy noted, "the patient may be conscious of the movement of the [post-operative] air when the head is turned, but its presence is without any other effects."

The first 20 cases in which Dr. Dandy used ventriculography, moreover, were all children with internal *hydrocephalus*—that is, an abnormal accumulation of cerebrospinal fluid in the ventricles. The pressure of this excess fluid leads to brain damage, often irreversible. Thus, tapping the ventricles and removing some of the excess fluid was a common therapeutic procedure. What Dr. Dandy accomplished in effect during these first 20 trials was to relieve at least temporarily the excess pressure within the brain, and incidentally, in the course of the therapeutic procedure, to admit enough air into the ventricles to make possible X-ray visualization.

The results exceeded his expectations. "Air and water in a ventricle," he explained, "behave exactly as they would in a closed flask. Following any change in position the fluid gravitates to the most dependent part and the air rises to the top." Thus, by altering the position of the patient's head, Dandy was able to maneuver the air bubble to any desired portion of the ventricular system. A series of plates could be made visualizing in turn each of the brain-ventricle boundaries.

Often when a new procedure is developed, it must be used repeatedly before practical results are achieved. Dr. Dandy had better luck.

"Even in the few cases here reported," he wrote in his announcement of the new procedure, "ventriculography has proven of great practical value. For the first time we have a means of diagnosing internal hydrocephalus in the early stages. Internal hydrocephalus is one of the most insidious diseases of the brain and is rarely diagnosed before a considerable amount of cortical destruction has resulted.... With exact visualization of the ventricles the findings are pathognomonic"—that is, decisive both in cases where the disease is present and in cases where it is absent. "Not only the existence of hydrocephalus but its degree and the amount of brain destruction are at once evidenced from the ventriculogram."

Dr. Dandy went on to cite several striking examples. In one case, a 3-year-old child had "remained drowsy for several days after apparent recovery from an attack of epidemic cerebrospinal meningitis. The spinal fluid was clear and contained no organisms. The ventricular fluid was turbid and organisms were present; the ventriculogram demonstrated a greatly enlarged ventricle. The diagnosis of obstructive internal hydrocephalus, clinically unsuspected, was made with absolute certainty from the ventriculogram....

"One of the most interesting diagnoses, made possible only through the ventriculogram, was in a colored child 8 months old. The head was definitely larger than normal, indicating the probability of an internal hydrocephalus. Over the anterior fontanelle, but slightly to one side, was a protruding tumor suggesting a meningocele, and this diagnosis had been made. Air injected into the lateral ventricle passed directly into the tumor. In the lateral ventriculogram the tumor was seen to arise from the greatly distended ventricle by a narrow neck. An anteroposterior ventriculogram showed this communication to be unilateral. The diagnosis of a ruptured cortex with a (false) ventricular hernia was established...."

Most of these early cases were infants and young children whose fontanelles (skull openings) had not yet grown together. Dr. Dandy had selected these cases for his first trials because the air needle could be introduced into the ventricles through the open fontanelles; in older children and adults, it would be necessary to drill a small hole through the skull in order to admit the needle. This operation he expected to perform on adults later.

"Several possibilities are anticipated from ventriculograms in adults," Dandy predicted in his initial paper. "(1) The enlarged ventricles in internal hydrocephalus should be absolutely defined. (2) Tumors in either cerebral hemisphere may dislocate or compress the ventricle and in this way localize the neoplasm. (3) Tumors growing into the ventricles may show a corresponding defect in the ventricular shadow. (4) A unilateral hydrocephalus may be demonstrable if the air cannot be made to enter the opposite ventricle." [19]

All of these predictions were subsequently to be confirmed in clinical practice.

Pneumoencephalography

While Dandy was engaged in his initial explorations of ventriculography, he had a second flash of insight leading to the discovery of a second air-contrast procedure of at least equal importance.

Dandy's initial concern, as has been noted, was to visualize the brain ventricles and the boundaries separating them from brain tissues. Quite early in his series of cases, however, he noted that the air which he injected into the ventricles could also be manipulated into other portions of the cerebrospinal system.

This system is remarkably complex. The cerebrospinal fluid, it is generally believed, initially enters the system through the two lateral ventricles. It flows from these ventricles through passageways known as *foramina* into the third and fourth ventricles, then through additional foramina or aqueducts into reservoirs or *cisternae* located near the base of the brain, where the spinal cord emerges. The largest and most important of these cisternae is the cisterna magna. From it, the fluid flows down the spine, then upward again, so that the spinal cord and nerves are bathed in slowly circulating fluid. Cerebrospinal fluid from the cisterna magna also migrates into the *sulci*—small channels along the surface of the brain. Because the cisternae, spinal cord, and sulci are enclosed in a delicate membrane called the *arachnoid,* they are sometimes jointly known as the *subarachnoid space.* What Dandy noted early in his trials of ventriculography was the exciting fact that the air he injected into the ventricles sometimes migrated into the cisternae, the sulci, and other portions of the subarachnoid space, thus outlining other brain boundaries.

Dandy reported this essential finding in the *Annals of Surgery* for October 1919, just 15 months after his first announcement of ventriculography. "These observations," he explained, "at once gave promise of new possibilities in intracranial diagnostic study. Many lesions of the brain affect part of the subarachnoid space directly or indirectly. In hydrocephalus of the communicating type, adhesions at the base of the brain obliterate the cisternae and the cerebrospinal fluid cannot reach the sulci over the cerebral hemispheres; a local area of subarachnoid space may be obliterated by a tumor situated on or near the surface of the brain; a defect in the brain due to atrophy must necessarily be filled with cerebrospinal fluid, which may maintain communication with with the subarachnoid space. These, and no doubt many other conditions, should be demonstrable by the absence or by the presence of air over the cerebral hemispheres." [10]

To exploit fully this approach to intracranial diagnosis, however, the injection of air into a ventricle proved lamentably inadequate, for the amount of air which could be injected was limited by the size of a ventricle. In Dandy's words, "The problem therefore before us was: How can we in every case be sure of obtaining a *complete* injection of the subarachnoid space?"

Once Dandy had thus formulated the problem, the answer was ready at hand: "The solution lies in the direct injection of air into the spinal canal." Air thus injected rises to the cisternae and sulci, while additional cerebrospinal fluid gravitates downward and can be withdrawn in its turn. "By this method the influence of the ventricular system is entirely eliminated; the air passes directly into the cisterna magna and thence into the ultimate ramifications of the subarachnoid space.

"The technic is essentially similar to that . . . for intraventricular injections. A small quantity of spinal fluid is withdrawn and an equal amount of air injected into the spinal canal. This process of substitution is repeated until the fluid ceases to appear on aspiration." To avoid excessive air injection and hence excessive pressure within the system, Dandy left the needle open for a few minutes after the last injection so that the intraspinous pressure became equalized with the atmospheric pressure.

"I have injected air intraspinously into eight patients—four children and four adults—from Professor Halsted's service without any bad effect," Dandy reported in his October 1919 paper. "The amount of air has varied from 20 to 120 c.c. . . .

"What becomes of the air? Air disappears from the subarachnoid space quite rapidly. It is absorbed as from other spaces and undoubtedly passes directly into the blood. Usually no air is demonstrable in the roentgenogram 24 hours after the injection. Absorption from the subarachnoid space is many times faster than from the ventricles." As the air is absorbed, fresh cerebrospinal fluid enters the system to replenish the supply.

In his first eight cases, Dandy reported with pardonable pride, "the location of the lesion has been accurately determined in three." In the remaining five cases, moreover, the subarachnoid space proved normal, a finding which was itself of great diagnostic value. "In the three patients in whom the lesion was located by means of intraspinous air, other methods had entirely failed."

In one of these three early cases, moreover, a discovery of major pathological importance was made. Hydrocephalus was at that time a condition surrounded by considerable mystery. The dire symptoms are caused by the accumulation of too much cerebrospinal fluid—but why does the excess accumulate? It might be because too much fluid was being added to the system, or because the absorption of the fluid somewhere in the system was being blocked. Dandy's X-ray negatives led him directly to the correct solution. The major sites of absorption, Dandy's findings revealed, are the channels along the surfaces of the cerebral hemispheres—the sulci. If the fluid is blocked from reaching the sulci, absorption is prevented and excessive fluid pressure builds up.

Almost immediately Dandy was able to put his new theory of the pathogenesis of hydrocephalus to the test. "... A boy of 19 ... was suffering from intracranial pressure. An internal hydrocephalus was discovered. But what had caused the hydrocephalus? From his symptoms a tentative diagnosis of a cerebellar tumor was made, and since the signs and symptoms pointed to both sides equally, a vermis tumor seemed most likely. After a thorough cerebellar exploration I was unable to find any trace of the tumor. The foramen of Magendie was normal." Three weeks after the operation, another neurological test was made which suggested an obstruction somewhere between the third ventricle and the foramen of Magendie—but where? An air injection of 120 c.c. was tried. The air "was stopped in the anterior end of the cisterna pontis; none reached the cerebral sulci. These findings could admit of only one interpretation —the pressure of a tumor in the region of the aqueduct of Sylvius, which had occluded it and the cisterna pontis." At operation, a tumor as large as a hickory nut was found at the indicated site. The passageway or aqueduct "had been completely obliterated by the tumor."

At least one of these early cases had a happy ending:

> [The patient was] a boy of 18. Hydrocephalus of a year's standing had followed an acute illness which had been diagnosed as measles. At operation the hydrocephalus was found to be due to closure of the foramina of Luschka and Magendie by dense adhesions. I made a new foramen of Magendie and wanted to be sure that it was functioning

before allowing the patient to go home. Six weeks after the operation, air injected into the ventricles passed through the new foramen of Magendie and filled the cisterna magna and many of the cerebral sulci. We now could feel certain not only that the foramen of Magendie was patent, but also that all the subarachnoid space was receiving cerebrospinal fluid for absorption. The boy has since resumed his studies in college.

Dandy noted in conclusion, "The practical value of intraspinous injections has been thoroughly established by the results in the few cases here reported." Thus, his second procedure, pneumoencephalography, was a suitable companion to the injection of air into the ventricles—"an analysis of the signs and symptoms of the individual case enabling us to determine which should be tried first. From the data obtainable from the combination of intraventricular and intraspinous injections it is difficult to see how intracranial tumors can escape localization." [10]

This final expression of optimism, although understandable, was no doubt a bit premature. Many years of patient work with ventriculography and pneumoencephalography were to be required before the full meaning of the shadows on the X-ray negatives could be interpreted with precision. Other radiological techniques, including the visualization of the system of cerebral arteries supplying the brain, were to be developed along with improved air-injection techniques. Yet the methods of intracranial diagnosis in common use today remain in many respects the methods Walter E. Dandy pioneered at the Johns Hopkins in 1918 and 1919.

The remarkable successes scored by ventriculography and pneumoencephalography led to renewed interest in air injection for the visualization of other bodily organs, and to additional applications of the air-injection principle. Thus, in July 1962, when Dr. Harold O. Peterson of the University of Minnesota Hospitals reviewed in the *American Journal of Roentgenology, Radiation Therapy, and Nuclear Medicine* 57 "special procedures" then recognized as important in diagnostic radiology, 10 of the 57 were based on the injection of air or other gases:

Name of Procedure	Portion of Body Visualized
Encephalography	Brain
Ventriculography	Brain and spinal canal
Myelography	Spinal canal
Arthrography	Joints
Cystography	Bladder
Retroperitoneal	Abdominal organs
Intraperitoneal	Abdominal organs
Pneumomediastinum	Chest
Cardiography	Heart
Pyelography	Kidneys

Soluble Iodine Compounds

Contrast Media in the Veins and Arteries

Neither the heavy contrast media like bismuth and barium nor air and other gases could be safely used as contrast media in the circulatory system of the living human body. For safe injection into the bloodstream it was necessary to find some nontoxic chemical compound opaque to the X rays yet readily soluble and readily absorbable. Generally such compounds depend for their X-ray opacity on the presence in each molecule of atoms of iodine, bromine, or some similar opaque element.

The first known use of such a compound in the human circulatory system was reported in April 1919 by an Argentinian radiologist, Dr. Carlos Heuser (1878–1934):

> When the vein in the leg of a dog is injected with 0.5 potassium iodide diluted with 5 c.c. of distilled water, the proximal end of the limb is tied, and a radiograph of the limb is taken, there is observed great opacity in all the veins of the limb.
>
> This has induced me to perform in a case in which it was indicated the injection of potassium iodide intravenously, to make a radiograph of the arm at the moment of injecting a solution of potassium iodide into the dorsal veins of the hand, and I have observed that the veins of the forearm and arm have been made more visible. In a child with lesions of congenital syphilis, I have seen the iodine in the radiograph of the heart. To those who have hospital services, I commend this method, for here is a new method for examining the pulmonary artery and vein.[11]

Dr. Heuser's recommendation was not followed up, however, so far as is known—no doubt because it appeared only in Spanish in an Argentinian publication, *La Semana Médica*. Hence, it was necessary for the principle to be rediscovered.

One rediscovery occurred at the Mayo Clinic in Rochester, Minnesota, where a young resident in medicine, Dr. Earl D. Osborne, was studying the physiology and clinical use of sodium iodide injections in 1921 and 1922. Syphilologists at the time and before had been accustomed to inject enormous doses of sodium iodide into the bloodstream when treating patients suffering from syphilis; young Dr. Osborne's project was to study the fate of the sodium iodide after it was injected. In a series of papers published begining in 1921,[12] he showed, among other things, that the injected sodium iodide was promptly picked up out of the bloodstream by the kidneys and excreted in the urine.

Dr. Leonard G. Rowntree, chief of medicine at the Mayo Clinic, pounced on that particular clue in the reports of his young resident. Dr. Rowntree was concerned with the diagnosis of diseases of the kidneys and of the urinary tract, and he knew well the difficulty of visualizing these organs in the manner then customary—by introducing bismuth, barium, or other opaque substances through a catheter in the urethra. Dr. Rowntree also knew, of course, that sodium iodide is opaque to the X rays. The Osborne studies thus naturally led him to consider the possibility that, if Dr. Osborne's patients were X-rayed following their sodium iodide injections, "roentgenograms of the kidneys, ureters, and bladder might be secured without the need of catheterization." [13]

Testing Dr. Rowntree's hypothesis proved absurdly simple. Dr. Osborne's patients, who were already receiving the sodium iodide injections therapeutically, "were informed of our interest in this problem, and many of them volunteered to undergo the roentgen-ray studies." All that was necessary was to X-ray them at the right time.

Dr. Osborne and Dr. Rowntree were assisted in this work by one of Dr. Carman's radiologists, Dr. Charles G. Sutherland, and by a Canadian-born Mayo Clinic urologist, Dr. Albert J. Scholl. The results far exceeded expectations. The four men reported in the *Journal of the American Medical Association* for February 10, 1923, that:

> 1. By the method described, it is possible to obtain roentgenograms of the urinary tract during the excretion of sodium iodide following its intravenous or oral administration.
> 2. The method uniformly gives excellent and accurate shadows of the urinary bladder and renders reliable information relative to its size, shape, and location.
> 3. It has been partially successful in depicting the renal pelves and the ureters in a limited number of cases.
> 4. In a number of cases it assists in revealing the kidney itself through intensifying the renal shadow.
> 5. It has been proved a success in revealing the existence of residual urine in the bladder and in furnishing approximate information of the amount, thus eliminating the necessity of catheterization and its attendant dangers of infection.
> 6. Oral administration of the drug will prove satisfactory for routine use in making roentgenograms of the bladder, while for shadows of the ureters and kidneys intravenous injection of large doses of sodium iodide is desirable.

The Osborne-Sutherland-Scholl-Rowntree paper describing these results constituted a major contribution to urinary tract diagnosis, but it helped in addition to lay the foundations for X-ray visualizations of the veins and arteries. For the investigators had used the fluoroscope when injecting the sodium iodide, and had noted that the vein into which it was injected had "the appearance of steel wire" as the iodide passed through it.

Well aware of the importance of this incidental finding, seen almost accidentally in the course of looking for something very different, the four Mayo Clinic investigators staked out broad claims at once. Important results might be obtained with sodium iodide injections, they predicted, "with regard to the venous returns and the peripheral arterial circulation. In the study of aneurysm and of arteriovenous anastomosis, it should also be of value." They concluded, "The method described offers numerous possibilities in the field of research, not only with regard to the urinary tract, but also with regard to other organs, systems, and tissues."

Confirmation of these predictions came later in 1923 from Dr. Barney Brooks of the department of surgery at Washington University Medical School and Barnes Hospital in St. Louis. Whether or not he was familiar with the Mayo Clinic report of February 10, 1923, he did not say, but on September 23, 1923, Dr. Brooks injected 10 c.c. of a solution of sodium iodide into an artery in the leg of a patient and then made X-ray negatives.[14]

Dr. Brooks's patient was a woman of 62. Twenty years before, Dr. Brooks reported, she had contracted childbed fever. After she got up, ulcers developed on both legs. "The ulcer on the left leg healed. The ulcer on the right leg had been open continuously ever since." Now, after 20 years, the condition had grown worse. Dr. Brooks no doubt injected the sodium iodide hoping that the X-ray negatives would help him decide whether or not to amputate. The films, when developed, revealed in beautiful detail the major blood vessels of the leg.

Dr. Heuser's 1919 discovery that water-soluble iodine compounds render the veins and arteries opaque to the X rays was also independently rediscovered by two German investigators, Drs. Lasar Dünner and Adolph Calm of the Roentgen Institute, Moabit Hospital, Berlin. Drs. Dünner and Calm presented their findings at the March 14, 1923, meeting of the Berlin Medical Society,[15] 1 month after publication of the Osborne-Sutherland-Scholl-Rowntree paper. They stated, however, that their work had been completed 2 years earlier and that publication had been delayed "because of unforseen circumstances."

Thereafter, progress was rapid in developing new contrast media which could be safely injected into the blood stream, new methods of injecting these substances, and new techniques for recording and interpreting their shadows on films or fluoroscope screens. By 1962, in his *American Journal of Roentgenology, Radiation Therapy, and Nuclear Medicine* review of special X-ray diagnostic procedures, Dr. Peterson of Minnesota was able to list 21 procedures then in common use which relied on "water-soluble or absorbable contrast media." His list follows:

Cardiography (I.V.—Selective-Retrograde Catheter-Transthoracic)
Aortography (Direct Puncture-Catheter-I.V.)

Selective Arteriography (renal)
Peripheral Arteriography (extremities)
Cerebral Angiography
Peripheral Venography
Venacavography
Intraosseous Venography
Splenoportography
Myelography
Discography
Cystourethrography (retrograde and voiding)
Retrograde Urography
Nephrotomography
Seminal Vesiculography
Renal Cyst Injection
Bronchography
Arthrography
Hysterosalpingography
Lymphography
Percutaneous Transhepatic Cholangiography

Gallbladder Diagnosis

The Osborne-Sutherland-Scholl-Rowntree paper of February 10, 1923, on the use of sodium iodide as a contrast medium was followed almost immediately by efforts at Washington University in St. Louis to find a contrast medium for visualization of the gallbladder.

"One day in the early spring of 1923," Dr. Warren H. Cole of Washington University later recalled, "Dr. Evarts Graham asked me to come to his office to discuss my activities for the following year." [16] Dr. Cole was then 25 years old and a 2nd-year resident in surgery at the Washington University School of Medicine; Dr. Graham was 40 and professor of surgery there; both were also on the staff at Barnes Hospital. Dr. Cole was at first concerned that the call to Dr. Graham's office meant he would not be reappointed for the coming year, but "Dr. Graham's greeting was unusually friendly, and . . . he said he had a laboratory experiment in mind which he hoped I would be willing to work on the following year, beginning July 1." The experiment would be the injection of a phenolphthalein compound into dogs or other laboratory animals to determine whether the gallbladder could thus be visualized.

Several earlier clues had led Dr. Graham to decide this hypothesis was worth testing. As an authority on the gallbladder, he knew of work at the Johns Hopkins in 1909[17] showing that a number of phenolphthalein compounds, including several containing iodine, are excreted by the liver into the bile instead of into the intestines. This had been discovered by Dr. John J. Abel and his young associate Dr. Leonard G. Rowntree—the same Dr. Rowntree who had been co-author of the paper on sodium iodide as a contrast medium, published a few weeks before Dr. Cole's visit to Dr. Graham. Further, Dr. Graham was familiar with the 1921 work of Drs. Peyton Rous and Philip D. McMaster of the Rockefeller Institute[18]; they had shown that the bile, after leaving the liver, enters the gallbladder and is there concentrated eight-fold or ten-fold by extraction of the fluid it contains. Thus, the possibility was opened up that a phenolphthalein compound made opaque to the X rays by iodine or perhaps bromine atoms attached to it might travel with the bile from the liver to the gallbladder, might be concentrated there, and might produce a far clearer X-ray image of the gallbladder than could otherwise be achieved.

For their supply of phenolphthalein compounds, Drs. Graham and Cole turned to a nearby chemical company which had had long experience in supplying contrast media to radiologists, the Mallinckrodt Chemical Works in St. Louis. Mallinckrodt was asked "if they could make or supply us with several halogenated phenolphthalein compounds for experiments on a mechanism of visualizing the gallbladder." The firm "expressed a keen interest in the problem," Dr. Cole reported, "and assigned Dr. N. Drake, a chemist in their Research Department, to cooperate with us in the manufacture and procurement of compounds." [16]

Drs. Graham and Cole especially wanted tetraiodophenolphthalein, one of the compounds with which Abel and Rowntree had worked in 1909, and which had once been in use as an antiseptic dusting powder. This compound, they believed, would prove particularly opaque to the X rays because of the four iodine atoms attached to each phenolphthalein molecule. However, none was immediately available. "While waiting for it to arrive," Dr. Cole recalled in 1960, "we injected sodium phenoltetrachlorphthalein intravenously into some dogs"—with negative results.

Thereafter, as additional compounds became available, "for several months, one after another, we tried the sodium, calcium and strontium salts of tetrabromphenolphthalein and tetraiodophenolphthalein, confining the injections to dogs and rabbits. The first sample of tetraiodophenolphthalein was more toxic to our dogs than was tetrabromphenolphthalein. Therefore, for a time we concentrated on the latter drug.

"I must have injected as many as 200 dogs and rabbits without obtaining a single gallbladder shadow. We knew that it would require six to ten hours after injection of the solution for the gallbladder to concentrate it to a maximal degree. Therefore, if we started our injections at 8:30 A.M. or 9:00 A.M. it would be undesirable to take roentgenograms much before 5:00 P.M. We had no X-ray equipment in our laboratory so we had to transport the animals across the street (via a tunnel) to the X-ray room at the hospital; this transportation fell to my lot since our laboratory assistants stopped work at 5:00 P.M. sharp. . . . I shall always be grateful to our hospital X-ray technician, Miss O'Brien, who stayed overtime so often and made sure that we had good films before she left for the day. Without her complete and congenial cooperation the experiment would have been more difficult and discouraging."

Two hundred failures in a row might have been enough to discourage many experimenters, but Drs. Graham and Cole went on. It is probable that they were influenced to continue by the success achieved at just this time by their colleague in the department of surgery at Barnes Hospital, Dr. Barney Brooks, whose startlingly successful visualization of a patient's arteries and veins by means of sodium iodide (see above, page 232) occurred at Barnes Hospital on September 23, 1923, in the midst of the Graham-Cole experiments.

In November 1923, after 4½ months of uninterrupted failure, Dr. Cole at long last succeeded in securing a single film on which he could clearly see what seemed to be the shadow of a dog's gallbladder. "As soon as I saw the film," Dr. Cole recalled in 1960, "I called Dr. Graham, who was working late as usual. We stood there admiring the dripping film with a white blob in the center, as if we had found a treasure chest full of gold. After a few moments of silence he slapped me on the back and announced enthusiastically, 'Well, Warren, we have a muskie on the line, and if the line doesn't break or the boat capsize we should land him.' "

However, "landing the muskie" did not prove easy. The next few injections into dogs produced no gallbladder shadows on the films whatever.

Perhaps a mistake had been made. To recheck, Dr. Cole returned to the Radiology Department and looked once more at his only successful film "to be certain that we were not misled by some round bone or other object the dog might have swallowed accidentally." A Barnes Hospital radiologist, Dr. Walter Mills, soon reassured him on that score.

"As I was standing near the view box studying the film," Dr. Cole later recalled, ". . . out of the corner of my eye I saw Dr. Mills come through the door. . . . He was wearing his dark glasses and peering straight ahead in his rush to get to the adjacent room. I heard him walking rapidly and then suddenly skid to a stop." Despite his hurry, Dr. Mills's sharp eye had noted on the film something he had never seen before.

"Young fellow, where did you get that film?" Dr. Mills asked. Dr. Cole explained, and added that he was afraid the shadow might be a bone or something. Dr. Mills's reply left no room for doubt: "Don't be silly, young man; *this is a shadow of the gallbladder.* . . ." [19] *

As experiments on other dogs continued to produce negative results,

------

* Italics added.

however, Dr. Cole became increasingly distressed. Why did only one dog display a visualizable gallbladder? "Finally, in desperation, I looked up Bill (the animal caretaker) and asked him if he had done anything to that particular dog which he had not done to the others. Was there anything abnormal about him?

"Bill hesitated, stammered a bit, and finally announced that he could think of no way in which that animal differed from the others. However, his expression of apprehension melted considerably when he learned that that dog was a favored one and very meekly, as if fearing a sharp reprimand from me, muttered, 'Well, Dr. Cole, there was one thing somewhat different. I forgot to feed that dog the morning you injected him.' " [16]

Now everything clicked into place in Dr. Cole's mind. "The lack of food during the test with this dog represented a definite difference from the routine carried out with the other dogs, and I was willing to assume it might be a vital point. Besides, a short time previously, [Dr. E. A.] Boyden of [the] Harvard [Medical School] had reported[20] at the annual meeting of the American Society of Zoologists that feeding, especially fat, was an important item in the filling and emptying of the gallbladder." Cole accordingly rushed at Bill, the animal caretaker, "trying to slap him on the back and grasp his hand in appreciation at the same time. He retreated hastily, no doubt thinking I was going to manhandle him. However, I quickly convinced him I was merely trying to express my appreciation for the great favor he had unknowingly conferred upon me."

Experiments during the next few days showed that the canine gallbladder could quite readily be visualized on the X-ray film if the phenolphthalein compound was injected into *unfed* dogs. Accordingly, Drs. Graham and Cole proceeded without delay to administer the compound to their first human patient. The date was November 26, 1923, and the compound used was a phenolphthalein salt, with four atoms of bromine attached to each molecule.

The 200 dogs and rabbits injected prior to the first canine success were an important factor in making possible so prompt a clinical trial, for the lack of severe toxic reactions in the animals indicated that the injections were safe. If the first visualization of the canine gallbladder had come earlier in the animal series, the first human trial might have had to be delayed for toxicity studies.

During the initial clinical trials on human patients, the muskie again almost got away. The first patient received a very small dose to check for toxic reactions; the dose was too small to permit visualization of the gallbladder. The next four patients received gradually increasing doses; the subsequent patients received still larger doses. Roentgenograms on the fifth patient did show a "very slight shadow," Dr. Cole later noted, but it was "too faint to be of definite diagnostic aid." Throughout their first 15 cases, he and Dr. Graham "did not obtain a really good shadow."

In retrospect, Dr. Graham and Dr. Cole were later able to guess why. The patients who received adequate doses without gallbladder visualization were no doubt suffering from gallbladder disease. The gallbladder did not appear on the negative because bile containing the compound had failed to enter it—a major diagnostic sign. However, as the first 15 patients were one by one injected and then X-rayed with negative or doubtful results, Drs. Graham and Cole could not be sure whether they were in fact demonstrating diseased gallbladders unable to take up bile or were merely proving the worthlessness of contrast-medium cholecystography. Some of the patients, moreover, developed reactions to the injection, ranging from mild to quite severe.

The 16th patient turned the tide—but almost turned it in the wrong direction. She was a nurse at Barnes Hospital, with symptoms so clearly suggesting gallbladder disease that the surgeons were planning to remove her gallbladder. But first, Dr. Cole tried the as-yet-unsuccessful Graham-Cole test on her.

"I mixed the solution...at 7 A.M. as usual," he later reported, "allowing time to sterilize and cool it before beginning the injection at 9 A.M. This was on February 21, 1924. I had already learned that rapid injection of this solution tended to increase the reaction. Accordingly, I gave the injection very slowly, hoping to avoid a reaction completely. However, my hopes were blasted.... After injection of slightly over half of the solution the patient began complaining of nausea, followed shortly by pain in the back and elsewhere. I stopped the injection and waited ten minutes; the nausea disappeared so I renewed the injection." Retching and generalized pain followed. Dr. Cole considered giving up, but as he later reported, "I had been watching her pulse and blood pressure closely and since they had remained practically normal, I had the courage to proceed." By starting and stopping repeatedly, Dr. Cole was "finally able to complete the injection of the entire amount, although it required over an hour...."

Before exposing the first X-ray plate, the plan called for Dr. Cole to wait 4 hours while the compound passed through the liver to the gallbladder. The wait must have seemed interminable—and it was during this wait that the muskie almost got away again.

Sixteen patients had now been injected over a period of 3 months. In not one of the first 15 had the gallbladder been visualized with sufficient clarity to assure diagnostic reliability. Several patients had had reactions, and this 16th patient, on whom Dr. Cole had lavished particular care, since she was a nurse at his own hospital, had had a severe reaction. If the X-ray film in this case, too, had revealed no shadow of the gall-bladder, Dr. Cole later declared, "after seeing [her] in such misery with severe nausea, retching, and generalized pain, I doubt that I would have had the courage or the 'cruelty' to continue with injection of other patients."

In so uncomfortable a situation, with 8 months' work at stake, young Dr. Cole can surely be forgiven for having exposed the first X-ray plate 3¾ hours after completing the injection instead of waiting the full 4 hours. But now his luck had changed, and Dr. Cole must have recorded his findings with growing elation as the subsequent hours rolled by:

> At 3¾ hours, gallbladder probably outlined, but exceedingly faintly.
> At 7½ hours, gallbladder definitely outlined and distended. . . .
> At 24 hours, *gallbladder spectacularly outlined.* . . .[21]†

Following a radiological diagnosis of "normal gallbladder," the Barnes Hospital nurse was saved from an unnecessary operation for gallbladder disease, and her symptoms were later traced to her kidney. Dr. Graham and Dr. Cole were encouraged to continue their series.

Without waiting for this first major success, however, Drs. Graham and Cole had submitted to the *Journal of the American Medical Association* a "Preliminary Report" on their animal experimentation and their first group of human cases. This paper—which appeared February 23, 1924, two days after Dr. Cole's harrowing vigil with the Barnes Hospital nurse—was illustrated with two X-ray negatives showing the faint outlines of a human gallbladder.

Among the many radiologists and other physicians who must have read that first paper with fascination was Dr. Carman at the Mayo Clinic. He had just written a paper on the *need* for improved gallbladder diagnosis which was appearing almost simultaneously in the February 1924 issue of *Radiology*. Dr. Carman traveled to St. Louis from Rochester, Minnesota, shortly after the Graham-Cole paper appeared, to see those gallbladder shadows for himself. "I had, of course, heard much about him," Dr. Cole later recalled, "and felt highly complimented that he would come to St. Louis to talk to us about our work." Dr. Cole explained the technique to Dr. Carman. Dr. Carman looked "quite perturbed" at the 4 hours required per patient, Dr. Cole later wrote, and remarked, "That's fine, young man, but how are we going to conduct these injections on 25 patients in one morning?"[19]

Nevertheless, Dr. Carman sent Dr. Virgil S. Counsellor, a Mayo Clinic

---

† Italics added.

fellow in surgery, to St. Louis to master the "Graham test" technique, and at the September 1924 meeting of the American Roentgen Ray Society, the two Mayo Clinic physicians were able to confirm the Graham-Cole findings and report 178 cases of their own.[22]

A Barnes Hospital radiologist, Dr. Glover H. Copher, joined with Drs. Graham and Cole in February or March, 1924. With a grant from Edward A. Mallinckrodt, Jr., the three St. Louis researchers now had abundant opportunities to continue their work and report to fellow surgeons and radiologists eager to improve their own gallbladder diagnosis. They read a paper before an American Surgical Association meeting in April 1924,[23] and another before the Radiological Society of North America in June 1924.[24] They published a third article in the *Journal of the American Medical Association* for May 31, 1924, a fourth in the *Journal* for January 3, 1925, and a fifth in the *Journal* for April 18, 1925. Dr. Cole published a paper on his related experimental work in the *American Journal of Physiology* for March 1925, and the three men delivered the Charles Lester Leonard Prize paper at the September 1925 meeting of the American Roentgen Ray Society, published in the December 1925 issue of the *American Journal of Roentgenology and Radiation Therapy*.

The worldwide machinery for distributing information through radiological organizations and journals was well developed by 1924 (see pages 301–327 below), and the Graham-test technique soon spread to other radiological centers. By the time of the January 1925 meeting of the American Roentgen Ray Society, barely 14 months after the first canine gallbladder was visualized, Dr. William H. Stewart of New York City was able to state, "We have no doubt that [contrast-medium cholecystography] has been used in at least a thousand cases." Dr. Stewart himself had tried it in 36 cases—using a gas X-ray tube instead of a Coolidge tube, for reasons he did not explain. By September 1925, speakers at an American Roentgen Ray Society meeting could report that "cholecystography is now a routine diagnostic procedure in many clinics." [25]

Radiologists in other countries also reported their confirmation of the Graham-Cole-Copher findings. Thus, two French physicians, Drs. Tuffier and Nemours-Auguste, presented a paper on contrast-medium cholecystography at the January 1925 meeting of the Societé de Chirurgie in France[26]; Drs. Henry Cohen and R. E. Roberts reported in the *British Medical Journal* for July 11, 1925; Drs. P. Kaznelson and F. Reimann of the German University of Prague, Czechoslovakia, published on the subject in the *Klinische Wochenschrift* for July 16, 1925; and Dr. J. A. Saralegui told the September 1925 meeting of the American Roentgen Ray Society that since 1924 he had used the technique in 182 cases at the Rivadavia Hospital in Buenos Aires.[27] Radiologists from all over the world attending the July 1925 meeting of the First International Congress of Radiology in London were no doubt impressed when Dr. Carman informed them that "during the last 15 months more than 1,100 patients have been examined at the Mayo Clinic by cholecystography." [28] (During the next 3 months, one of Dr. Carman's Mayo Clinic associates examined an additional 1800 cases!)[29]

A number of improvements in the technique of cholecystography were reported during 1924 and 1925, several by Drs. Graham, Cole, and Copher themselves. They tested at least 32 different chemical compounds and found that ten of these had "the power of making the gallbladder visible" under the X rays.

The compound which Graham and Cole had used on their first patients—a calcium salt of phenolphthalein with four bromine atoms added to each molecule to render the compound opaque to the X rays—was also used initially by others. It was the lack of solubility of this salt which required so large and so prolonged injection. Then Drs. Graham, Cole and Copher, and perhaps others as well, discovered that the sodium instead of the calcium salt of this compound could be used with equally good results, and could be diluted in a much smaller quantity of water, thus reducing the volume and duration of the injection.

For some of their early animal experiments, Drs. Graham and Cole had used a phenolphthalein compound with iodine instead of bromine atoms attached to provide X-ray opacity, but they had abandoned the iodine compound because it seemed to make their dogs sick. Later it was learned that the symptoms were due to impurities. Purifying the iodine-phenolphthalein compound proved a difficult problem. Drs. Lester R. Whitaker and Gibbs Milliken of the Peter Bent Brigham Hospital in Boston, however, secured a highly purified supply of the iodine compound from the Eastman Kodak Company and ran a comparative trial.

"To further the comparison, I took the test myself," Dr. Whitaker reported at a meeting of the Radiological Society of North America, "both the bromine and iodine salts intravenously at various times. With the bromine salt there was a marked reaction, with vomiting and prostration. The iodine salt produced no symptoms except a slight drowsiness and weariness. We immediately began to use the intravenous injection of sodium tetraiodophenolphthalein clinically, and by it have obtained strikingly good results. In 28 cases, proved at operation, the diagnosis has been correct in 93 percent. Reactions are very rare indeed. In the last 20 cases just one patient had nausea and vomiting, but that was not severe." [30]

In a report given initially to the Harvard Medical Society on November 11, 1924, Drs. Whitaker and Milliken noted that the iodine compound permitted a smaller dose and had other advantages over the bromine compound.[31] They also published a report on the superiority of the iodine compound in *Surgery, Gynecology, and Obstetrics* for June 1925.

Drs. Graham, Cole, and Copher secured a purified form of the iodine compound at about the same time and reported in the *Journal of the American Medical Association* for January 3, 1925, that with a relatively small dose of it they could "get [gallbladder] shadows with practically no toxic effects."

Thereafter other radiologists also switched from the bromine to the iodine compound with excellent results. Dr. James T. Case of Battle Creek, Michigan, for example, told the September 1925 meeting of the American Roentgen Ray Society that he used it and that "the last 350 injections have been done in the office between five and six o'clock and the patients have gone about their affairs. Of that number a few have felt 'grippy,' and we have had them lie down on a couch. . . . But they were all able to leave within about half an hour and very few of them made any complaint." [29]

A second advance was the oral administration of the contrast medium in place of intravenous injection. In their paper of January 3, 1925, Drs. Graham, Cole, and Copher had called attention to this possibility. "Ideally," they noted, "it would be desirable to have a substance that could be given by mouth." They added, "A new method of administering tetrabromphenolphthalein by mouth is being tried, but as yet sufficient data are not available."

The data were soon forthcoming. At Peter Bent Brigham Hospital in Boston, the radiologist Dr. Merrill C. Sosman had made an interesting observation. Three days after performing the "Graham test" on a patient, he had run a routine gastrointestinal series of X rays. When he read the films of the latter examination, he noted that the shadow of the patient's gallbladder, which had disappeared after 24 hours, had reappeared at 72 hours. Some of the opaque salt excreted by the bile system, he realized, must have been *reabsorbed from the alimentary tract,* and after circling through the liver again must have reached the gallbladder a second time. Dr. Sosman appreciated the significant point in this cycle—the likelihood that if the opaque salt were administered orally, it would also be absorbed through the alimentary tract—and he pointed this out to the two young Peter Bent Brigham physicians who were already working on iodine salts for cholecystography, Drs. Whitaker and Milliken.

They and their radiologist associate, Dr. Edward C. Vogt of Peter Bent Brigham, made their first report on oral administration at the January 27, 1925, meeting of the Harvard Medical Society,[32] and Dr. Sosman, with Dr. Whitaker and Dr. P. J. Edson, read a further report at the September 1925 meeting of the American Roentgen Ray Society.[33] After preliminary experiments indicated that dogs fed the iodine form of the compound suffered no ill effects except vomiting, the compound was given orally to a human subject—no doubt one of the researchers. "There was a slight iodoform taste with an astringent quality," the subject reported, and the researchers added: "The gallbladder shadow began to appear after six hours and was very distinct in 12 hours.... The advantages of the oral method are that it relieves many patients of the hospitalization necessary for the intravenous method, and that it causes them very little inconvenience and few unpleasant symptoms."

Independently, meanwhile, two other radiologists were making the same observations at about the same time. They were Drs. Thomas O. Menees and H. C. Robinson of the Blodgett Memorial Hospital in Grand Rapids, Michigan, and they reported their results, a few weeks after Whitaker and Milliken, at the February 1925 meeting of the American Roentgen Ray Society.[34] They were still using the bromine form of the contrast medium, and were distressed by "occasional severe reactions" when it was injected intravenously. So they administered oral doses to three of their medical colleagues, whose names they gratefully recorded: Drs. L. A. Brunsting, J. D. Miller, and W. J. Jonker. Their report, too, concluded that oral administration was safe and effective.

Improved contrast media for cholecystography, both oral and intravenous, have been introduced since 1925, and other minor refinements in technique have been developed. But in principle, this exceedingly useful test remains today very much the same as the test which the pioneers developed during the first 2 years. Many patients each year are relieved of gallbladder distress by means of surgery, and many others are spared an unnecessary gallbladder operation, as a result of the Graham-Cole test.

Nonabsorbable Contrast Media: Lipiodol

The introduction of oily contrast media marked another major step forward in diagnostic radiology. This technique was pioneered in France in 1921, and its subsequent history constitutes an object lesson in international radiological cooperation.

Just as sodium iodide was often injected into the body as a treatment for infectious disease, so iodine-containing oils were often used in Europe. One of these oils, Lipiodol, was developed in 1901 and was particularly opaque to the X rays because it contained, in some formulations, as much as 40 per cent of iodine by weight. When injected under the skin or into a muscle, moreover, the Lipiodol sometimes lingered for months or even years, casting a very dark shadow on the X-ray plate which could readily be confused with some pathological condition. Lipiodol shadows were often seen by radiologists during the 1900's and 1910's; indeed, it became necessary to publish a warning against misinterpreting them.

Among the physicians who noted Lipiodol shadows was Jean-Athanase Sicard, professor of medicine at Paris and physician at the Necker Hospital, and Dr. Sicard went on to draw the obvious conclusion. "Lipiodol once injected into muscle," he jotted down in his journal in 1909, "leaves opaque spots on X rays. *Try to use its opacity in radiology.*" [35]‡

Twelve years went by before that note bore fruit. Then in 1921 a young interne, Jacques Forestier, visited Sicard's home one evening to discuss future research projects, and Sicard showed him his journal containing many research suggestions. The note on Lipiodol interested Forestier at once, and he declared he would like to try it. Sicard smiled and said, "You will do as the others did. I have spoken to three or four of your predecessors; nobody has followed up on this project."

But Forestier did not do as the others did. "Next day," he recorded, "I got a sample of the precious drug and started it on animals, making injections everywhere, under the skin, into the muscle, into the peritoneum." [35] Out of this work, pursued intensively by Sicard and Forestier during the next few years, grew a number of important new diagnostic procedures based on Lipiodol and other non-absorbable contrast media.

Lipiodol Myelography

Dr. Sicard had a special interest in diseases of the spine and spinal cord; it was therefore natural that one of the first uses of Lipiodol he and Dr. Forestier explored was for the localization of spinal cord tumors.

The method was quite simple. They injected Lipiodol into the subarachnoid space containing the spinal fluid. Because it was an oil, it did not mix with the fluid. By stretching the patient out and then tipping the bed back and forth, they could follow the migration of the Lipiodol up and down the spine. If a tumor or some other lesion blocked the Lipiodol, it could be readily located on the X-ray plate.

News of this Sicard-Forestier procedure received at first a lukewarm reception in the United States. Among the first Americans to try it were Drs. James B. Ayer and William James Mixter of the Massachusetts General Hospital in Boston. At a meeting of the Boston Society of Psychiatry and Neurology on December 6, 1923, they reported that they had for 3 months been experimenting on cats with the Sicard-Forestier oil "and with a number of similar oils made up for us" by the Massachusetts General Hospital chemist. Their findings were hardly encouraging. "The irritability of the oil was obvious in all of the six animals injected with the French oil. The cats were usually 'groggy' for one, two, or three days.

---

‡ Italics added.

As an index of irritation of the meninges, it may be noted that in one cat the cell count in the spinal fluid was 4,420, mostly polymorphonuclear leukocytes, on the third day after oil injection. . . . One animal went into convulsions immediately after injection and died; at necropsy there was no evidence that the needle [as distinct from the oil] had injured the brain." [36]

Despite these ominous animal findings, Drs. Ayer and Mixter went on to try intraspinal Lipiodol on two humans—terminal cancer patients whom they described as "hopeless paraplegics from metastatic spinal disease." The site of the spinal block in both cases was successfully demonstrated, and the patients experienced no neurological side effects, though this might be accounted for by the completeness of their paralysis. Dr. Ayer accordingly concluded that while the iodized oil might be of diagnostic value, "its considerable irritating qualities within the spinal subarachnoid space must be reckoned with; its very slow absorption may also be an important disadvantage. It would seem, therefore, unwise to use this diagnostic procedure as a routine measure; it should be reserved for cases in which clinical and other laboratory methods are insufficient." [37]

Dr. Mixter was even less enthusiastic. ". . . I should rather make it a little stronger that I am dissatisfied with the procedure as it stands," he declared during the discussion that followed the Ayer-Mixter paper.

Dr. Percival Bailey of Dr. Harvey Cushing's celebrated neurological clinic at the Peter Bent Brigham Hospital in Boston also indicated during the discussion that he was dissatisfied with the procedure, and would not use the oil even though he had some on hand. "I am familiar with the French experimenters," he stated. "I was present when Sicard read the [1923] article referred to. We have some [iodized oil] locked up at the Brigham Hospital which we have not used." [37]

These Boston views differed markedly from the findings of Sicard and Forestier in Paris—perhaps because the oils used in Boston differed from the Parisian Lipiodol.

Despite the *caveats* voiced by the Boston neurologists in December 1923, a Philadelphia neurologist ventured a few months later to inject Lipiodol into the spinal canal of a patient. The neurologist was Dr. Ethel C. Russell of the Philadelphia General Hospital, and, as will be seen, she had no feasible alternative.

Dr. Russell described her patient as "a white man, aged 25, a dental mechanic," admitted to Philadelphia General in May 1922 complaining of paralysis of both legs.[38] Cerebrospinal fluid drawn through a lumbar puncture appeared to be normal, and no organic cause of his paralysis could be found. So he remained in the hospital convalescent ward, confined to a wheelchair, from May 1922 until February 1924. During this period urinary incontinence made its appearance, and then partial fecal incontinence.

On February 21, 1924, the dental mechanic's case was "reconsidered," and further tests were ordered. These tests established beyond any possible doubt that the spinal fluid was blocked somewhere between the cisterna magna and the lumbar region—but where? None of the available tests made precise localization possible. The block might be anywhere along 15 inches of spine.

To explore surgically a single inch of that stretch, it would be necessary to chisel away the protecting bone, then cut through the dura and the arachnoid membranes; to explore the entire 15 inches was an obvious impossibility. Yet if the block could once be found, the odds were excellent that it could be relieved and a permanent cure achieved. In sum, here was the ideal case in which to try out the Sicard-Forestier technique of myelography. Localization of the block was essential, and localization by all other available means had proved impossible. Dr. Russell resolved to risk Lipoidol.

"Accordingly," she wrote, "2 c.c. of iodized oil was introduced into the cisterna magna, and roentgenograms were taken of the thoracic spine." The result was definite localization. The lipiodol descended to the level of the fifth dorsal vertebra and remained there, localizing the block precisely. "The conclusion was thus made of an obstruction at the fifth dorsal vertebra or seventh thoracic segment of the cord, and surgery was recommended." The patient suffered no convulsions, rise of temperature or other clinical ill effects from the oil.

Dr. John Stewart Rodman operated on April 23, 1924, and found a tumor "at the level indicated." It lay within the subarachnoid space, and was 4 or 5 centimeters long; it appeared to be a benign fibroma and therefore not likely to recur. "Although exceedingly friable, it was readily separated from the cord, with no evident injury to it." [38]

Dr. Russell disclaimed any pioneering in her report of the case. "I have personal knowledge," she wrote, "of the use of this method in two other cases with no untoward results." Yet if she was not the first American to perform Lipiodol myelography, she was at least among the first to admit it in print, in the face of the Boston warnings.

Major credit for opening the American door to Lipiodol myelography belongs primarily to Dr. Dandy at the Johns Hopkins. Following his introduction in 1919 of pneumoencephalography based on the injection of air into the spinal canal through a lumbar tap, Dr. Dandy continued to use air as a contrast medium for both cerebral and spinal diagnosis. By 1924 he had collected a series of 36 cases of spinal cord tumor, all but two of them confirmed by operation.[39] In a number of these cases, he was able to show that air injections helped in the diagnosis or in the localization. Then, as his series was almost complete, he learned of the use of Lipiodol by Sicard and Forestier. At first, no doubt, he was dubious, recalling his own uniformly fatal results whenever he had injected iodine compounds and other substances into the cerebrospinal fluid of animals (see above, page 223). But after trying Lipiodol himself, he gave glowing praise to the French pioneers.

"This communication was originally intended," he wrote in the *Annals of Surgery* for January 1925, "to present the results obtained from a series of intraspinous injections of air, but the brilliant discovery of Sicard makes necessary a reconsideration of the entire subject. What seemed impossible has been accomplished"—that is, the discovery of an X-ray-opaque contrast medium readily tolerated within the subarachnoid space.

He had tried Lipiodol 10 times, Dandy went on to report, and had found that "the iodine is so well protected by the oil that no noticeable irritation of the cord follows its introduction. . . . I have seen no harm result from the oil. Aside from a temperature reaction lasting over two weeks in one patient, I have seen no ill effect. There has been no pain either at the time of injection or subsequently."

Dandy did note a few objections to the Sicard-Forestier technique; in particular, he was concerned that the oil remained for months or even years as a sort of foreign body in the spinal canal, perhaps capable of causing trouble later if not initially. But he quickly added: "The value of Lipiodol in cases where it is indicated overwhelms these objections which then become of minor concern. If a tumor is present it can always be located with absolute precision by Lipiodol. The density of the shadow is most striking. Its employment makes the diagnosis and localization almost foolproof. . . . And doubtless one can *exclude* spinal cord tumors with equal certainty when the passage of Lipiodol is unobstructed. It would be difficult to imagine that a tumor which gave symptoms could be present if Lipiodol passed freely from the cisterna magna to the caudal end of the spinal canal." [39]

With this warm welcome from Dandy, Lipiodol myelography gradually established itself as a recognized special procedure in the United States, including Boston. Indeed, Drs. Mixter and Ayer, whose initial comments had been so negative, went on to accept the Sicard-Forestier procedure and to adapt it to the diagnosis of an additional disease—rupture of an intervertebral disk.[40]

Lipiodol Bronchography

Along with their use of Lipiodol in the diagnosis of spinal diseases, Sicard and Forestier in 1922 announced the successful use of the oil in visualizing the bronchial tree.[41] This announcement naturally aroused much interest at Jefferson Hospital in Philadelphia, where Dr. Chevalier Jackson had from time to time since 1905[42] been visualizing the bronchi by blowing dry bismuth powder into them through a tube. This method had not won wide acceptance, however, because of reports of bismuth poisoning. Accordingly, Dr. Jackson and his associates, including Dr. Willis F. Manges and Dr. Louis H. Clerf, launched competitive clinic trials of the Jackson method, the Sicard-Forestier method, and other methods. Dr. Clerf reported the findings at the May 1925 meeting of the American Laryngological, Rhinological, and Otological Society.[43]

"The methods of choice," he concluded, "are the insufflation of dry bismuth subcarbonate or the injection of Lipiodol, and these are now used exclusively at the Bronchoscopic Clinic [of Jefferson Hospital]."

Dr. Clerf reported also a new method of injecting the Lipiodol "through a Jackson aspirating tube which is introduced through a previously inserted bronchoscope and passed into the bronchus to be outlined. At the Bronchoscopic Clinic this method of bronchoscopic instillation is used in preference . . . , since it permits of a more definite localization of the liquid to the areas to be outlined and can be carried out as a part of the diagnostic bronchoscopy." And Dr. Clerf went on to describe six important functions of bronchography, performed with either bismuth or Lipiodol:

1. In foreign body work it has a distinct field of usefulness to localize a foreign body "around the corner," to establish the relation between a peripherally located foreign body and the nearest accessible bronchus, to determine the relative position and size of the nearest bronchus in a case of penetrating foreign body, and to ascertain whether a suspected shadow is a foreign body in a bronchus or a calcareous deposit in the parenchymal tissue.

2. Lung abscesses are rarely seen bronchoscopically but can be definitely outlined and localized by mapping.

3. In bronchiectasis the degree and extent of the bronchial dilatation and the presence of terminal abscesses can be readily diagnosticated by the introduction of a radiopaque substance and valuable data can be obtained for the surgeon. The presence and location of a bronchial stricture can be definitely ascertained as demonstrated in Luken's case.

4. Helpful data can often be supplied in a case of suspected bronchopleural fistula.

5. The extent of involvement of a primary malignant growth of the bronchus can often be accurately determined for the information of the surgeon as was so clearly shown in Chevalier Jackson's case.

    6. In addition other infiltrating processes can often be demonstrated.[40]

Much greater enthusiasm for Lipiodol was voiced by two Canadian investigators at the Royal Victoria Hospital in Montreal. One of them, an otolaryngologist, Dr. David H. Ballon, published his preliminary report in the *Canadian Medical Association Journal* for October 1925 and gave a fuller report at the November 1925 meeting of the Montreal Medico-Chirurgical Society.[44]

Dr. Ballon called the introduction of Lipiodol by Sicard and Forestier "an event of far-reaching importance to medicine." Like Chevalier Jackson's group in Philadelphia, he preferred the injection of the Lipiodol through the bronchoscope to the techniques used in France, and he stressed the safety and comfort of the procedure: "The patients suffer little if any pain at the time of the injection and there are scarcely any after effects. It is remarkable how tolerant the lung is to Lipiodol. Some patients are very little distressed even with 30 c.c. of Lipiodol in their lungs. One normal volunteer, another volunteer who had been gassed during the war, and a third bronchiectatic patient went home the same day and were at work the next day. . . .

"That Lipiodol has no irritating effect is evident by the fact that in spite of its presence in the lung for considerable time as demonstrated by X-rays, it produces scarcely any cough in the normal individual." On the basis of 50 cases of Lipiodol injection, Dr. Ballon concluded:

> The topography of normal trachea and bronchi are clearly shown, and stand out in marked contrast to the pathologic.
> Bronchial stenosis is recognizable.
> True lung abscess which remains either partially or wholly unfilled is readily differentiated from a bronchiectatic abscess or a tuberculous cavity which fills readily.
> Bronchiectasis is diagnosed at a glance. . . .
> In pulmonary tuberculosis, cavities are localized; the presence and extent of associated bronchiectasis and normal lung are demonstrated. . . .
> Bronchial fistulas and empyema cavities are clearly defined.
> Respiratory studies show the changes occurring in the bronchi and bronchioles during respiration.

Dr. Ballon noted further that Lipiodol bronchography can provide the thoracic surgeon with "a useful means of deciding whether or not to operate, the extent of operative interference, and the prognosis." This point was illustrated in an accompanying paper by Dr. Ballon's Royal Victoria Hospital colleague, Surgeon-in-Chief Edward Archibald, which presented three surgical case histories.[45] In all three, Lipiodol provided the surgeon with relevant pre-operative information not otherwise available.

Following the lead of Chevalier Jackson and Dr. Ballon, many American centers used the bronchoscope for injecting Lipiodol directly into a bronchus; European centers tended to use less effective injection techniques. In a 1928 book on Lipiodol diagnosis, Drs. Sicard and Forestier explained why: "... Intrabronchial injections ... call for great ability on the part of the operator, who must be specially trained in the use of the bronchoscope. In Europe capable bronchoscopists are far less numerous than in the United States, where the pioneer work of Chevalier Jackson has created a galaxy of remarkably efficient specialists." [46]

At the September 1925 meeting of the American Roentgen Ray Society, two papers on Lipiodol bronchography—one by Major Henry W. Grady, M.D., of the Army Medical Corps and Walter Reed General Hospital,[47] and the other by a radiologist, Dr. Preston M. Hickey, and an otolaryngologist, Dr. A. C. Furstenberg[48]—reported diagnostic advantages of the procedure. The *Journal of the American Medical Association* for April 10, 1926, carried an enthusiastic article based on more than 600 bronchial injections by Drs. Stuart Pritchard, Bruce Whyte, and J. K. M. Gordon of Battle Creek, Michigan. A visit of Dr. Forestier to the United States in the spring of 1926 won further adherents. Finally, both the technique of Lipiodol bronchography and the technique of Lipiodol myelography may be said to have achieved full American acceptance at the "Symposium on the Use of Lipiodol" held in Milwaukee from November 29 to December 4, 1926, under the auspices of the Radiological Society of North America.

In addition to their pioneering of Lipiodal myelography and Lipiodol bronchography, Sicard, Forestier, and their associates explored the possible uses of their oil for a number of other diagnostic purposes. By 1928 they had reported on the use of Lipiodol in the uterus and Fallopian tubes, the seminal vesicles, the vas deferens, the bladder, the urethra, the ureters and renal pelves, the blood vessels, abscesses, sinuses, lacrymal ducts, salivary glands, joints, and other tissues and organs. Some of these procedures have fallen into disuse; others are used only rarely; further uses have been developed since 1928; and other nonabsorbable contrast media have been introduced. Thus, when Dr. Peterson drew up his list of special procedures commonly recognized in 1962, eight were based on the use of Lipiodol and other "oily or non-absorbable" contrast media[49]:

Name of Procedure	Organ Visualized
Bronchography	Lung and bronchial passageways
Myelography	Spinal cord
Cystourethrography	Bladder and urethral passageways
Seminal vesiculography	Seminal vesicles
Hysterosalpingography	Uterus and Fallopian tubes
Lymphography	Lymph ducts and nodes
Thorotrast for liver and spleen	Liver and spleen

CONTRAST-MEDIUM CATHETERIZATION

In addition to the enormous diagnostic progress achieved through the exploitation of varied kinds of contrast media—air, watery iodides, iodinated oils, phenolphthalein compounds, and other more recently developed substances—diagnostic radiology was benefited greatly since 1929 from the pioneering of unusual methods of introducing contrast media.

An early step in this direction was announced in 1929 by a 25-year-old physician-in-training at a small hospital in Eberswalde, Germany. The problem young Dr. Werner Forssmann (1904–   ) hoped to solve was the administration of drugs in adequate quantity to the heart itself. If a drug were merely injected into one of the veins leading to the heart, it became diluted before reaching the heart with additional blood entering from other veins. Radiologists, too, were troubled by this unfortunate fact of circulatory physiology; when they injected a contrast medium into a vein, it was similarly diluted too much to portray clearly the heart and the great vessels leading from it.

Forssmann began his search for a solution by working with cadavers. He soon mastered the delicate art of introducing a thin, lubricated catheter into a vein near the elbow, then working it up toward the shoulder and down again until the tip actually entered the heart. Through a catheter thus placed, he could introduce drugs directly into the heart in any desired concentration—into the heart of a cadaver, that is.

Could this procedure of cardiac catherization also be applied to the living human heart? Dr. Forssmann resolved to find out. "First, in a preliminary experiment," he reported in the German *Klinische Wochenschrift* for November 1922,[50] "I allowed a colleague of mine, who kindly placed himself at my disposal, to puncture my right elbow vein with a thick needle. I then introduced, as in the experiments with the cadavers, a very well-oiled ureteral catheter through a cannula in the vein. The catheter passed very easily to a length of 35 cm. [14 inches]. Since it seemed to my colleague as though further insertion of the catheter might be dangerous, we stopped the experiment, at the end of which I felt perfectly well. After a week, I undertook another experiment alone. I administered local anesthesia, and since venepuncture with a thick needle is technically very difficult to accomplish, I performed a venesection on my left elbow vein and passed the catheter without resistance its entire length of 65 cm. [25 inches]. This distance seemed to me after measuring on the surface of the body to be equal to the distance from the left elbow to the heart.... During a sudden movement, the catheter pressed on the superior and posterior wall of the axillary vein and I experienced an intense warmth behind the clavicle; simultaneously, perhaps because of irritation of the vagus nerve, a slight urge to cough."

Assured by these inner sensations and by the length of tubing introduced that the catheter had indeed reached his heart, Dr. Forssmann then "observed the path of the catheter by means of a mirror which was held by a nurse in front of the fluoroscopic screen," and he also exposed an X-ray plate. The plate showed the catheter tip in the right atrium of the heart. "The length of the catheter was not sufficient for it to be inserted further," Dr. Forssmann explained, apparently in an effort to apologize for not having pushed the catheter on down into one of the vessels leaving the heart.

Dr. Forssmann's initial clinical use of such a catheter in the heart of a patient was to administer a therapeutic infusion to a "patient in very poor condition" with what appeared to be "a severe circulatory disturbance" following a ruptured appendix. On November 29, 1930, moreover, he reported to the Medical Society of Eberswalde that he had reintroduced the catheter into his own heart a number of times, and on two occasions had injected contrast media in an effort to visualize with X rays the heart and great vessels.[51]

Dr. Forssmann received the Nobel Prize for Medicine in 1956 for his work 27 years earlier on heart catheterization, but for technical reasons he never did achieve a clear X-ray negative of his own heart. Others working in Portugal, Sweden, France, and Italy did succeed, however, and cardiac catheterization became one of the accepted ways of achieving X-ray visualization of the heart and the great blood vessels associated with it. Later investigators learned to continue the passage of the catheter through the heart and on into the blood vessels serving the lungs; indeed, they could select the particular vessel best suited to visualize a particular portion of the lungs—a procedure now known as selective angiopneumonography.

Building on these foundations, techniques were also developed for introducing contrast media through arterial as well as venous catheters, and by means of puncture injection into various blood vessels and organs, giving rise to such specialized procedures as angiocardiography, thoracic aortography, cerebral angiography, and many more. The lymphatic system as well as the blood-circulatory system was opened to investigation by these new procedures. Thus, it is fair to say that by the 1960's, not a single organ or region in the body remained unexplored or unexplorable by the X rays, either directly or through visualization of the blood vessels supplying them and the lymphatic channels draining them; for many bodily regions (including the brain and the gallbladder), powerful combinations of methods were available to record both an organ's direct shadows and the shadows of its opacified blood supply.

MAMMOGRAPHY

In marked contrast to the diagnostic advances described above, the X-ray diagnosis of breast lesions, and particularly of breast cancer, has reached a stage of notable effectiveness without a single major discovery.

The foundations for radiography of the breast were laid by a German surgeon, Albert Salomon, who published in 1913 a monograph in which he compared his findings based on X-ray plates of female breasts following their surgical removal with the pathological findings.[52] During the following decades, many radiologists in many countries used X rays for study of the breast and reported their findings; important American contributions were published by Dr. Stafford Warren of Boston in 1930 and 1932, Dr. Frederick Hicken of the University of Nebraska in 1937, Dr. J. Gershon-Cohen and his associates at the Albert Einstein Medical Center and Temple University Medical School in Philadelphia from 1938 to date, and others.[53] The injection of contrast media, including air, into the breast was tried but abandoned; stereoscopic projection proved helpful in some medical centers; but as late as 1960 the finding of breast cancers by means of the X ray prior to their clinical appearance on manual examination had still not won general acceptance as a routine diagnostic procedure.

Since cancer of the breast is the commonest form of cancer in women, and since, in a high proportion of cases, these cancers cannot be clinically diagnosed until it is too late for cure, the need for improved diagnosis was most urgent. Then, in *Radiology* for December 1960, Dr. Robert L. Egan of the University of Texas-M. D. Anderson Hospital and Tumor Institute, now at Emory University Medical School in Atlanta, published a startling paper.

From 1956 to 1959, he reported, he had X-rayed 1000 female breasts with no knowledge whatever of the patient's medical history or of the findings on physical examination.

In 240 of these breasts, cancer was present. Dr. Egan, on the basis of the X-ray films alone, spotted 238 of the 240. One of the two cancers he missed was in the tail of the breast and was early in the series, prior to his introduction of a side view designed to reveal cancers in that area. In 20 cases, the cancer could not be located by palpation even after it was seen on the film, but was shown to be there at biopsy or operation. There were no false positive diagnoses in Dr. Egan's series, and few cases in which benign lesions were mistakenly identified as cancer. In a subsequent series of 2000 cases, Dr. Egan's diagnoses were 97 per cent accurate.

How had he achieved so remarkable a record? No scientific "breakthrough" was responsible. Rather, *careful attention to all of the details* lay at the heart of his method.

A good mammogram, Dr. Egan explained, should be capable of visualizing fibrous bands "as thin as a spider's web," and calcium deposits less than $\frac{1}{250}$ inch in diameter—so small that to see them, the radiologist must examine the film through a magnifying lens. In many cases, moreover, the pathologic tissue being searched for differs only very slightly in X-ray opacity from the normal tissue surrounding it. Hence, the utmost care must be taken to secure the best possible results at every stage in the process.

Most diagnostic films are made with a pair of intensifying screens (see above, page 205). These screens have many advantages, including a shortening of exposure time and a reduction of dose to the patient, but in mammography, Dr. Egan learned, they make it impossible to see those details which are as fine as a spider's web.

Ordinary X-ray film, moreover, while excellent for ordinary use, has a "graininess" which appears when the film is viewed through a magnifying lens. Hence, Dr. Egan switched for mammography to a slower, more fine-grained, *industrial* type of film.

Again, most diagnostic X-ray films are exposed at relatively high voltages—perhaps 70,000 volts or more. This is appropriate for most kinds of diagnosis, but in mammography, because the tissues involved are all soft and because there is so slight a difference in opacity between normal and pathological tissue, Dr. Egan used much lower voltages (as low as 20,000 volts). Selecting exactly the best voltage also proved to be important; a change of as little as 2000 volts—a variation considered trivial in most X-ray work—could significantly improve or impair the quality of a mammogram, Dr. Egan found.

Using slow film without intensifying screens, and low voltage as well, meant that the *time* of exposure was greatly lengthened. This could be partially compensated for by operating the X-ray tube at the highest amperage which it could safely stand, but even so, exposures of as long as 6 seconds were required for some angles of exposure. The slightest movement of the breast during those 6 seconds would blur the spider-web shadows he was seeking. Accordingly, Dr. Egan developed simple but effective techniques for holding the breast motionless. It was supported in such a way, for example, as not to rise and fall with the patient's breathing, and the patient was instructed to hold her breath throughout the exposure.

The shortest possible distance between the breast and the X-ray film also proved essential for sharp mammograms; hence, Dr. Egan placed the filmholder directly up against the breast.

Filtration of the X-ray beam is useful in most kinds of X-ray diagnosis, but Dr. Egan found that in mammography it impairs results; hence, he removed the filter from his apparatus before making a mammogram. He used an efficient cone, however, to limit the diameter of the beam to the area of diagnostic interest, thus reducing exposure to the patient and cutting off "stray rays." He paid careful attention to the *processing* of the film after it was developed, to make sure that as much as possible of the information recorded on the film would be visible when it was later viewed through the magnifying lens.

Finally, Dr. Egan learned to "read" the resulting films accurately— to spot the specific shadows which meant specific types of lesion, and to interpret the meaning of these shadows.

None of these minor changes in technique was revolutionary. All were based on principles long known to radiology. However, the results of combining these refinements of detail in each film exposed did prove revolutionary and led to Dr. Egan's 97 per cent diagnostic accuracy.

Could the Egan technique be taught to others? To find out, 35 radiologists were gathered at the M. D. Anderson Hospital and Tumor Institute for a 5-day indoctrination course in mammography. They made diagnoses based on 9743 consecutive mammograms with 88 per cent accuracy in cancer diagnoses and 94 per cent in benign lesions.[54] By 1964 Dr. Egan was able to report, "The widespread and mushrooming interest in mammography, following the publication of a single article on the subject in 1960, is almost unbelievable, but most heartening."

Much of this interest arose from a project sponsored by the U.S. Public Health Service, during which a radiologist from each of 24 medical centers in the United States—none of which had had previous experience in mammography—received Dr. Egan's 5-day training course. When they returned home they used the Egan method in their practice, without knowledge of the clinical findings, and mailed their reports to the Public Health Service. The surgeons independently mailed their findings. When the two sets of findings were collated, excellent agreement was found.[55] By 1964 more than 200 radiologists from all over the country had received Dr. Egan's training course, and had in turn indoctrinated their colleagues upon their return home. Thus, within a few short years mammography was established as a routine diagnostic procedure—not because of any scientific "breakthrough," but as a result of subtle refinements of technique, first mastered and then taught to others.

The diagnostic procedures reviewed in this chapter, it should be stressed, are only a selection from the many developed since 1913. Dr. Peterson of the University of Minnesota, in the 1962 paper cited above, listed many more which are used today in exploration of the heart and major blood vessels, the brain and spinal cord, the genitourinary tract, the gastrointestinal tract, the lungs, joints, liver, spleen, abdominal cavity, and other organs and sites[49]:

I. Circulatory System
   A. Heart and Great Vessels
      1. Intravenous angiocardiography
      2. Right-sided catheterization and selective cardiography
         (a) Wedge arteriogram
      3. Retrograde catheterization into left ventricle
      4. Transbronchial auricular [atrial] puncture
      5. Transthoracic left auricular puncture
      6. Transthoracic left ventricular puncture
      7. Retrograde brachial or subclavian aortography
      8. Coronary artery catheterization
      9. Injection of root of aorta through catheter
         (a) Cardiac arrest and Valsalva maneuver
     10. CO_2 injection of right auricle
   B. Lumbar Aortography
      1. Catheterization
      2. Direct needle puncture
      3. Intravenous aortography (with dextran)
   C. Renal Angiography
      1. Selective catheterization or ring catheterization
      2. Direct lumbar aorta puncture
      3. Intravenous aortography and nephrotomography
   D. Peripheral Arteriography (Extremities)
   E. Peripheral Venography
   F. Venacavography
   G. Splenoportography
      1. Needle or catheter technique
   H. Hepatic Angiography
   I. Intraosseous Venography
   J. Lymphography
II. Central Nervous System
   A. Cerebral Pneumography
      1. Encephalography
      2. Ventriculography
   B. Cerebral Angiography
     a. Arterial Injection
      1. Carotid puncture
      2. Vertebral puncture
      3. Subclavian puncture
      4. Retrograde brachial puncture
      5. Arterial catheterization via subclavian, brachial and femoral vein
     b. Dural Sinus Venography
   C. Myelography
      1. Gas

   2. Water soluble opaque media
   3. Nonwater soluble opaque media (Pantopaque, Lipiodol, etc.)
  D. Discography
III. Genitourinary Tract
  A. Retrograde Urography
  B. Cystourethrography
  C. Seminal Vesiculography
  D. Retroperitoneal Air Studies
  E. Renal Cyst Injection
  F. Hysterosalpingography
IV. Gastrointestinal Tract
  A. Sialography
  B. Percutaneous Transhepatic Cholangiography
 V. Miscellaneous
  A. Bronchography
  B. Pneumoperitoneum
  C. Pneumomediastinum
  D. Arthrography
  E. Thorotrast Studies of Liver and Spleen
  F. Retroperitoneal Air Studies

For the original papers announcing a number of the major diagnostic procedures not covered in this chapter, readers are again referred to André J. Bruwer's 2059-page sourcebook, *Classic Descriptions in Diagnostic Roentgenology* (1964). Enough has perhaps been presented here, however, to illustrate the nature of progress in diagnostic radiology, the drama of discovery, and the major American contributions to what was in fact a worldwide undertaking.

REFERENCES

1. *Acta Med. Scand., 55:* 555–564, 1921.
2. *Amer. J. Roentgen., 1:* 83–87, 1913; *J. Nerv. Ment. Dis., 40:* 83–87, 1913.
3. *JAMA, 66:* 954, 1916.
4. *Surg. Gynec. Obstet., 24:* 362, 1917.
5. *Amer. J. Roentgen., 5:* 384, 1918.
6. *Amer. J. Roentgen., 6:* 12, 1919.
7. *Ibid.,* p. 190.
8. *Johns Hopkins Hosp. Bull., 27:* 224–311, 1916.
9. *Ann. Surg., 68:* 5–11, 1918.
10. *Ann. Surg., 70:* 397–403, 1919.
11. *Semana Méd. (Buenos Aires), 26:* 424, 1919.
12. *JAMA, 76:* 1384–1386, 1921.
13. *JAMA, 80:* 368–373, 1923.
14. *JAMA, 82:* 1016–1019, 1924.
15. *Fortschr. Roentgenstr., 3:* 635–636, 1923.
16. *Amer. J. Surg., 99:* 206–222, 1960.
17. *J. Pharmacol. Exp. Ther., 1:* 231–264, 1909–1910.
18. *J. Exp. Med., 34:* 47–73, 1921.
19. *Radiology, 76:* 354–375, 1961.
20. *Anat. Rec., 24:* 388–389, 1923; *30:* 333–363, 1925.
21. Cole notebook.

22. *Amer. J. Roentgen., 12:* 403–413, 1924.
23. *Ann. Surg., 80:* 473–477, 1924.
24. *Radiology, 4:* 83–88, 1925.
25. *Amer. J. Roentgen., 14:* 495–503, 1925.
26. *Presse Méd., 1:* 348–353, 1925.
27. *Amer. J. Roentgen., 14:* 511, 192⁵
28. *Lancet, 2:* 67–69, 1925.
29. *Amer. J. Roentgen., 14:* 511, 1925.
30. *Radiology, 5:* 211–221, 1925.
31. *Surg. Gynec. Obstet., 40:* 646–653, 1925.
32. *Ibid.,* pp. 847–851.
33. *Amer. J. Roentgen., 14:* 495–503, 1925.
34. *Amer. J. Roentgen., 13:* 368–369, 1925.
35. *Médecine, 10:* 466–470, 1929; translated in Bruwer, A. J., *Classic Descriptions in Diagnostic Radiology,* pp. 943–944. Charles C Thomas, Publisher, Springfield, Illinois, 1964.
36. *Arch. Neurol. Psychiat., 11:* 499–500, 1924.
37. *Idem.*
38. *JAMA, 82:* 1775–1776, 1925.
39. *Ann. Surg., 81:* 223–254, 1925.
40. *New Eng. J. Med., 213:* 385–393, 1935.
41. *Bull. Soc. Med. Hôp. Paris, 46:* 463–469, 1922; translated in Bruwer, *op. cit.,* pp. 1467–1471.
42. Jackson, C., *Tracheo-bronchoscopy, Esophagoscopy and Gastroscopy,* p. 69. Laryngoscope Co., St. Louis, 1907.
43. *Surg. Gynec. Obstet., 41:* 722–727, 1925.
44. *Arch. Otolaryng., 3:* 401–422, 1926.
45. *Canad. Med. Ass. J., 15:* 1000–1002, 1925.
46. Sicard, J.-A. and Forestier, J., *The Use of Lipiodol in Diagnosis and Treatment,* p. 108. Oxford University Press, London, 1932.
47. *Amer. J. Roentgen., 15:* 65–70, 1926.
48. *Ibid.,* pp. 227–230.
49. *Amer. J. Roentgen., 88:* 4–20, 1962.
50. Translated in Bruwer, *op. cit.,* pp. 508–511.
51. *München. Med. Wschr., 78:* 489–492, 1931; translated in part in Bruwer, *op. cit.,* pp. 512–519.
52. *Arch. Klin. Chir., 101:* 573–668, 1913; translated in part in Bruwer, *op. cit.,* pp. 422–430.
53. Gershon-Cohen, J., in Bruwer, *op. cit.,* pp. 414–491.
54. *Ann. N.Y. Acad. Sci., 114:* 794–802, 1964.
55. *Amer. J. Roentgen., 90:* 356–358, 1963.

19   Improvements in Diagnostic Equipment

The Coolidge tube, the Potter-Bucky grid, improved power supplies, and X-ray films, as noted above, opened the door to modern diagnostic radiology, but inventive ingenuity did not stop there. A number of later devices contributed notably to diagnostic progress.

BODY-SECTION RADIOGRAPHY[1]

The 1896 pioneers had recognized at once a major shortcoming of the X rays for diagnosis: the fact that as the rays pass through the human body, the shadows of one dense object in their path—a bone, for example—blot out the fainter shadows of tissues above and below it. This appeared to be an insuperable obstacle, but proved in fact quite easy to overcome.

The modern technique, known generally as body-section radiography but also as laminography, stratigraphy, tomography, and planigraphy, depends upon imparting a reciprocal motion to the X-ray tube and film, so that when the tube is moving from left to right with respect to the region of interest in the patient being X-rayed, the film is moving in a parallel plane from right to left, and when the tube moves back or forward, the film moves forward or back. The movement of the tube blurs the shadows cast by the portion of the patient's body close to it; the movement of the film similarly blurs the shadows cast by portions of the body in its vicinity. Only the structures in between cast unblurred shadows, which can thus be "read" on the film without interference from the shadows of overlying and underlying structures.

Monographs by two radiologists—Dr. J. Robert Andrews[2] and Dr. James D. Bricker[3]—have traced in detail the history of this ingenious solution to a major radiological problem. Their findings are here briefly summarized.

1. In 1914 a Polish radiologist, Dr. Carol Mayer, sought to visualize the heart without the distracting shadows cast by the ribs. So he moved the X-ray tube back and forth. This blurred all of the images on the plate, but since the heart was farther from the tube, its shadow was less blurred than the rib shadows.

2. In 1915 an Italian, C. Baese, applied for an Italian patent on a device for linking an X-ray tube and fluoroscopic screen in such a way as

to impart to them a proportional, reciprocal motion. Baese's purpose, however, was to locate bullets and other foreign objects; apparently he did not realize that his device could "erase" unwanted shadows.

3. In 1921 a Frenchman, André-Edmund-Marie Bocage, applied for a patent on a device for moving both an X-ray tube and a plate reciprocally and proportionately. His invention had almost all of the essential features of modern devices. Bocage did not succeed, however, in having such a device built until 17 years later.

4. In 1921 two Frenchmen, F. Portes and M. Chausse, applied for a similar patent.

5. In 1927 a German, E. Pohl, also applied for a patent.

6. None of these early proposals, however, led to the manufacture of a device which would really record one plane clearly without interference from structures above and below it, and none of them was known to a 31-year-old victim of tuberculosis named Jean Kieffer, who in 1928 and 1929 became the American inventor of body-section radiography.

Born in France, Kieffer was a self-taught technician who, after recovering from a bout of tuberculosis himself, secured employment in the X-ray department of a Connecticut tuberculosis sanitarium. During a relapse in 1928, he spent many months in bed. His own lesions lay in his mediastinum—a region impossible to visualize because of overlying and underlying bones. Kieffer spent his time in bed inventing a device which would X-ray his mediastinum.

The device that he dreamed up had a number of important features. Tube and film were linked together by a pivoted system somewhat resembling a teeter-totter. By moving the pivot-point or fulcrum in one direction or the other, he could "bring into focus" any desired plane of the object under study. The linked tube and film, moreover, could be moved back and forth, or in a circle, or along a sine curve or spiral, or in any combination of these paths; the motions remained always reciprocal and proportional. This wide variety of motions made possible a more complete erasure of the unwanted shadows under varying circumstances. The thickness of the unblurred section could be changed by varying the amplitude of the movement; the more ample the motion of tube and film, the thinner the section recorded on the film without blurring and the more complete the erasing of shadows cast by objects above and below that plane. Kieffer even worked out a way to combine his device with a Potter-Bucky grid.

Kieffer named his invention the "X-ray focusing machine," and he applied for a patent on it in 1929.[4] "For the next two or three years," he told a reporter for the Hartford *Courant* (May 23, 1937), "I tried to get people to build [such] a machine. . . . My proposals met with sharp skepticism. I went to X-ray manufacturers only to be turned away with the assurance that the method probably wouldn't work. The head of one of the largest firms said: 'It doesn't seem as if there could be anything to this idea of yours or our own engineer would have discovered it.' " Reminiscing in 1937, Kieffer wrote, "On account of poor health, the then beginning depression, and skepticism on the part of the men I tried to interest, I was unable to have the machine built. . . ." [5]

Surely this skepticism was at least in part understandable. Kieffer was merely a self-educated technician in the X-ray department of a state sanitarium, lacking even a high-school diploma. His invention, moreover, was like a perpetual motion machine; it lacked *prima facie* plausibility. The problem that it was designed to solve was so obviously insoluble as to discourage investment in an alleged solution. Kieffer's European predecessors had had similar difficulties.

On September 29, 1936, his 8-year-old invention still existing merely as an idea in his mind—and in the Patent Office files—Jean Kieffer picked up a copy of the *New York Times* and read a disturbing headline:

NEW X-RAY DEVICE 'DISSECTS' BY FILMS

Machine Makes Possible Photographs of Parts of Organs Unobscured by Tissue

TAKES 'SLICES' OF BODY

Shown at Roentgen Ray Meeting, It Enables Demonstration of Diseased Portion.

Under the headline was an Associated Press dispatch from Cleveland which began:

> A new X-ray machine which makes picture slices of the head or organs of the body was demonstrated today to early arriving members of the American Roentgen Ray Society.
>
> Known technically as a "tomograph," the device makes possible for the first time effective photography of separate parts of particular organs without such parts being obscured by shadows of intervening tissue.
>
> Dr. J. Robert Andrews and Robert J. Stava, of the Cleveland University Hospitals who perfected the machine, demonstrated with their X-ray pictures how sections of the human skull, for example, could be pictured clearly to show the presence or absence of diseased conditions. By a simple adjustment, sections could be made one inch back of the forehead, two inches back, or at any similar point. . . .

More than 3,000 members of the X-ray society were expected to attend the scientific sessions opening tomorrow....

Kieffer set off at once for the American Roentgen Ray Society meeting in Cleveland.

Dr. Andrews, who was exhibiting there a model of a machine which he called a "planigraph," clearly recalls Kieffer's arrival: "Toward the end of the 1936 meeting, an unassuming, unpretentious, and somewhat reticent chap presented himself to me while I was demonstrating our exhibit and told me, in almost these words, that he had been watching me for several days in order to 'size up' what kind of person I was and whether he would dare to approach me as he ... considered himself the inventor of this apparatus, and it now appeared as if I were getting all the credit. This was all very strange, and so I agreed to meet him privately in his room in the hotel after dinner." [6] There Dr. Andrews told Kieffer some very disappointing historical facts.

In addition to the pioneers listed above—Mayer in Poland, Baese in Italy, Bocage, Portes, and Chausse in France, Pohl in Germany—Europeans had gone right on reporting the "discovery" of body-section radiography *after* Kieffer had applied for his patent. Among them were (7) an Italian, Vallebona, in 1930; (8) and (9) two Dutch investigators working independently, Ziedses des Plantes and Bartelink, in 1931; and (10) a German, G. Grossman, in 1935.

11. Dr. Andrews himself, while a resident in radiology at the University of Pennsylvania, had happened upon an abstract of a paper in a European journal mentioning such a machine. "This abstract," Andrews recalled, "hinted at what was possible" without explaining how. " ... The article set me thinking about how 'focusing' could be accomplished by introducing a mechanical motion in the beam." Since Dr. Andrews was then a candidate for the degree of Doctor of Science in addition to his M.D., and was casting about for a subject for his postdoctoral thesis, he examined the European literature further; in 1936, after moving to the radiology department of the Cleveland University Hospitals, he and Robert J. Stava of the Picker X-ray Corporation, still ignorant of Kieffer's patent, constructed the first workable American apparatus for body-section radiography. It was this simple and relatively crude initial model which Dr. Andrews was exhibiting at the September 1936 meeting of the American Roentgen Ray Society. Dr. Andrews, of course, claimed no priority for his work.

The history of body-section radiography which Dr. Andrews outlined to Jean Kieffer in Kieffer's Cleveland hotel room on that October evening in 1936 must have come as a stunning blow to a man who had thought for 8 years that his invention was unique. However, all was not lost. If Kieffer's device was not the first, it was in any event the best. Jean Kieffer still had an important role to play in the history of body-section radiography.

Most of the radiologists who stopped at Dr. Andrews's exhibit at the 1936 American Roentgen Ray Society meeting had been unimpressed. "When a planigraphic film is first seen by an uninitiate who is familiar only with conventional radiography," Dr. Andrews explained, "it looks like pretty terrible technical quality." Instead of showing more, it seems at first glance to show much less than a conventional negative. One cannot even see the ribs in a chest exposure, for example. However, one of the passersby who grasped at once the significance of what he was seeing was Dr. Sherwood Moore, director of the Edward Mallinckrodt Institute of Radiology, Washington University School of Medicine, St. Louis. He stopped to talk with Dr. Andrews, and Dr. Andrews introduced Jean Kieffer to him. Dr. Moore was deeply impressed both with Kieffer personally and with his detailed plan for a flexible device capable of impressing a wide range of movements on tube and film. "When shown the design and told of my hope that it would prove of clinical value," Kieffer wrote in a paper prepared for the September 1937 meeting of the Fifth International Congress of Radiology, "he immediately realized the possibilities of the machine and obtained permission from the authorities of Washington University to finance its building at the Mallinckrodt Institute." [7]

Kieffer secured a brief leave of absence from the Norwich Sanitarium to supervise the construction, but there followed what Dr. Moore called "inevitable delays". Dr. Moore added, "collaboration with the inventor of the laminagraph, Mr. Jean Kieffer, has been most difficult because of the great distance of his residence (1,400 miles) from the place where the apparatus was being built and the limited amount of time at his disposal for the purpose of construction." [8] On-the-spot mechanical work was directed by R. H. Tontrup, and Kieffer was able to report, "The first test, made during construction, was so successful that the machine was soon put into clinical use." [9]

In a letter written to his wife from the Mallinckrodt Institute, on July 28, 1937, Kieffer gave a more intimate and exciting view of the moment he had been awaiting since 1928:

> I am so tickled at the machine and what it does that I would like to dance a jig! Dr. Moore and I almost did that yesterday morning when I got a film that he didn't think could be gotten . . . a picture of an abdominal aneurysm! The impossible! And it was also of very much importance because it absolutely proved the diagnosis, which

was questioned by some men. Boy-Oh-Boy! I was working on the machine when Dr. Moore came up with the film as it came out of the dark room. "Come and see this!" he literally yelled.... It definitely showed things you wouldn't even guess with regular X-ray film.... When Dr. Moore saw the long motion working (you know he was somewhat skeptical) he said, 'I won't believe it until I see it again' and he did. He was all smiles and shook my hand and said, 'Kieffer, we got them all licked.'... The [Potter-Bucky] diaphragm also works as I expected—improved the results a lot.[9]

Dr. Moore named Kieffer's device the *laminagraph*,[10] and described the Mallinckrodt Institute model as "a sturdily built table and rail-mounted tube stand of conventional type. The tube stand carries a platform on which are mounted a track for universal tube movement in a plane, a revolving disk containing a spiral cam, and suitable slots for employing a spiral, circular or transverse movement to the tube which is driven by a motor of multiple speed. A crossarm leads from the disk to the tube carriage and imparts the required movement to the tube. Another crossarm from the tube carriage connects with a rigid link which passes down to the film holder. This arm transmitting the tube movement to the film carriage passes through an adjustable fixed point in such a way that movement of these two structures [film and tube] is in synchronism and in opposite direction.... The minimum thickness of layer which can be laminagraphed is of the order of from 2 to 5 mm. The thickness of layer can be increased by decreasing the excursion of tube and film carriage...."[8]

From the beginning, the Kieffer machine proved its worth. "In 28 months of operation of the laminagraph," Dr. Moore told the September 1939 meeting of the American Roentgen Ray Society, "1,069 patients have been examined, an average of one a day.... The great majority of the cases were laminagraphed because of failure of other methods of examination."[11] A commercial model, known as the Kieffer laminagraph, was soon placed on sale by the Keleket Company of Covington, Kentucky.

"Up to the beginning of World War II," Dr. James D. Bricker of Windsor, Ontario, Canada, noted in his comprehensive review of body-section radiography, "the tomograph had been used mainly in the chest."[12] The conditions diagnosed and localized included tuberculous lesions, lung cancer, and cancer of the larynx. Dr. Moore in St. Louis also used Kieffer's machine for study of the temporomandibular joints, sinuses, and the upper cervical spine. Others used it to study calcifications and aneurysms in the abdomen. In more recent years, Dr. Bricker adds, many additional uses have been found.

IMAGE INTENSIFICATION

While much progress was made after 1913 in recording X-ray images on plates and films, fluoroscopy lagged behind. In a classic paper delivered at the December 1941 meeting of the Radiological Society of North America,[13] Dr. W. Edward Chamberlain of the Temple University Medical School detailed the shortcomings of the fluoroscopes then available in frank and distressing terms.

"For nearly half a century," Dr. Chamberlain noted, "physicists and engineers have devoted themselves to the advancement of roentgenology. Today we have access to apparatus which was undreamed of a few years ago. But these spectacular advances in method and equipment have practically all been in the fields of therapy and roentgenography. Fluoroscopy is much as it was when Carman's first edition appeared in 1917. In fact, there is remarkably little difference between the 1941 models of commercially available fluoroscopes and the one Bob Kelley sold my father back in 1912."

Dr. Chamberlain had first become aware of the shortcomings of the standard fluoroscopes, he reported, when he joined Dr. Chevalier Jackson's Bronchoscopic Clinic at Temple in 1930. During the next few years, with the help of a Temple University engineer, O. C. Hollstein, he introduced a number of improvements. In order to improve the quality of the image, for example, he trebled the distance from the tube to the screen. To protect the physician making the examination from excess radiation, he linked the fluoroscopic screen to the X-ray tube in such a way that the X-ray beam always fell on the protective lead-glass shield. He provided two levels of intensity for the X-ray beam, one a little dimmer than usual and the other substantially brighter. The high-intensity beam was of limited usefulness, for if used more than a few seconds, it would burn out the tube and deliver an excessive dose of rays to the patient. But "it at once became apparent," Dr. Chamberlain declared, "that when these high energies were used for one or two seconds at a time, a foreign body which was thus visualized often remained visible after a return to the lower energies. In other words, the brightness of the screen having been brought up to a high enough level so that perception was possible, a return to the lower level of energy input (and screen brightness) did not result in a disappearance of the observed details. We now knew what we were looking at and it remained visible in a very reassuring way." The net effect of these and other improvements was a notable increase in diagnostic effectiveness, accompanied by a marked reduction of radiation exposure to both patient and physician.

An important feature of Dr. Chamberlain's technique was to insist that the physician remain in the dark for a full 40 minutes before engaging in fluoroscopy, instead of the 5 or 6 minutes then considered long enough, in order to adapt his eyes as fully as possible for dark vision. To impress his 1941 audience with this point, Dr. Chamberlain told a story:

"A good many years ago a young man who has since become a very successful radiologist held the privilege of making fluoroscopic studies in my department, and one day he and I entered the fluoroscopic room together. After a few minutes he signaled for a patient, and I remarked that I was not yet dark-adapted. He expressed surprise and said, 'It's a pity that a man who does as much fluoroscopic work as you, Dr. Chamberlain, has to wait so long.' "

To teach the young man a lesson, Dr. Chamberlain told him that he had had a barium-meal examination a few weeks before, and asked him to examine his stomach for barium residue. The young man complied, and found none. Considerably later after both men's eyes were properly dark-adapted, he asked the young man to look for the barium again. "He was obviously rather surprised at my request," Dr. Chamberlain continued, "as he was convinced in his own mind that further fluoroscopy was unnecessary and would reveal nothing. Imagine his surprise when this additional fluoroscopic examination brought to light, very vividly, a definite barium residue in my appendix. With this lesson before him, he was better able to appreciate the importance of dark adaptation."

However, recent work at Temple by Dr. Chamberlain and a physicist, Dr. George C. Henny, had persuaded Dr. Chamberlain that neither minor improvements in equipment nor 40 minutes of dark adaptation would really solve the problem of safe, high-quality fluoroscopy. The human retina, he pointed out, contains two kinds of light-sensitive elements, the rods and the cones. The dim light emitted by the fluoroscope screen, even under the best conditions, required the radiologist to see only with his cones, and vision is much less effective under such circumstances. For normal rod-and-cone vision, the brightness of the fluoroscopic screen might have to be increased 1000-fold. Such an increase was clearly impossible, for, even if a tube could be built capable of emitting a beam of sufficient intensity, its rays would be fatal to the patient in less than a minute.

Was the problem therefore insoluble? On the contrary, Dr. Chamberlain announced dramatically, "in my own opinion [a solution] is just around the corner and when it comes it will put medicine and radiology through another revolution not very different from that which followed the advent of roentgenography and present-day fluoroscopy at the turn of the century." The solution Dr. Chamberlain proposed was to apply to medical fluoroscopy the techniques of *image amplification* (also known as image intensification) already adapted for use in the electron microscope and in television.

The idea, Dr. Chamberlain conceded, was not original with him; on the contrary, Dr. Irving Langmuir of General Electric had applied for a patent[14] on a device for intensifying the fluoroscopic image 4 or 5 years before. "It is a little hard to understand the delay in the creation of a practical device," Dr. Chamberlain noted. "Perhaps what is needed is a realization by the physicists and the engineers of the great need for brighter fluoroscopic images and the great advantage to humanity which their arrival would entail." [13]

Dr. Chamberlain's brilliant analysis provided precisely that awareness. World War II delayed the introduction of fluoroscopic image intensification, but during the 1950's a number of image intensifiers based on the principles Dr. Chamberlain had outlined came on the market. They proved to have many advantages:

1. The fluoroscopic images were so bright that they could be viewed in an undarkened room without prior dark adaptation—a notable saving in the valuable time of the radiologist.

2. Details could be seen which were invisible using conventional fluoroscopy.

3. The recording of the image on moving picture film or on magnetic tape became feasible. Many earlier systems of cinefluoroscopy, dating back to 1896, had been proposed and even tried, but the inherent dimness of the fluoroscopic screen made them of little value prior to the development of image amplification.

4. Stereoscopic fluoroscopy also became feasible.

5. The X-ray exposure of the examining physician was reduced almost to zero.

6. The X-ray dosage to the patient was also notably reduced, making possible types of examination previously impossible; for details, see below, page 429.

Phototimers and Other Steps toward Automation

While advances in equipment design notably improved the quality of the X-ray films which *could* be taken, they also made more complicated the consistent achievement of high quality.

Consider, for example, the problems faced by a radiologist or his technician when making a simple film of the wrist, chest, or other portion of the body prior to 1942. One decision which had to be made was the duration of the exposure. This depended upon a number of independent factors—the speed of the film, the kilovoltage applied to the tube, the milliamperage, the ray-absorbing characteristics of the Potter-Bucky grid used, the thickness and opacity of the part being X-rayed, the fatness or leanness of the patient, and so on.

Although charts had been prepared to guide radiologists with respect to kilovoltage, milliamperage, film speed, and grid, each exposure required the exercise of judgment with respect to the other factors. It is hardly surprising that many films emerged from the developer either underexposed or overexposed, even when taken by a radiologist of long experience. Training a technician to achieve consistently films neither too dense nor too thin was not a short or an easy process, and, as the volume of work required of each radiologist increased from year to year (see above, page 211), the need for some simpler way by which technicians could secure proper exposure consistently became increasingly pressing.

The first step toward a solution was announced in 1942 by a University of Chicago radiologist, Dr. Russell H. Morgan, in a paper entitled "A Photoelectric Timing Mechanism for the Automatic Control of Radiographic Exposures." [15] Dr. Morgan's device was ingenious but in principle quite simple. He mounted a fluorescent screen behind the film, so that X-rays from the tube, after traversing the patient being X-rayed and the film, caused the screen to fluoresce. Near the screen was a phototube—a device which emits a slight electric current when light falls upon its face. This current, after amplification, was fed to a condenser which stored it up. When a specified amount of electricity was stored in the condenser, it discharged, tripping a relay which terminated the X-ray exposure. Thus, the radiologist or technician in command of the X-ray apparatus no longer had to guess how long an exposure would be required to secure a film of the desired density; the phototimer automatically timed the exposure to achieve (at least in theory) the desired density.

The first Morgan phototimers were used after 1942 for filming of the gastric region at the University of Chicago, and for chest work at Army, Navy, and Public Health Service installations. One phototimer controlled more than 100,000 chest exposures during its first 2 years in use. However, the phototimer as initially designed had a number of significant shortcomings. Dr. Paul C. Hodges of the University of Chicago radiology department accordingly joined with Dr. Morgan and with University of Chicago engineers and technicians to develop an improved model. They reported notable progress at a joint meeting of the American Roentgen Ray Society and the Radiological Society of North America in September 1944.[16]

One problem with the initial model was the size and placement of the fluorescent screen used to sample the quantity of X rays passing through the film. A 2 by 2-inch screen was used initially; this proved too large for some purposes and too small for others; in both instances, the light striking the X-ray film and the tube might therefore be turned off too soon or too late.

To remedy this shortcoming, the improved 1944 Morgan-Hodges phototimer introduced a series of "stops" instead of a single fluorescent screen. Stop 1, for example, allowed the X rays to fall on the screen through a circular aperture 2 inches in diameter located at the center of the field; this provided satisfactory sampling of the X rays during exposure of the skull, gallbladder, and certain other organs. Stop 2 allowed X rays to reach the fluorescing screen through 16 aperatures, each 1 inch in diameter, located four in each corner; this stop permitted sampling of a wide area and was used for filming the chest, abdomen and pelvis. Stop 3 was similarly designed for filming the spine, and Stop 4 for the hand, wrist, fingers, and toes. By selecting the appropriate stop, the technician operating the apparatus could be assured that the exposure would be terminated at precisely the right time.

Many other modifications were required to adapt the phototimer to practical use in general radiography. How, for example, could the photoelectric unit be mounted under the radiographic table without interfering with the operations of the oscillating Bucky-Potter grid which also had to be mounted there? Was it necessary to alter the settings of the timing mechanism to compensate for different kilovoltages applied to the tube? How could the special problems raised by a rotating anode in the tube be solved? Some radiologists liked their films a little denser or a little thinner than customary, and denser or thinner films were sometimes desired for special diagnostic purposes; could an adjusting device be added to the phototimer to make possible these variations from the average or usual density? Solutions to these and other problems were described in the Hodges-Morgan 1944 paper. The result was a highly complex electronic circuit (Fig. 33).

With further refinements presented by Dr. Hodges and his associates in 1949,[17] the Morgan-Hodges phototimer became standard equipment in radiographic apparatus. The phototimer devices used today in many automatic-exposure cameras are in effect variations on the original Morgan phototimer.

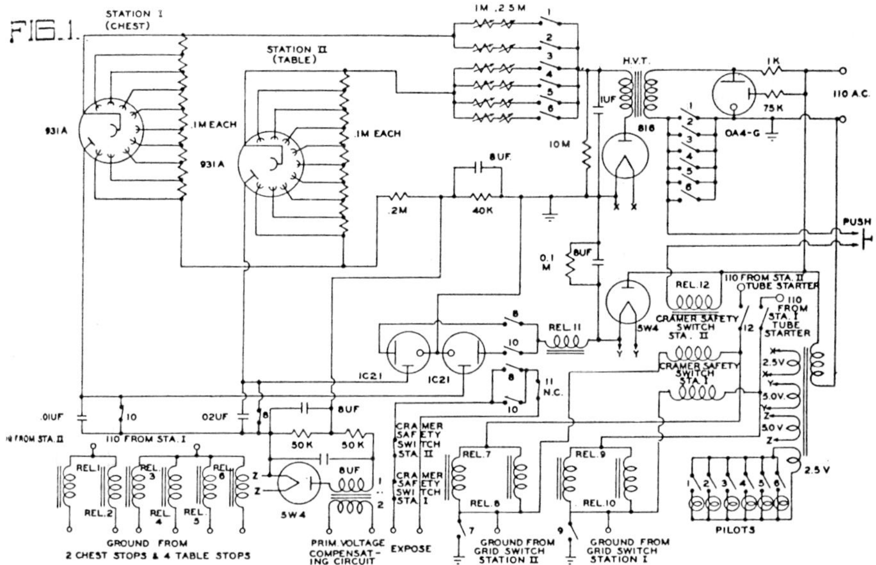

FIG. 33. From *American Journal of Roentgenology, 53:* no. 5, p. 475, May 1945.

Automation has also been applied to other aspects of radiology, notably the processing of films after they have been exposed, and the exposure of many films in rapid succession to catch the successive stages of a dynamic process (a procedure pioneered by Dr. Cole in the 1910's). These improvements added nothing which was in principle new to the practice of radiology, but they made it possible for radiologists and their staffs to maintain standards of quality during the rapid expansion of the radiological work-load described above.

REFERENCES

1. For a fuller account, see BRICKER, J. D., in BRUWER, A. J., *Classic Descriptions in Diagnostic Roentgenology*, pp. 1406–1430. Charles C Thomas, Publisher, Springfield, Illinois, 1964.
2. *Amer. J. Roentgen., 36:* 575–587, 1936, and *38:* 145–151, 1937.
3. BRICKER, *op. cit.*
4. U.S. Patent 1,954,321. Issued 1934.
5. Paper at Fifth International Congress of Radiology (1937), published in *Amer. J. Roentgen., 39:* 497–513, 1938.
6. ANDREWS, J. R., Personal communication.
7. *Amer. J. Roentgen., 39:* 497–513, 1938.
8. *Ibid.*, pp. 514–522.
9. Private papers in possession of Mrs. Jean Kieffer, Napa, California.
10. *Radiology, 33:* 605–614, 1939.

11. *Idem.*
12. Bricker, *op. cit.*
13. *Radiology, 38:* 383–412, 1942.
14. U.S. Patent 2,196,479, applied for March 13, 1929, issued April 10, 1934.
15. *Amer. J. Roentgen., 48:* 220–228, 1942.
16. *Amer. J. Roentgen., 53:* 474–482, 1945.
17. *Radiology, 54:* 64–73, 1950.

   Progress in Radiation Therapy

Just as the Coolidge tube ushered in a new era for diagnostic radiology after 1913, so the availability of substantial quantities of radium after 1913 ushered in a new era for radiation therapy.

During the years prior to 1913, as noted above (page 160), American radiologists lagged behind their European contemporaries in the therapeutic use of radium, especially for cancer therapy; one major reason was the lack of adequate radium supplies. The initial source of radium was uranium ore from mines in Austria; all of this ore was processed in Europe and almost all of it remained in Europe. Prices skyrocketed until as much as $180,000 per gram was being asked. After 1910, substantial new supplies of uranium ore were shipped from mines in Colorado, but this ore also went to Europe for processing, and failed to bring down the price—allegedly because of an international "radium trust" which maintained a monopoly

Credit for making radium available in the United States at relatively moderate prices must be shared by two enterprises:

1. The Standard Chemical Company of Pittsburgh, founded by Joseph M. Flannery, who purchased mines in Colorado in 1911 and began to market radium in 1913.

2. The National Radium Institute and the U.S. Bureau of Mines. The Institute was founded in 1913 by Dr. Howard A. Kelly of Baltimore and Dr. James Douglas of New York. Dr. Kelly, as noted above (page 159), was one of the first Americans to use radium therapeutically. In 1913 he had the largest American cache of it—$\frac{1}{3}$ gram, too little for a number of important applications. Dr. Douglas, head of the Phelps-Dodge Corporation, one of the world's largest copper suppliers, had a daughter with cancer and had had to take her to Paris—and to rent radium from the *Banc du Radium* at an exorbitant price—because adequate radium treatment facilities were not available in the United States. The Institute founded by these two men went into partnership with the U.S. Bureau of Mines at the suggestion of Dr. Charles L. Parsons of the Bureau, and by early 1917 it had refined $8\frac{1}{2}$ grams of radium. The Bureau of Mines's share went to government hospitals; Dr. Kelly's share went to the Kelly Hospital in Baltimore; and Dr. Douglas donated his share to Memorial Hospital in New York. The Institute also made public the details of the

radium-extraction process, so that several smaller companies were able to enter the field.

These augmented radium supplies were promptly put to good use by Dr. Kelly, by Dr. William Duane (a physicist) and his medical associates in Boston, by Dr. Henry H. Janeway and his colleagues at Memorial in New York, and by others at other leading medical centers.

CERVICAL CANCER IN BALTIMORE

Dr. Kelly was the first to report. In addition to his gynecological work at the Johns Hopkins, he had established a small private radium center, the Howard A. Kelly Hospital, in a converted mansion on Eutaw Place in Baltimore. At the June 1915 meeting of the American Medical Association[1] he and Dr. Curtis F. Burnam reported their results in 213 cases of carcinoma of the cervix and vagina treated between January 1, 1909, and December 30, 1914. "Although one of the cures dates from 1909," Dr. Kelly and Dr. Burnam explained, "it was not until December, 1912, that we secured sufficient radium and developed sufficient enthusiasm to employ it systematically. . . ."

Even the bare statistics of cases treated at the Kelly Hospital indicated significant progress. Radium investigators only a few years before had considered a single striking "cure" sufficient to warrant a paper in a medical journal—or even a whole series of papers (as in "Skinner's case" above, pages 143–145)—or they had lumped in a single paper their findings in a dozen or score of cases of several different diseases, benign as well as malignant. A report on 213 cases of a single type of cancer, carcinoma, all in a single anatomical region, and all treated with radium, marked a giant step toward statistically reliable findings instead of mere clinical impressions.

Of their 213 cases, Drs. Kelly and Burnam stated, only 14 were considered operable; the others were already too far advanced. In 10 of these 14, the cervix, uterus, and adjacent organs were surgically excised prior to radiation; radium was used only prophylactically following the operation. Clearly the Baltimore physicians did not yet have enough confidence in radium to rely on it in early cases where an operation was still possible.

The remaining 199 cases were deemed inoperable; they were "hopeless" by any criterion then known. "We have refused treatment to no inoperable case that has come to the hospital," the report proudly noted. If significant results could be achieved in these far-advanced cases, the future for radium—and for carcinoma of the cervix—looked bright indeed.

Highly promising results were in fact achieved. Of the four operable and 199 inoperable cases in which radium was the sole mode of therapy,

57 were "clinically cured"—that is, radiation was followed by "the complete disappearance of the cancer so far as palpation, curettage, or other method may disclose, associated with the apparent perfect general health of the patient."

Dr. Kelly conceded that "clinical cure" in this sense might fall short of permanent or 5-year cure; carcinomas are notorious for recurrence. However, there was reason to hope that many of these would eventually prove to be true cures; indeed, one "clinically cured" patient had already survived for 6 years without a recurrence, three for more than 4 years, 38 for more than 1 year, and the remainder for more than 6 months.

In addition to the 57 "clinical cures," 109 of the irradiated patients were scored as "markedly improved," which Drs. Kelly and Burnam defined as meaning "a definite betterment of the patient's condition. In the lesser degree this may consist of a cessation of hemorrhage and discharge, or a disappearance of pain which has resisted all drugs, including morphine. Among these, too, are placed twelve cases in which all local trouble disappeared, but the patient showed metastasis. . . ." In two patients, a hysterectomy was performed following clinical cure; the uterus, even when examined under the microscope, was found to be free of cancer cells. In two other patients, who died of metastases, the region actually irradiated was found to be free of cancer at autopsy. "We are convinced," Drs. Kelly and Burnam concluded, "that radium is of exceedingly great value in the treatment of cancers of the cervix uteri and vagina."

But there were *caveats*, too, in the Kelly-Burnam report. Thirty-seven patients were *not* improved, despite the fact that their carcinomas appeared to be of the same kind and received the same radium treatment. No explanation of these failures could be found. "The general strength of the patient is not of prime importance," the two investigators noted. "We have seen local disappearances in patients in the last stages of general carcinomatosis. Nor is the extent of local involvement of importance; large growths may disappear and small ones may fail to do so." The mystery of such failures remains in considerable part unsolved today.

There was danger, Drs. Kelly and Burnam stressed, that normal tissues might be damaged during the radiation. "The most easily injured normal tissue in connection with cervical and vaginal cancer radiation is the rectum. In our earlier cases, when we were less familiar with our agent and totally unacquainted with the tissue reactions, this complication was not uncommon, and in some cases led to such serious results as ulceration, fistula formation, and even death from infection. Such a complication manifests itself first in from ten days to two weeks after the application, by diarrhea and tenesmus. . . . In the severer grades the proctitis lasts two months or more, then disappears to recur about the beginning of the sixth or seventh month, with ulceration in the anterior rectal wall. This condition is very painful and takes from three to five months to heal. In the worst cases actual fistula formation takes place before healing. *We are happy to state that this complication can be avoided in every case.* We have not seen it for months." [1]*

Along with this Kelly-Burnam paper at the 1915 A.M.A. meeting, Dr. Henry Schmitz of Chicago described his radium therapy in 112 cancer patients treated since April 1914; 41 of the 112 suffered from cancer of the female pelvic organs.[2] Dr. Schmitz's results were generally similar to those of Kelly and Burnam. Both papers were published in the *Journal of the American Medical Association* for November 27, 1915, where they could alert the entire medical profession to the new and sounder phase into which radium therapy had entered.

Twenty-one years later, at the 1936 meeting of the American Radium Society, Dr. Burnam brought up to date his and Dr. Kelly's 1915 report on the cases that they had treated.[3] "What impresses me, in looking them over now," he remarked, "is the number of severe injuries *and* the number of permanent cures. From this period [1913–1915], there are living today [1936] patients who then had such conditions as mediastinal tumors, sarcomas of the neck, thyroid sarcomas, endothelioma of the brain, sarcoma involving the dorsal vertebra with complete paraplegia, a large abdominal malignancy due to testicular tumor. Of all these cases, perhaps the most striking is the cure of a very extensive intrinsic carcinoma of the larynx. This man, who received a very heavy single treatment, at a distance of an inch, to the larynx, and who had a severe burn going all the way down to the cartilage, had the growth completely clear up and never had a recurrence. However, he did have a long and painful period of convalescence from the burns and he, more than any other patient, impressed upon us the danger of over-radiation."

Thus, the basic dilemma of radiation therapy was clearly visible from the start: to risk an inadequate dose followed by a recurrence, or to risk damage to healthy tissues in the hope that the dose will be curative. Drs. Kelly and Burnam chose the former alternative; the case of the larynx burn, Dr. Burnam declared, "prevented us, for a number of years, from adequately irradiating other larynx cases for fear of a similar experience with burns."

Radium at Huntington Hospital in Boston

In September 1913, 9 months after large-scale trials of radium therapy were begun at Dr. Kelly's clinic, the Cancer Commission of Harvard

---

* Italics added.

University secured ⅕ gram of radium and inaugurated a therapeutic program at its own new cancer center, the Collis P. Huntington Memorial Hospital in Boston.

The Huntington Hospital program was directed by William Duane (1872–1935), a physicist who had studied at Harvard and had then taken his doctorate in physics at the University of Berlin in 1897. In that year Duane had visited the Curies in Paris, and his interest in radiation was kindled. In 1907, aged 35, he returned to Paris to serve for 6 years as radium research assistant in Mme. Curie's laboratory. Then, in 1913, the Harvard Cancer Commission brought him back to the Huntington. He was the first physicist to be employed full-time in an American radium center, and it was he who set the pattern of cooperation between physicists and physicians in radium therapy—a pattern which was to have the most beneficial consequences through the subsequent years.

Dr. Duane and Dr. Robert B. Greenough reported the results of the Huntington Hospital radium work at the June 12, 1917, meeting of the Section on Surgery, Boston Medical Society; their report was published in the September 13, 1917, issue of the *Boston Medical and Surgical Journal.*

During the period from September 1913 to January 1916, the Huntington investigators stated, 642 patients were treated with radium. Of these, 354 (55 per cent) "received definite benefit." [4]

Results varied widely with the type of cancer treated. Among 83 cases of carcinoma of the skin, for example, 33 (39 per cent) were apparently cured and showed no recurrence of the disease to the date of reporting; only 10 cases (12 per cent) "failed to obtain definite benefit." Good results were also secured, as in Baltimore, with carcinoma of the cervix, including several inoperable cases free of apparent disease for as long as 19 months after treatment. On the other hand, nine cases of cancer of the pharynx showed "no material benefit with the exception of one case which showed temporary improvement under prolonged treatment." For cancer of the breast, 49 cases received radium and 27 received X-ray treatment; only three of the radium cases showed even local improvement and "the internal progress of the disease was not affected. It is our opinion that X-ray treatment with massive doses offers more than radium in the palliative treatment of recurrent cancer of the breast."

At the Huntington, as at the Kelly hospital, patients had "suffered pain and inconvenience from the effects of radium burns in certain instances," but these were described as "of a temporary character." Nausea and depression, also temporary, were noted. "With continued and excessive dosage," the Huntington report continued, "very profound constitutional effects may be obtained. A serious diminution of white cells in the blood is observed after continued heavy dosage. This is a more lasting phenomenon, and may be of serious importance. . . . On this sub-ject we are not, as yet, ready to report."

In the past, the Huntington Hospital investigators pointed out, "the obviously extravagant claims of some of the earlier exponents of radium therapy served to arouse in the more conservative members of the pro-fession a natural pessimism, which led them to distrust its value al-together. As a fact, the real truth lies somewhere between these two extremes. Radium is not a cure for all kinds of cancer. There are many cases of cancer in which it can be said to be of no material benefit; but there are also many cases where its use prolongs life, relieves distressing symptoms, improves the general condition and the functional activities of the patient, and mitigates, as does no other agent which we have employed, the gradually progressive symptoms of advanced incurable cancer. . . .

"In the large group of cases in which radium has marked beneficial effect as palliative treatment, and in the smaller group in which its ef-fects are more permanent and complete in eradicating the clinical signs of the disease, radium had already justified the very considerable outlay necessary for its purchase, and the further difficulties and dangers of its effective administration." [4]

Memorial Hospital in New York

One of the motives which had led Dr. James Douglas to join forces with Dr. Kelly and the U.S. Bureau of Mines in exploiting the Colorado uranium deposits was his desire to secure a supply of radium for Memorial Hospital (now Memorial Center for Cancer and Allied Diseases). How-ever, Dr. Douglas was a patient man; he took only about $\frac{1}{30}$ gram of the 1914 production and $\frac{7}{10}$ gram of the 1915 production. It was not until 1916 that he took the lion's share—1.6 grams—for Memorial. Thus, Memorial lagged for a time behind the Kelly and Huntington hospitals, but by the end of 1916 it possessed one of the world's major supplies of radium, more than 2.3 grams. With this supply, and with subsequent additions to it, Memorial soon became the outstanding United States radium research center and took its place among the world's other great centers in France, England, Germany, and Sweden.

To head Memorial's new division of radium therapy, its chief, Dr. James Ewing, selected in 1912 a fellow surgeon, Dr. Henry H. Janeway. During the next 2 years Dr. Janeway prepared himself for his new responsibilities and for the expected arrival of Colorado radium by in-tensive courses in physics at Columbia University, and in 1915 he added to his staff a brilliant young physicist just graduated from Columbia, Gioacchino Failla (1890–1961). Thus, an effective integration of medicine with radiation physics was from the very beginning a hallmark of the Memorial approach.[5]

Dr. Janeway, Mr. (later Dr.) Failla, and Dr. Benjamin S. Barringer reported their 1915–1916 findings in a 242-page book, *Radium Therapy in Cancer at the Memorial Hospital,* published in 1917–one of the enduring classics in both radiology and cancer research. Mr. Failla dealt with the physical aspects, Dr. Janeway reported on principles, methods, and results generally, and Dr. Barringer covered the special field of bladder and prostate cancer.

During 1915 and 1916, Dr. Janeway noted, 424 malignant tumors were treated with radium at Memorial. Of these, 120 achieved "clinically complete regressions," defined as "a complete disappearance of the objective signs of the disease." Sixty-six of the complete regressions were in cancer of the skin, but 53 were in other sites, and in 21 cases out of these 53, the patients had already remained free from recurrence for 1 year or more at the time of reporting. Five cases had survived 2 years or more without a recurrence. "Familiarity with the character of the majority of retrogressions," Dr. Janeway added, "cannot fail to leave the impression that many of them will prove permanent." Thus, the early Memorial experience confirmed the findings in Baltimore and Boston.

However, it was in its detailed consideration of principles, its close observation of significant details, its ingenious techniques, and its efforts at quantitative measurement that the first Memorial report was outstanding.

The heart of the matter, Dr. Janeway noted early in his part of the report, is the fact that "tissues of malignant tumors are more susceptible to the influence of the radiations of radium than the normal tissues." The evidence for this seemed clear. "...Superficial epitheliomas of the skin can be made to disappear by appropriate exposures to radium without more than the slightest degree of erythema to the surrounding tissues." The cancer cells "are destroyed with a dose which has a negligible action upon the normal epithelium." This was true despite the fact that, as compared with some other kinds of cancer, many skin cancers are relatively resistant to radiation.

"The clearest examples of the selective action of radium on tumor tissue are furnished by the cellular teratomas and lymphosarcomas," Dr. Janeway continued. "These tumors seem to melt away with the greatest rapidity whenever, one might almost say, radium is anywhere in their vicinity."

A 10-year-old girl, case S. R., was one of several seemingly miraculous examples. She was operated on in Panama in March 1916 for advanced teratoma of the ovary. A mass of hard, nodular tumor tissue as large as her head was found in her abdomen—so large that nothing could be done surgically and "the operation resolved itself into a mere exploratory incision."

Young S. R. was accordingly brought north to Memorial, and on April 30, 1916, she received a 6-hour radium treatment applied to the skin over her abdomen. "Following this treatment," Dr. Janeway noted, "the tumor entirely disappeared within a few weeks' time." Nor was the retrogression short-lived. Two follow-up examinations were reported:

> *Jan. 20, 1917:* No growth palpable in abdomen. General health excellent.
> *March 16, 1917:* Condition unchanged.

This result was achieved, moreover, with a radiation dose too small to provoke more than a temporary reaction in the skin through which it passed.

Dr. Janeway made several efforts to achieve a quantitative estimate of this difference in sensitivity to radiation between normal and cancer tissues. The comparisons were difficult and the measurements were very rough, but Dr. Janeway thought it "safe to draw the conclusion" that, when all the radiation except the hard gamma rays has been filtered out, the dosage required to destroy normal skin cells "is probably two to four times that required to destroy epidermoid carcinoma." He thought that a 4:1 ratio "is roughly true for the majority of malignant growths, certainly including the tumors of the breast and rectum, and is at least a conservative conclusion, the actual difference being probably greater." Thus, the hope of radium therapy lay in exploiting this fourfold variation "by such a distribution of the source of radiation and by such a dosage that a complete destruction of the malignant tissue is accomplished with a negligible damage to the normal tissues."

It sounded easy, but in practice, Dr. Janeway frankly conceded, it often proved exceedingly difficult—in large part because of the difficulty of securing "uniform distribution of the radiation throughout the affected tissue. By approaching as nearly as possible to such a uniform distribution there will be little difference between the dose received by the cancer tissue and the surrounding normal cells; and it will be possible to furnish the cancer cells with a maximum fatal dose without at the same time producing an injury to the normal tissue. This is a matter of the greatest importance because the injury to the normal tissues which radium produces is not one which heals readily." Radium injuries "not only cause the patient severe pain but also frequently a serious impairment of the function of the part." In an eloquent warning to his fellow investigators, Dr. Janeway added, "The disastrous effects of overexposure are so serious, and they inflict on patients already pitiable so much additional suffering, that too great care cannot be taken to avoid it. It takes at least two or three months to know the full consequences of some of these more deeply penetrating exposures, and before the operator is aware of it, he will be deeply regretting the fact that instead of relieving suffering he has increased it." [6]

USE OF RADIUM SPREADS

The preliminary Kelly, Huntington, and Memorial reports, several others which accompanied them, and comparable reports from the major European radium centers firmly established radium as the treatment of choice for many inoperable cases of cancer and for some operable cases. Soon other American hospitals and physicians in private practice were securing radium supplies of their own.

The extent of this spread was described at the 1931 meeting of the Radiological Society of North America by Dr. R. R. Sayers, chief surgeon of the U.S. Bureau of Mines.[7] The Bureau had sent a radium questionnaire to all hospitals and physicians in 1931, with the following results. Of the hospitals and clinics, 287 reported that they had supplies of radium. Of these, 128 hospitals and clinics had substantial supplies— 75 milligrams or more. The radium held by hospitals and clinics totaled nearly 86 grams. Of the physicians, 414 reported that they had radium, and of these, 171 had 75 milligrams or more. The total reported by physicians was more than 33 grams. Five commercial laboratories had 5 grams of radium; this radium could be leased by physicians, or radon extracted from it (see below, page 280) could be purchased and used therapeutically. New York State had by far the largest supply— nearly 30 grams; Pennsylvania was second with nearly 13 grams. Thus, one-third of all the therapeutic radium reported was in these two states. But only one state—Wyoming—reported no radium available for therapeutic use.

In 1929, Dr. Sayers noted, about 112,000 deaths from cancer were reported in the United States. His questionaire returns indicated that about 80,000 patients annually were being treated for cancer with radium. Thus, a substantial proportion of all cancer victims were securing radium treatment in 1931. The need for more radium, however, remained acute; indeed, 700 hospitals and physicians owning 126 grams of radium reported a need for an additional 117 grams.

MODES OF APPLICATION

The earliest pioneers in radium therapy had mostly used flat applicators of one kind or another, and simply strapped them close to the lesion being treated. During the years after 1913, countless improvements on this primitive technique were developed.

Radium Emanation

One of the earliest and most interesting was proposed by William Duane while he was still an assistant in Mme. Curie's laboratory in Paris. Radium itself, Duane knew, emits only alpha rays or particles—the nuclei of helium atoms. These alpha particles are of no therapeutic value because they lack penetrating power; even an ordinary sheet of paper blocks them completely. In the process of emitting an alpha particle, however, a radium atom is transmuted into an atom of a radioactive gas, now called radon but known before 1923 as *radium emanation*. Each atom of this gas in turn is transmuted into an atom of radium A, which is transmuted into radium B, and so on through a series of other "daughter elements." In practice, the radium used in therapy is sealed up in a glass or a metal container so that the daughter elements accumulate; it is the daughter elements, especially radium B and radium C, which emit the therapeutically useful beta and gamma rays. Duane's ingenious proposal, said to have been advanced as far back as 1908, was to draw off the emanation gas from the radium, seal it into containers, and use these instead of radium containers for therapeutic purposes.

Methods of extracting emanation from radium were known, but they required that the emanation be frozen at exceedingly low temperatures. Duane designed in 1909 a more practical apparatus which made possible the collection of the emanation at room temperature. "As an ionizing agent," he wrote in 1911, "I have been employing the rays emitted by radium emanation. This emanation is extracted from more than 300 mg. of radium chloride, generously placed at my disposal by Mme. Curie in her laboratory. The emanation is sealed in tiny gas spheres having a volume of less than half a cubic millimeter." [8]

The first therapeutic use of radium emanation in the United States no doubt occurred at the Kelly Hospital in Baltimore back in 1911. In that year Professor Benjamin B. Boltwood of the Yale physics department visited Baltimore to advise Drs. Kelly and Burnam. He brought with him a small emanation-collecting apparatus and set it up for Dr. Kelly. Only 30 milligrams of radium were available for use in the Boltwood model, however, so that only homeopathic amounts of emanation could be secured. [9]

Dr. Duane set up the first full-scale radium emanation plant at Huntington Hospital soon after his arrival there in 1913, and helped set up a second at Memorial 1 year later. Early in 1915 Dr. Kelly secured a full-sized emanation plant to replace the Boltwood model; Walter Lantsbury, one of Ernest Rutherford's technicians, brought it over from England with him when he came to work at the Kelly Hospital.[9] Radium emanation proved to have a number of advantages over radium for certain therapeutic purposes:

1. The radium itself could be kept safely in a single large container in the extraction plant instead of risking loss through handling small containers in hospital rooms and doctors' offices.

2. The radium could be kept adequately shielded.

3. Because the emanation is a gas, it could be sealed into very small containers of various sizes and shapes, and very conveniently handled after sealing.

4. Although the radiations were otherwise identical, a given volume of emanation emitted far more intense radiation than the same volume of radium. Tubes, needles, and "seeds" containing emanation could thus be fabricated small enough to be buried directly in tumor tissue, with a minimum of trauma during the insertion.

5. Radium is very long-lived; hence, if it was buried in diseased tissue it must be removed again. In many cases this required a second operative procedure. Seeds containing emanation lose half of their strength in 3.8 days and almost all of it in a few weeks: they could in some situations be left in the tissue permanently.

6. Doctors and hospitals unable to afford radium could buy from commercial companies adequate supplies of emanation at relatively moderate cost as needed.

Radium emanation, like radium itself, was used during the 1910's and 1920's in three distinctive ways: applied at or close to the surface of the skin (*external radiation*); by means of containers or applicators inserted into the nose, mouth, rectum, or vagina and uterus (*intracavitary radiation*); or by means of small seeds or needles inserted directly into the diseased tissue (*interstitial radiation*). Later a fourth means of application was developed: the radium *pack* or "bomb," containing several grams or more of radium—enough so that it could be placed several inches from the skin and could therefore provide a high "depth dose" to underlying tissue with a minimum of skin reaction.

The 1917 Memorial Hospital report described the equipment used for these various modes of treatment in more detail.

First of all, there were the sealed glass tubes containing radium emanation. The tubes were $\frac{3}{8}$ to $\frac{1}{2}$ inch long and less than $\frac{1}{50}$ inch (0.5 millimeter) in diameter. These emanation tubes could be lodged in a body cavity or laid on the skin surface. They delivered, of course, both beta and gamma rays.

Next came thin tubes of aluminum or silver into which the glass emanation tubes could be inserted. The metal tubes protected the glass tubes from breakage, and also filtered out some of the beta rays.

Third came heavier platinum tubes of various sizes and shapes to provide more effective filtration. Platinum was used to hold down the size; a platinum tube with walls 1 millimeter thick, for example, had the same filtering effectiveness as a tube with lead walls of 2 millimeters and, as Dr. Janeway reported, "permit the emergence of only very hard, practically homogeneous gamma rays." Small hooks could be threaded to the ends of these tubes, so that "the tube may be hooked upon almost any ulcer or mucous surface, and can be counted upon to retain its position." Hollow needles in which the glass tubes could be lodged were also available; these needles could be threaded, inserted into tumor tissue, and then withdrawn again at the end of the treatment by pulling on the thread. Also in common use were glass "seeds"—tiny emanation-filled containers about $\frac{1}{10}$ inch long and $\frac{1}{100}$ inch in diameter—which could be implanted directly in tumor tissue and left there permanently.

Dr. Janeway also reported on the use of moulds made of wax or dental compound to hold the radon tubes in place. A mould or "moulage" of the tumor or other tissue to be radiated was made first, and the tubes were inserted into the body of the mould; the mould could then be placed in position against the tissue, assuring a proper geometric alignment of the tubes.

For surface radiation, plaques $\frac{1}{2}$ or 1 inch square were fashioned, containing the emanation tubes placed side by side. These plaques, in turn, could be combined into larger surfaces. Thus, a flat surface of any desired size and shape could be radiated, using any desired filter or combination of filters. Other variations were also possible.

Initially the flat plaques were placed directly on the surface to be radiated, but Dr. Janeway and his Memorial associates soon found that holding the plaques 1 or 2 inches away "practically eliminated a radium inflammation, and yet permitted the administration of doses sufficient to produce retrogression of deep-seated tumors, as, in some instances, metastatic epidermoid tumors of the lymphatic glands of the neck." The gradual evolution of these various forms of application, Dr. Janeway declared in 1917, was "responsible for a continuous improvement in the results as time went along." [6] Far more sophisticated equipment was developed in subsequent years, but the basic principles of tiny seeds for burial in tissue, applicators for use in body cavities, plaques for surface radiation, and adequate filtration of the softer rays were reasonably well understood by 1917.

Failla's Gold Seeds

The early work on modes of application was almost entirely empirical; a new idea was tried out on patients and, if it seemed to work well, its use spread. By the 1920's, however, experimental methods were developed at Memorial and elsewhere for testing a new idea before trying it out on patients. One example among many of these new experimental methods was the development of the implantable gold seed, announced by Dr. Failla at the 1926 meeting of the American Radium Society.[10]

Two major methods of burying radiation sources in tumor tissue were then in common use, Dr. Failla explained. One was the Memorial method, using glass seeds containing radon (radium emanation). The other was the Radium Institute of Paris method, developed by Claude Régaud, using platinum needles filled with radium which were sewn into place and then withdrawn again.

The main advantage of the Régaud method was that the platinum filtered out the beta rays; hence, there was much less painful and hazardous necrosis in the overdosed tissue immediately surrounding the implant. The main advantage of the Memorial method was the fact that the radon seeds could be left permanently in place. Hence, the problem was set: could a permanent implant be devised which nevertheless protected the nearby tissues by filtering out the beta rays?

Drs. A. C. Heublein and Douglas Quick at Memorial had tried one approach to a solution. "Knowing that tissue necrosis is practically limited within a few millimeters around a bare tube," Dr. Failla explained, "Heublein conceived the idea of surrounding each tube in the tissue with a comparable thickness of bismuth paste." The paste was injected into the tissue through a specially designed syringe after the glass seed was in place. Alas, extensive tests of the new method showed that the paste did not distribute itself evenly around the implanted tube and remained too long in the tissue.

Dr. Failla's own first approach was simply to enclose the glass radon seeds in a platinum tube and insert the tube by means of a hollow trocar. "We used platinum of different thicknesses (0.15 to 0.4 mm.) and conducted animal experiments with the cooperation of Dr. [Eugene] Leddy. In this work some tubes were left in the animal until it was sacrificed, and others were removed at various intervals. The results showed that the amount of necrosis could be greatly reduced by using platinum filters. Of necessity, however, the filtered implants were considerably larger than the glass tubes, and the trocar had to be considerably larger in diameter. The question of trauma, therefore, assumed greater importance. In order to make filtered implants of the smallest possible size, it was evident that the radon should be collected directly in a metal tube, and we directed our efforts toward that ideal."

But what metal should be used? "It is well known," Failla noted, "that the most effective filter is one having the highest atomic weight and density. Of the available metals, iridium, platinum, and gold are the most suitable for this purpose." The problem of selecting one of these three metals was turned over to one of Dr. Failla's closest associates, Dr. Edith H. Quimby. "Experiments conducted in our laboratory by Quimby to determine the absorption of radium emanations by different metals showed that equal thicknesses of platinum and *pure* gold had the same absorbing power, within the limits of experimental error. This being the case, gold is preferable because it is about one-fifth as expensive as platinum. Accordingly we had some capillary gold tubing made by Baker and Company."

It was relatively easy to fill foot-long sections of this tubing with radon gas, using the same equipment used to fill the glass seeds. But once a long, thin, gold tube has been filled, how could it be divided into short lengths, each length tightly sealed at both ends to prevent the escape of the radioactive gas? "This part of the problem gave us considerable trouble," Dr. Failla reported with some amusement, "but we finally succeeded in making gastight seals by a very simple device. Pure gold being quite soft, and the bore of the tubing being very small, we found that a gastight seal could be made by simply pinching the tubing." The gold seeds thus prepared were carefully tested for leakage and it was found that they could "be boiled for one hour or more without loss of radon."

Next another curious problem of detail was encountered. It was found that when a long gold tube was filled with radon and pinched step by step into short sections, beginning at one end and proceeding toward the other, the last sections to be pinched off contained more than their share of radon. The solution was simple; the first pinch was made in the middle of the long tube; then each of the two halves was pinched in the middle, and so on—a method assuring equal distribution of the radon.

How thick should the gold walls of the seeds be? Dr. Quimby's filter experiments had shown that, to absorb the beta rays completely, 0.5 millimeter of gold was necessary. However, this would make necessary a very large trocar for insertion and cause greater damage to the tissue. Hence, experiments were run with gold filters ranging in thickness from

0.02 to 0.5 millimeter. The law of diminishing returns made a startling appearance. Gold walls a mere 0.02 millimeter thick, it was found, blocked 73 per cent of the beta rays; and walls 0.2 millimeter thick blocked more than 99 per cent. At first blush, accordingly, it would seem that little benefit could be achieved by walls thicker than 0.2 millimeter.

But radium is a tricky substance. If even 1 per cent of the beta rays were allowed to pass through the gold walls of the tube, beta rays continued to constitute a considerable proportion of the total radiation emitted. Indeed, calculations showed that, even though gold walls 0.2 millimeter thick blocked more than 99 per cent of the beta rays, the remaining fraction of 1 per cent of the beta rays constituted 22.5 per cent of the emitted radiation. Increasing the wall thickness from 0.2 to 0.3 millimeter reduced the proportion of beta rays from 22.5 per cent to 8.8 per cent. Accordingly, subsequent experiments were run comparing both 0.2- and 0.3-millimeter gold tubes with the glass tubes previously in use.

One set of experiments used butter as the test object—a method developed at Memorial a little earlier. "It has been found by Segiura that radium emanations bleach ordinary butter," Dr. Failla explained. "When a tube containing a sufficient amount of radon is placed on the smooth surface of a block of butter (which is kept on ice) one can observe an area of discoloration which increases in size for a number of days. The outline of this region is quite sharp and can be measured with fair precision. The physical conditions which determine the distribution of the radiation around the tube are quite comparable when butter and tissue are used as the media. Accordingly, some definite information can be obtained by measuring the area of discoloration around tubes of different strength and different filtration." [5]

Next, rabbit muscle was used in testing. Seeds of various types, sizes, and strengths were buried in the dorsal muscles of living rabbits for varying periods. At autopsy, the changes occurring in the surrounding tissue were examined under the microscope. Combining both the butter data and the rabbit muscle data with other calculations and experimental results, Dr. Failla was able to conclude that gold tubes with walls 0.3 millimeter thick were somewhat superior to those with walls only 0.2 millimeter thick, and vastly superior to glass tubes.

Through countless series of experiments of this kind, carried on at major centers both in the United States and in other countries, the basic principles of radium therapy were gradually discovered, new techniques were devised, and new equipment was developed. The cooperation between physical research, technological development, and clinical medicine was no doubt as close in the field of radium therapy as in any other branch of medicine. Indeed, radium therapy may have been one of the early models for the free interplay of basic science, applied science, and clinical practice which is so familiar today.

PROBLEMS OF RADIUM DOSAGE

Specifying the amount of radiation used in radium therapy seemed in the beginning a simple problem.[11] A unit of radiation, the *curie,* had been defined by international agreement in 1912 as the amount of radiation emitted by 1 gram of pure radium and its daughter elements under specified conditions. Since early radium therapists generally used much less than 1 gram of radium, they expressed the amount in terms of *millicuries*—thousandths of a curie—and since the length of time to which a tumor was exposed to radiation was as important as the amount of radiation, they talked in terms of *millicurie-hours.*

However, this primitive method of specifying the quantity of radiation soon proved utterly inadequate, for it described only the radiation leaving the source. What was needed was some method of measuring or calculating the amount of radiation reaching each bit of tissue being irradiated—or better yet, since some of the radiation reaching a tissue may pass through it and emerge again without producing an effect, some method of specifying the dose of radiation *absorbed* by each cubic centimeter of tissue.

One important factor in translating quantity of radiation emitted into dose absorbed, of course, is the distance between source and target tissue. Thus, a radium source which delivers 1000 units of radiation to tissues $\frac{1}{10}$ inch away will deliver only 250 units to tissues $\frac{2}{10}$ inch away, 40 units to tissues $\frac{1}{2}$ inch away, 10 units to tissues 1 inch away, and so on.

This calculation, however, assumes that the radiation is passing through a vacuum. If it is passing through air, water, or tissue, some of the rays are absorbed along the way, and others are "scattered"—that is, they emerge from the tissue in a direction different from the direction in which they entered. In the process, moreover, new "secondary" rays are emitted. As a result of these factors of absorption, scattering, and secondary radiation, and of other factors less clearly understood, the amount of radiation actually reaching a distant tissue may differ quite substantially from the amount calculated on the basis of distance from the source alone.

Absorption, scattering, and secondary radiation depend, moreover, on the type and quality of radiation. The beta rays of radium, for example, are absorbed and scattered quite differently from the gamma rays, and the hard gamma rays emerging from a thick filter are absorbed and scattered differently from the mixture of hard and soft rays emerging from a thinner filter.

The shape of the source also has a notable effect on the dose reaching distant tissues. Radiation from a tiny sphere will produce one pattern of distribution in tissues an inch away; radiation from a needle or seed will produce an altogether different pattern, and radiation from a flat plaque will distribute itself in yet another way. A plaque 1 inch square will show a pattern of distribution different from a plaque 2 inches square.

The curie was of no use as a unit for expressing these differing distributions; it could be used only to compare two sources of radiation. To compare the radiations reaching a tissue, some other unit was required.

The primary effect of radiation on living tissue and on other substances is ionization—that is, the breaking up of atoms or molecules into positively and negatively charged ions. Hence, an excellent way, in theory, to determine the amount of radiation reaching a given region is to place a small device known as an ionization chamber in that region and thus to determine the number of ions produced within the region. Ionization chambers were used during the 1910's and 1920's to measure both X-ray and radium radiation, but the methods were crude and were particularly unreliable when applied to the highly penetrating gamma rays from radium.

Even if the ionization could have been accurately measured, moreover, problems might remain. Suppose that a given quantity of hard gamma rays and a given quantity of mixed hard-and-soft gamma rays produce the same number of ions in an ionization chamber. Will they also produce the same effects in a cancer cell? No one knew the answer in the 1920's, and some questions of this kind remained unanswered today.

In lieu of ionization measurements, many investigators during the 1910's and 1920's accordingly sought some *biological* test for measuring the relative amounts of radiation of various kinds delivered to or absorbed by tissues. Thus, Failla, Quimby, and their associates at Memorial devised the "threshold erythema dose" (T.E.D.), defined as the amount of radiation of any kind sufficient to produce a slight reddening or tanning of the skin of the forearm in 80 per cent of patients and no noticeable effect in the other 20 per cent. Many thousands of patients were tested at Memorial under varying conditions to determine the T.E.D. for various sources of radiation, and the doses delivered to deeper tissues could thereafter be specified as fractions or multiples of the

T.E.D. However, since other centers used other biological tests for comparing different radiations, the basic difficulty was not overcome. Also, the T.E.D. remained suspect for the same reason that ionization measurements were suspect; how could anyone be sure that two doses of different kinds of radiation which yielded the same T.E.D. would also produce the same effects in cancer cells?

A major step forward occurred in the 1930's, when Dr. Quimby[12-14] in the United States, and Ralston Paterson and H. M. Parker in England,[15, 16] began publishing long series of tables showing, for applicators of various sizes, shapes, and strengths, and with filters of varying thickness, the relative amounts of radiation delivered at specified distances from the applicators. Separate tables were prepared for surface applications, interstitial applications with buried seeds or needles, and intracavitary applications.

The importance of these Quimby and Paterson-Parker tables in helping to convert radiation therapy from an art to a science can hardly be overestimated. During the early years, radiation therapists had gradually developed a skill in arranging the source of radiation so as to secure the desired results, but the skill was almost wholly intuitive. There was no way to teach the art to others or to duplicate precisely the methods of one laboratory in another. With the new dosage tables, distributing a specified dosage of radiation uniformly through a tissue became a learnable technique.

An exceedingly simple example will illustrate the new principle. Suppose that a radium therapist desires to irradiate through the skin a tumor 4 centimeters square lying 1 centimeter below the surface of the skin. How should he arrange his radium to secure as uniform a distribution as possible of radiation reaching the tumor?

Using intuitive methods, the therapist might select four radon needles, each 4 centimeters long, and arrange them 1 centimeter apart, parallel to one another—a common arrangement in the early days—or he might arrange the same four needles as the four sides of a square (Fig. 34).

To the untutored eye, it might appear that the two arrangements of the needles were roughly equivalent. However, by referring to the Quimby and the Paterson-Parker tables, it was possible to determine that the effects were remarkably different. With the four needles placed parallel, the tissue 1 centimeter below the skin receives a maximum of 40 units of radiation at the center but a minimum of only 21 units at the corner. With the four needles arranged in a square, the radiation is far more uniform: 27 units at the point of maximum intensity and 22 units at the point of minimum intensity.[17]

Once these dosage tables were available, other steps could be taken

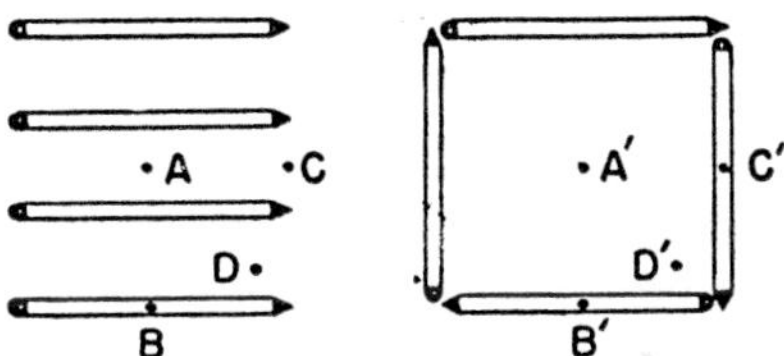

Fig. 34. From Glasser, O., *et al.*, *Physical Foundations of Radiology*, Ed. 2, p. 334. Hoeber Medical Division, Harper & Row, New York, 1952.

toward effective, uniform radiation of tumor tissue with minimum radiation to surrounding tissues. The "Ernst applicator" for radium therapy of the cervix was an example. Developed by Dr. Edwin C. Ernst of St. Louis in the 1940's, the applicator had nine compartments for radium or radon, three introduced in a row into the uterus through the cervix, the other six remaining in an arc in the vagina.[18] The compartments were on flexible mounts, so that they could be adjusted to optimum positions after introduction. Each compartment could be loaded with 10, 20, or 30 units of radium, or could be left unloaded; in all there were 4096 symmetrical ways of loading the applicator. By means of simple charts, it was possible to determine, for each cubic centimeter of tissue in each direction from each compartment, the amount of radiation delivered with any pattern of loading. Thus, a pattern of loading could be tailored to deliver the desired dosage to all portions of the tumor while minimizing the dosage to the bladder, rectum, and other nearby tissues.

X-Ray Therapy Catches up

The increasingly successful use of radium during the years after 1913 tended to overshadow the therapeutic use of X rays. Between 1910 and 1920, as Dr. Ewing of Memorial later recalled, "there was little conception of the possibilities of roentgen therapy," except for superficial skin conditions. "Roentgenologists who engaged in therapy were looked upon with suspicion. It was difficult to enlist the interest of any qualified roentgenologist in this questionable field." [5] Unlike the gamma rays from radium, which penetrated deep into tissues, the 100,000-volt X rays of that period were for the most part absorbed in the superficial tissues. (Methods of overcoming this limitation by placing the tube farther away from the body were not yet fully understood.)

Many years later, Dr. James T. Case of Battle Creek, Michigan, described how this problem was solved. Dr. Case was one of the few reputable radiologists using X rays for therapy in the 1910's and was therefore given an important opportunity.

"In 1913," Dr. Case recalled, "Dr. Coolidge brought out his hot-cathode tube, and at that time he sent half a dozen of these tubes to Lewis Gregory Cole in New York to test for their roentgenographic behavior and he personally brought to me in Battle Creek a shipment to test their behavior in radiotherapy. He was soon satisfied that the rays emanating from the hot-cathode tube were not therapeutically different from the rays generated in the old 'conventional' gas tubes, and after that I continued to use the Coolidge tubes for therapy...." [19]

Beginning about 1916, however, Dr. Case began to hear of remarkable work in Germany using tubes of higher voltage, and therefore capable of emitting more penetrating X rays, than the early Coolidge tubes manufactured in the United States. He accordingly had a transformer built which was capable of delivering 196,000 volts to a tube, and with this transformer he began operating Coolidge tubes far above their rated capacity. Some of the original Coolidge tubes, he learned, "would tolerate as much as 160,000 volts for a month or two." The results made him eager to try even higher voltages.

General Electric also heard of the wartime German work with high X-ray voltages, and, after World War I, Dr. Coolidge began to develop a high-voltage hot-cathode tube for GE. Dr. Case saw this tube in operation at the GE plant in Schenectady, New York, and later described it as "a large tube, nearly a yard long and with a much larger bulb than usual and therefore requiring a much larger lead-glass bowl" to cut off stray rays. Dr. Case was naturally eager to get such a tube, but he was told that "it was not yet on the market and would not be for nearly a year."

Then one day, Dr. Case told attendants at the 1953 Annual Banquet of the American Radium Society, "a gentleman brought his wife to me from Fort Wayne, Indiana, having been sent for the special X-ray treatment that the physicians there had heard I might be able to give. The patient had a recurrence of mammary carcinoma with positive biopsy of the supraclavicular glands"—and, by a remarkable coincidence, the husband was the manager of the General Electric plant in Fort Wayne.

The opportunity was too good to be missed. Dr. Case told his visitor about the new Coolidge high-voltage tube, and "the gentleman remarked that he would get Dr. Coolidge on the telephone and have one of the tubes for me 'day after tomorrow.'... True to his promise, I had my tube within the 48 hours."

But alas, disaster promptly followed. As soon as Dr. Case hooked up the new tube to his 196,000-volt transformer, the transformer burned out.

"The gentlemen found me almost weeping over the loss of the 196,000-volt transformer," Dr. Case told the banqueters, "but after listening to my explanation, he assured me that he would have another one of 300,000-volt capacity 'the day after tomorrow,' and sure enough, he had one trucked up from Fort Wayne and we had it in operation on the third day.

"This first patient survived nearly eight years, all but the last few months in comfort and general good health, but finally succumbed to pleural malignancy. I went on with this deep roentgen therapy, receiving patients from far and near, and working days and evenings. . . ."

As was the case in the introduction of other new equipment and procedures, harm as well as good was done initially. "At first we gave very large doses," Dr. Case recalled, ". . . so large in fact, and within so short a time, that most of the patients were forced to take to their beds for a week or so, and some of them were really prostrated. We often gave blood transfusions, and other supportive treatment." From the point of view of the clinic staff, too, Dr. Case noted, "we had not yet reached the stage of providing proper protection against the higher voltage tubes." [19]

In 1921, shortly after Dr. Case received his first high-voltage Coolidge tube, similar tubes were secured by Dr. Traian Leucutia at the Harper Hospital in Detroit and by others at other centers. Recalling the disastrous effects of overexposure when the low-voltage tubes were first introduced, and familiar with Dr. Case's unfortunate experiences, Dr. Leucutia did not immediately make use of the new tubes in therapy; instead, as he later reported, "the preliminary efforts were directed to construction of devices for protection from both electrical and radiation hazards. . . . Mr. Clifford Sherratt, electrical engineer and pioneer designer of high-voltage radiation protection . . . aided immeasurably in solving these contemporary problems, so that at the beginning of 1922 routine clinical therapy was made possible."

The first Harper Hospital installation had two tubes, energized by a single transformer. Each was housed for safety in a suspended lead drum. Two patients could be treated simultaneously, one by each tube.

While the voltage was high, however, the quantitative output of these early Coolidge deep-therapy tubes was low, necessitating very long treatment times. Hence, in a rebuilt Harper Hospital unit, "the two tubes were housed in lead boxes and used for the treatment of the same patient through two opposite ports simultaneously; one box was placed beneath the treatment table and the other was suspended above it. . . ." [20] When water-cooled and later oil-cooled tubes with much higher outputs became available, the apparatus was again redesigned, so that a single transformer and tube were used for treating each patient.

Dosage Problems with X Rays

Establishing a sound system of measuring and specifying dosage proved somewhat simpler for X rays than for the rays emitted by radium. Hence, by the end of the 1920's, at least the basic principles of X-ray dosage were well understood and in general use.

Ionization chambers were developed capable of determining quite accurately the quantity of ions produced in a given quantity of air by a specific beam of X rays. In 1928 a unit of measurement was agreed upon—the "roentgen," or r—defined by international agreement as an amount of radiation sufficient to produce a specified amount of ionization in a specified quantity of air under specified conditions.

Water-filled "phantoms" were developed to aid in dosage determinations. They were based on the principle that X rays are absorbed and scattered, and secondary radiations generated, in very much the same way whether the medium traversed is water or living tissue. Thus, by placing an ionization chamber at a given location in a water-filled phantom, and beaming X rays at the phantom, the amount of radiation (measured in roentgens) reaching a comparable location in the human body under comparable conditions could be determined. Moreover, "isodose curves" could be drawn on the basis of these phantom studies, showing how the radiation was distributed, and treatments could thereafter be planned on the basis of these isodose curves without repeating the measurements in phantoms. The early work with phantoms was done in Europe; workers in the United States who contributed to these developments included Dr. Otto Glasser and Dr. Failla and his associates.

Simple techniques were also developed for determining the quality, "hardness," or penetrating character of X rays. The softer rays which penetrate only a little way into the tissue, it was learned about 1912, are characterized by relatively long wavelengths and low frequencies. The harder rays, emitted only by tubes operated at a higher voltage, are characterized by shorter wavelengths and higher frequencies. Ways of measuring the wavelengths directly were developed in Europe after 1912, and it became possible to determine what proportion of rays emitted by a given X-ray tube under given conditions was being emitted in each band of wavelengths.

Such determinations were difficult and cumbersome, but a highly practical shortcut came into common use. The amount of radiation reaching a region at a given distance from an X-ray tube was measured in roentgens. Then the thickness of a filter of a given metal necessary to cut the intensity of the beam in half was determined. If a copper filter 3 millimeters thick cut the intensity in half, for example, the beam was said to have a *half-value layer* or h.v.l. of 3 millimeters of copper. In general, the thicker the layer of filter required to cut the intensity in half, the harder or more penetrating the beam. For practical purposes, the half-value layer could be used instead of the much more cumbersome wavelength determinations to specify hardness of X-ray beams.

Combining these two measurements, it became possible for a therapist to specify X-ray dosage quite adequately by recording the half-value layer of the radiation he was using plus the number of roentgens of radiation delivered to the tumor and surrounding tissues as shown by the isodose charts. He could then duplicate the same dosage in other cases, and therapists in other centers could duplicate his methods.

Crossfiring and Rotational Therapy

The isodose charts made it clear that increasing the voltage of the X-ray tube and filtering out the softer rays increased the dose of radiation which could be delivered to underlying tissues without increasing the skin dose. However, they also made it clear that even the heavily filtered beam from an X-ray tube operated at 250,000 volts could deliver only a relatively small dose to deep tissues without delivering a much larger dose to the skin. Hence, other ways were sought, in addition to high voltage and filtration, to increase the relative depth dose without increasing the skin dose.

The simplest way, it was learned quite early, was to increase the distance between the X-ray tube (or radium applicator) and the skin. This reduced the dose to the skin, of course, but it did not reduce the depth dose proportionately. As the distance between the radiation source and the skin was increased, the number of roentgens which could be delivered to the deeper tissues for a given dose to the skin increased significantly.

"Crossfiring" was a second means of increasing the depth dose without an excessive skin dose.[21] It consisted essentially in beaming radiation at the tumor from two or more angles. The tumor might receive only 40 per cent of the skin dose through one angle, 30 per cent through a second, and 20 per cent through a third, to consider a simple example, yet when the treatment was completed, the tumor would have received 90 per cent of the skin dose—enough, perhaps to eradicate it without damage to the skin.

A major limitation of crossfiring, however, was the difficulty of limiting the region of overlap—the region receiving radiation from two or more beams—to the tumor itself and to nearby tissues not easily damaged. To minimize this limitation, *rotational therapy* was developed.[21] Either the X-ray tube or the radium source was rotated around the patient, or the patient was rotated in the radiation beam. Rotational therapy was, at least in theory, roughly the equivalent of crossfiring from an infinite number of angles.

As early as 1925, in his textbook, *Principles and Practice of Roentgen Therapy*, Dr. I. Seth Hirsch of Bellevue Hospital in New York City made clear the theoretical advantages of rotational therapy. Suppose, he suggested, that a filtered beam of X rays be aimed at a roast of beef 8 inches in diameter. If the intensity of radiation at the surface (skin) was 118 units, the intensity at the center would be only 5 units. If the tube were rotated around the beef, however, the radiation reaching the center could be doubled—from 5 to 10 units—while simultaneously the radiation to any point on the surface was reduced from 118 units to only 5 units.

Such calculations were impressive for roasts of beef. It was not until isodose curves became available, however, that full advantage of the principles of crossfiring and rotational therapy could be taken in the treatment of living patients. By preparing isodose curves for each angle of radiation beamed at the tumor, and by using comparable techniques for rotational therapy, the dose of radiation actually delivered to the skin, to each portion of the tumor, and to the nearby organs could be charted on paper in advance. Even so, much additional development was required before the ability to plan an effective course of therapy on the basis of isodose charts became translatable into an ability actually to deliver that dose to a living human patient in accordance with the plan.

The problem of dosage was further complicated, for both X-ray and radium therapy, by the problem of dose-time relationships. It was discovered quite early that a given dose of radiation delivered in a period of minutes had a quite different effect on both normal and diseased tissue from the same dose delivered more slowly, over a period of many hours. Similarly a dose delivered in a single day had a different effect from the same dose delivered in small fractions over a period of many days. In general, the slower the rate at which the dose was delivered and the greater the number of days over which it was fractionated, the less damage to skin and other normal tissues and the larger the total dose that could be safely delivered.

But did prolonging and fractionating the dose really improve the results in cancer therapy? Or did the larger total dose made possible by fractionation have a lesser effect on cancer cells as well as on normal tissue? For many years a debate on this point raged, during which some therapists delivered massive or "hypermassive" doses over a short period of time while others used a prolonged and fractionated dosage schedule.

One rationale for fractionation arose out of a famous "law" announced back in 1906 by two French investigators, Jean Bergonié and L. Tribondeau. Immature cells and cells in an active state of division, the law of Bergonié and Tribondeau suggested, are more sensitive to radiation than other cells. This led to the hypothesis that the damage done to cells by radiation is done during a particular phase of cell division. If this were true, the problem of killing *all* the cells in a cancer might resolve itself into the problem of radiating over a long enough period so that all of the cells engaged in division during the irradiation.

A second rationale for fractionation was also frequently advanced during the 1930's. "The advantages of prolonged irradiation of low intensity or fractionated cumulative treatments are probably explained by the differential recuperation of normal and neoplastic [cancer] tissues," Dr. George T. Pack of Memorial Hospital told a meeting of the New York Academy of Medicine in February 1935.[22] "Presumably normal tissues have much greater power of recuperation than do neoplastic tissues, i.e., their rate of recuperation is faster." Thus, if doses are properly fractionated, the normal tissues may recover between treatments while the cancer tissues continue to retrogress.

Methods of fractionation and prolongation were particularly urged by Claude Régaud,[23] Henri Coutard,[24] and other French investigators, and came to be more and more accepted in the United States during the 1920's and 1930's. It was quite generally agreed, however, that a limit should be set to fractionation, for, if radiation were extended over *too* many weeks, even radiation-sensitive tumors gradually became radiation-resistant. The theoretical principles underlying fractionation have still not been fully developed, but, on the basis of clinical experience, the methods of fractionation worked out in the 1920's are still in general use.

COMBINED THERAPY

With both radium and X rays available for treating deep-seated tumors, many trials were made of "combination therapy." X-ray therapy might precede or follow radium therapy, and either X-ray or radium therapy might be used before or after surgery. In seeking to evaluate the results, however, many difficulties were noted.

An investigator wishing to try out a new technique or combination of techniques must first select a type of tumor on which to try it. Several years would no doubt elapse before he had treated enough tumors of this particular type in the new way to warrant a judgment. Then he would have to wait 5 more years for followup studies. In many cases, 8, 10, or even 12 years might elapse between the inauguration of a new treatment and a final report on its efficacy. During those years, of course, changes in equipment and other factors might render the findings quite irrelevant.

A report by Dr. Robert B. Greenough presented to the 1926 meeting of the American Radium Society[25] was one example among many. Back in 1918, Dr. Greenough explained, some of the surgeons at Massachusetts General Hospital had decided to try X-ray treatments before and after operations for cancer of the breast. The treatments were given by Dr. George W. Holmes. About half the patients seen were given X rays before or after operation or both; the other half were given none.

Did the X-ray therapy help? Following up, years later, the 134 primary cases of breast cancer treated at Massachusetts General in 1918–1920 proved a prolonged task, and, when it was completed, the conclusions were slender indeed. Pre-operative and post-operative radiation, Dr. Greenough reported in 1926, did "not appear to have been of value as an adjunct to surgical operation" [25]—*but* the series of cases was too small to warrant firm conclusions. By the time that the study was completed, of course, the introduction of the new high-voltage tubes had profoundly altered the outlook. Many more years would have to elapse before *their* pre-operative and post-operative effects could be evaluated. For the radiation therapist, then as now, patience was indeed a major virtue.

Stage and Grade of Malignancy

As techniques improved and studies multiplied, moreover, it gradually became apparent that results in radiation therapy were dictated only in part by the methods used and doses administered. Even more depended upon the tumor itself.

If the cancer were limited to a single, cleanly delineated site, of course, the chances of success were high. If it had already metastasized to other sites, the chances of cure were greatly diminished. Efforts were made to irradiate the adjacent lymph nodes and other areas to which cancer cells were most likely to spread; these proved successful in some cases, but metastatic cancer cells lodged in lymph nodes were usually found to be more resistant to radiation than those in the primary tumor. Soon the division of tumors into those which had metastasized and those which had not proved inadequate; the classification of tumors into four "stages" was introduced.[26]

The classification into stages further complicated evaluation of radiation results. The fact that one medical center reported a higher cure rate than another did not necessarily mean that its radiation techniques were superior. It might mean instead that it received patients at an earlier stage in their disease. The only comparisons that could be relied on must be based on the stage of the cancer in each case—and this meant a further delay in evaluation while sufficient cases in each stage accumulated.

The *grading* of tumors soon followed.[26] It was learned, for example, that cancers of the cervix—even those in the same *stage* of development— are not all alike. Some are composed of cells that multiply only slowly and are unlikely to metastasize; others are composed of much more malignant cells which multiply very rapidly and are very likely to spread. By examining a group of cells under the microscope, their grade of malignancy could be roughly estimated.

Here a significant observation was reported. In general, the low-malignancy tumors were relatively resistant to radiation while the most malignant varieties were the ones which seemed to "melt away" when exposed to even modest doses of X rays or radium. This was an encouraging indication. Soon standard "grades" of malignancy were established for many kinds of tumor, and the choice between operation and radiation was based in part on the grade.

However, the grading of tumors, when added to the staging, introduced a further complication in evaluating radiation results. Furthermore, grading, while it remains today an important part of the planning of radiation therapy, has proved to have several shortcomings. For example, the grading depends upon which particular group of cells happens to be selected for microscopic examination. A tumor graded in one way following the examination of one biopsy specimen may be graded differently if a second specimen is taken. Also, the relation between the apparent grade of a tumor on microscopic examination and its behavior when irradiated proved to be far from simple. Some tumors, although their microscopic appearance suggested high malignancy and therefore sensitivity to radiation, proved to be quite resistant when the radiation was in fact applied.

The net effect of all this was a further requirement for radiation therapists. In addition to a thorough groundwork in the physics of radiation and a mastery of the art and science of using radiation, they had to master vast quantities of information concerning the life histories of particular types of tumor at particular sites.

The inevitable result was further specialization. One therapist might treat only cancers of the cervix and uterus, another only cancers of the oral cavity. The textbooks of radiation therapy came to be organized in chapters, site by site. While individual physicians and small hospitals continued to use X rays and radium in the treatment of malignant conditions, the best work came more and more to be done in the major cancer centers where an array of therapists, each specializing in his own anatomic region, had available the ever-widening range of equipment and knowledge relevant to his particular subspecialty.

The complex interplay through the years of various modes of radiation, and of radiation with surgery, and the gradually improved cure rates resulting from this interplay and from other factors are illustrated by a series of 1958 cases of cervical cancer treated at Harper Hospital in Detroit between 1922 and 1954, and reported by Dr. Leucutia at the 1960 meeting of the American Roentgen Ray Society.[27] Dr. Leucutia divided this 32-year era into five periods of 5 years each, plus a sixth period from 1952 to 1954.

During all six periods, Dr. Leucutia noted, irradiation alone was the treatment most commonly used; in most cases it consisted of a combination of intracavitary radium treatment plus external X-ray treatment. During the first period, 1922–1927, however, a number of early cases were treated by pre-operative radiation followed by surgery. Because of poor results, this method was abandoned after 1928, to be revived in carefully selected cases during the fifth and sixth periods (1947–1954). Surgery *followed* by radiation was used during all six periods. Radiation for recurrences of cervical cancer was quite common in the first period but became increasingly rare during the later periods. The net effect of these changes, plus improvements in both radiation and surgical techniques, and perhaps earlier diagnosis, was a steadily rising rate of 5-year cervical cancer cures over the 32-year period:[27]

1922–26	15 per cent 5-year cures
1927–31	20 per cent 5-year cures
1932–36	30 per cent 5-year cures
1937–41	31 per cent 5-year cures
1942–46	40 per cent 5-year cures
1947–51	49 per cent 5-year cures
1952–54	50 per cent 5-year cures

For cases diagnosed early, of course, the 5-year survival rate was much higher than 50 per cent during the more recent periods.

RADIATION FOR BENIGN CONDITIONS

While the most important progress was being made in cancer therapy, radiologists and other physicians continued to use both radium and X rays in the treatment of a very wide range of benign conditions as well. Dr. George M. MacKee of the New York Post-Graduate Medical

School and Hospital, for example, listed in 1933 more than 100 "skin diseases in which roentgen rays and radium have been found useful." [28] The benefit achieved resulted in many cases from the anti-inflammatory effects of radiation and the resulting relief of pain and discomfort. The use of radiation in benign diseases has been curtailed in recent years as the potentially deleterious effects of radiation came to be more fully understood and as antibiotics, steroids, and other potent weapons against inflammation came into general medical use (see pages 430–431).

While the X-ray and radium therapists were concerning themselves in their day-to-day activities with the problems and achievements described above, world-shaking discoveries were being made in European and American physics laboratories. Great atom-smashing machines, beginning with the cyclotron and continuing through the betatron, the synchrotron, the linear accelerator, and many others, were being invented, and ways of producing artificially radioactive substances—radioisotopes—were being discovered. The impact of these new machines and new substances on the subsequent history of radiation therapy is described in Part IV below (pages 343–362 and 399–401).

REFERENCES

1. *JAMA, 65:* 1874–1878, 1915.
2. *Ibid.,* pp. 1879–1885.
3. *Amer. J. Roentgen., 36:* 437–452, 1936.
4. *Boston Med. Surg. J.* (now *New Eng. J. Med.*), *177:* 359–365 and 787–799, 1917.
5. *Amer. J. Roentgen., 31:* 153–163, 1934.
6. JANEWAY, H. H., BARRINGER, B. S., AND FAILLA, G., *Radium Therapy in Cancer at the Memorial Hospital.* Paul B. Hoeber, New York, 1917.
7. *Radiology, 20:* 305–310, 1933.
8. HAWES, LLOYD E., M.D., unpublished data.
9. *Amer. J. Roentgen., 36:* 437–452, 1936.
10. *Amer. J. Roentgen., 15:* 1–35, 1926.
11. Discussion of radium dosage based chiefly on QUIMBY, E. H., in *Amer. J. Roentgen., 45:* 1–16, 1941.
12. *Amer. J. Roentgen., 31:* 74–91, 1934.
13. *Amer. J. Roentgen., 33:* 306–316, 1935.
14. *Radiology, 43:* 572, 1944.
15. *Brit. J. Radiol., 7:* 592–632, 1934.
16. *Brit. J. Radiol., 11:* 252–313, 1938.
17. GLASSER, O., QUIMBY E. H., TAYLOR, L. S., WEATHERWAX, M. A., AND MORGAN, R. H., *Physical Foundations of Radiology,* Ed. 3, p. 341. Hoeber Medical Division, Harper & Row, New York, 1961.
18. *Transactions of the Fourth International Cancer Research Congress,* St. Louis, 1964; *Radiology, 49:* 425–428, 1947; *Radiology, 52:* 46–62, 1949; *Radiology, 60:* 583–587, 1953; *Amer. J. Roentgen., 85:* 940–948, 1961; also ERNST, E. C., *Dosage Measurements in Radium Therapy.* Ansco, Binghampton, New York, 1957.
19. *Amer. J. Roentgen., 70:* 487–491, 1953.
20. *Amer. J. Roentgen., 85:* 3–20, 1961.
21. WACHSMANN, F., *et al., Moving Field Radiation Therapy.* Chicago, 1962.
22. *Amer. J. Roentgen., 36:* 233–244, 1936.

23. *Amer. J. Roentgen., 21:* 1–24, 1929.
24. *Amer. J. Roentgen., 28:* 313–331, 1932.
25. *Amer. J. Roentgen., 16:* 439–443, 1926.
26. *Ibid.,* pp. 30–42.
27. *Amer. J. Roentgen., 85:* 3–20, 1961.
28. MacKee, G., in Glasser, O. (Ed.), *The Science of Radiology,* pp. 291–304. Charles C Thomas, Publisher, Springfield, Illinois, 1933.

  Radiological Organizations and
Publications

In the development of any new branch of science or medicine, some means must be promptly found to bring investigators and practitioners together and to establish channels of communication among them. Indeed, progress may be as severely impaired by communications lags or gaps as by failures in laboratory and clinic. The failure of Father Gregor Mendel's classic papers on Mendelian inheritance to reach an interested audience for three decades after their publication is one example among the many with which the history of science is strewn.

Fortunately, American radiology almost from the beginning escaped this kind of communications failure. Radiological organizations and periodicals of high quality were founded in abundant quantity to meet the need—or even in advance of the need. Some of the major landmarks in this development are traced below.

American X-Ray Journal (1897–1904)

Among the physicians attracted by Roentgen's initial announcement of the X rays was Dr. Heber Robarts of St. Louis, who secured a Crookes tube and exposed his first plates in February 1896. In May 1897, Dr. Robarts launched as a personal venture the *American X-Ray Journal*, described as "a monthly journal devoted to practical X-ray work and allied arts and sciences," and as "a monthly devoted to the practical application of the new science and to the physical improvement of man."

"In starting the *American X-Ray Journal*," Dr. Robarts subsequently recalled, "I did not consult anyone about the propriety or wisdom of my course. If I had, it would have been swallowed up by the historic monster of disapproval." [1]

During its first 5 years of publication, Dr. Robarts' *Journal* filled a useful purpose. It disseminated news of X-ray developments and reprinted extracts from radiological papers initially published in the longer-established medical periodicals. Despite the editor's whole-hearted enthusiasm for the new rays, its columns were open to reports of damage resulting from their misuse—an important service—but the issues were thin. Most of the leading investigators of the period preferred to report their work initially in the established journals, and increasingly Dr.

Robarts was forced to pad out his pages with materials not directly related to radiology.

In 1902 his *Journal* passed to other hands—"Dr. Robarts lost the journal to the professional electro-therapeutic highjackers," according to a history of the American Roentgen Ray Society written by Dr. Edward H. Skinner of Kansas City in 1950.[2] The *Journal's* office was moved to Chicago, and Drs. T. Proctor Hall and H. Preston Pratt became editors. In December 1904 the *American X-Ray Journal* took over the *Archives of Electrology and Radiology,* and in January 1905 the joint publication began appearing as the *American Journal of Progressive Therapeutics.*[3]

ROENTGEN SOCIETY OF THE UNITED STATES (1900–1902)

More significant in the early history of radiology than his ill-fated *Journal* was Dr. Robarts's role in founding the first American *organization* devoted to radiology.

Early in 1896, Dr. S. H. Monell of New York City, later the author of *A System of Instruction in X-Ray Methods* (1902), had proposed that an X-ray society be formed, but "he found no encouragement and no meeting was held."[1] The idea was revived in January 1900 by Dr. J. Rudis-Jicinsky of Cedar Rapids, Iowa, in a letter to Dr. Robarts. "At my request," Dr. Robarts later reported, "Dr. Rudis-Jicinsky wrote to 40 physicians with similar inquiry."[1] Following this initial round of correspondence, a meeting was held in Dr. Robarts' office in St. Louis on March 26, 1900, where Dr. Robarts was elected president and Dr. Rudis-Jicinsky secretary of the newly organized Roentgen Society of the United States. According to the minutes, nine states were represented: New York, Ohio, Illinois, Missouri, Iowa, Nebraska, California, Kentucky, and Texas. The names of those attending have not been preserved. It was arranged to hold the Society's "first annual meeting" at the Grand Central Palace in New York City on December 13 and 14, 1900.

From the very beginning, however, a shadow of dissension hung over the new society. Dr. Robarts himself reported in veiled phrases that following the mailing of Dr. Rudis-Jicinsky's initial proposal to the 40 physicians, "the answers were against the individual organization. Ex-Presidents of the American Medical Association and others therein interested modestly suggested its feasibility, *provided* it was agreeable to the great parent. Its existence was deemed only possible when it was accepted by and made contributory to their great association. A few, however, agreed that a society was timely."[1] What was at stake beneath this strained verbiage was a major issue: should the new organization be affiliated with the A.M.A., and should membership be limited to physicians in good standing with the A.M.A., or should non-physicians and physicians at odds with the A.M.A.—for example, electro-therapeutists—be eligible as well? Drs. Robarts and Rudis-Jicinsky decided to go ahead without the blessing of the A.M.A. "... We need the assistance of physicists in our meetings," Dr. Robarts explained at the first annual meeting, "which could not be, as members of the American Medical Association." [1]

The first meeting was held on schedule, and the *American X-Ray Journal* reported that it was a notable success. "The literary program ... contained 25 papers. The educational possibilities of such a program and full discussion by experts can hardly be grasped by anyone not present. ..." Another feature was the commercial exhibits. "Without any doubt there was exhibited in the 2,600 square feet of space devoted to apparatus the finest collection of X-ray appliances yet brought together anywhere in the world. The immense value of comparison as an educational value was here apparent. Side by side were seen competing instruments of the most varied types and construction. The strides that had been taken in mechanical improvements were visible on every hand. Two hours in this room were worth more to the incipient X-ray operator in search of information than two years of price list study." [1]

Five new committees were established at the first annual meeting, suggesting that responsible clinicians and medical investigators had a clear voice in the society's deliberations:

> Committee on Standards
> Committee on Medico-Legal Status
> Committee on Scientific Research
> Committee on X-Ray Therapeutic Investigations
> Committee on Revision of the Constitution

However, the dissension which had preceded organization of the Society continued at this first annual meeting. There were 150 in attendance, according to Dr. Skinner's history of the Society. The new organization had been repeatedly publicized in the *American X-Ray Journal* and "all those wishing to become charter members" were invited to do so by sending $5.00 annual dues to Dr. Rudis-Jicinsky; the $5.00 included an annual subscription to the *American X-Ray Journal*. The initial constitution specified that members "shall be physicians and surgeons, dentists, investigators, authors on X-ray topics, inventors, radiographers, or their assistants in hospitals, military or State institutions, technical electricians, chemists, teachers of chemistry and physics, specialists and experts in electro-techniques, qualified by at least one year experience with radiant matter, its application or therapeutic use." One of the few limitations was a warning in the *American X-Ray Journal*, *"No quacks or fakes of whatsoever sort need apply,"* [4] but no definition was promulgated of "quack" or "fake." With the doors thus opened very wide, it is hardly surprising that the first meeting attracted dubious participants, or that there was a demand for amending the constitution. "None of the Eastern roentgenologists who were already contributing brilliantly to our new specialty even attended this first meeting," Dr. Skinner wrote in 1950.[2]

The second annual meeting of the Roentgen Society of the United States was held in Buffalo, New York, September 10 and 11, 1901, and the name was changed to the Roentgen Society of America so that Canadians would feel included. Dr. Robarts reported that 105 members attended and paid dues.

The first two annual meetings "must have been chaotic affairs," Dr. Skinner declared later. "The documentary evidence, mostly within the columns of the issues of the *American X-Ray Journal,* seems to show that a fringe of electro-therapists attempted to either control or sabotage this poorly organized society, much to the embarrassment of Dr. Robarts. They attempted to euchre the editor out of his journal and finally succeeded."[2] Dr. Skinner described "the desperate plight in which Dr. Robarts seemed engulfed" at these early meetings, "with electro-therapists to the left of him, jealous X-ray neophytes to the right of him, upstart manufacturers in front of him, and colleagues at home pulling his coat tails. . . . Dr. Robarts, together with Dr. [J. P.] Girdwood of Montreal, Canada, Dr. [Mihran] Kassabian of Philadelphia, and Dr. [Arthur W.] Goodspeed, also of Philadelphia, fought a losing battle for the control of the Society policies. . . ."[2]

Then Dr. Skinner added: "Within two years, however, our Society was rescued from its despoilers and detractors, and the improvement and progress [have] been constant ever since."

AMERICAN ROENTGEN RAY SOCIETY (ARRS) (1902 TO DATE)

Reform, or perhaps a compromise, seems to have been achieved at the third annual Society meeting, held in Chicago on December 10 and 11, 1902. The electro-therapeutists gained control of the *American X-Ray Journal,* while physicians aligned with the American Medical Association gained control of the Society. They changed its name to the American Roentgen Ray Society, and they amended the constitution and by-laws. About 15 new members were admitted at this meeting, Dr. Skinner reports, "and many of them became familiar figures in the Society, fighting for a clean, ethical society and later making names for themselves in American radiology. Eight of these 15 new members were elected to the presidency of the Society in due course. At the 1903 meeting in Baltimore, Maryland, another 15 names were added to the list of members and six of these later became president of the Society after working their way up through committees and by contributing scientific evidence of merit." [2]

Membership as recorded on the Society's rolls[5] remained relatively stable for the next few years: 222 members in 1902 and 237 in 1906. There is reason to believe, however, that the figures after 1902 were somewhat inflated. In 1905, for example, only 83 members paid dues and only 71 attended the annual meeting. Then the membership list was weeded out; many Western members, in particular, either resigned or were dropped for nonpayment of dues, so that the ARRS became increasingly an Eastern society.

In 1911 admission standards were raised. Applicants were required to have a medical degree, 2 years of X-ray work following graduation, and three letters of recommendation—two from ARRS members in good standing and one from a physician or surgeon residing in the applicant's immediate vicinity. They were also required to "submit a scientific paper to the Executive Committee, which if approved, may be published in the Proceedings of the Society." The Executive Committee was empowered to "hold over for further consideration any applications that are . . . not entirely satisfactory to the Committee," and "to reject any application upon which they find good reason not to report favorably." On May 1, 1913, the Society had only 155 active members, 67 fewer than in 1902. Almost all were physicians specializing full-time or part-time in radiology; the few exceptions were physicists or engineers like H. Clyde Snook, who had contributed notably to the progress of radiology.

Despite the limited membership, the annual meeting of the American Roentgen Ray Society was—and remains today—an outstanding event of the radiological year. Nonmembers as well as members attend. Notable research findings are presented, and radiologists have an opportunity to exchange information and opinions. Manufacturers exhibit their latest equipment. Younger radiologists meet their seniors, old friendships are renewed. At each annual meeting the Caldwell Medal, named in honor of Dr. Eugene W. Caldwell, is awarded to an outstanding radiologist who gives the Caldwell Lecture. In 1921, the Society recognized radiology's long-forgotten debt to that obscure Boston dentist, Dr. William Rollins, whose many contributions have been described in Part II above, by electing Dr. Rollins to honorary membership.

"One of the traditions of the American Roentgen Ray Society from early years," Dr. Arthur C. Christie of Washington, D.C., wrote in 1956, "has been its insistence upon the complete integration of radiology into the practice of medicine. This was doubtless due in part to the fact that nearly all of the pioneer radiologists were originally practitioners of medicine, but this ideal has been maintained within the Society and among its members down to the present time. The Society has jealously guarded the ideal that the practice of radiology is the practice of medicine; that its practitioners must be broadly trained in general medicine; that they, like other physicians, must maintain a close personal relationship with their patients; that the relationship to physicians referring patients to them is that of a medical consultant; and that in all hospital and clinic relationships the radiologist must preserve his own freedom and autonomy as a practicing physician." [6]

Membership in the Society in 1967 is still limited to American and Canadian diplomates in radiology who have completed their residency training and a subsequent period of specialization in radiology. Applicants are still required to submit an acceptable scientific communication on a radiological topic. Despite the strict entrance requirements, membership in 1967 exceeded 850, and attendance at the annual meeting exceeded 2500.

Transactions of the American Roentgen Ray Society (1902–1908)

One of the advances made in 1902, when the Roentgen Society of America became the American Roentgen Ray Society, was the publication of the *Transactions* of the Society. Fifteen hundred copies of Volume I of these *Transactions,* covering the third annual meeting (1902), were published in 1903 by the Courier-Journal Job Printing Company of Louisville, Kentucky. Further volumes were published to cover the annual meetings for 1903, 1904, 1905, 1907, and 1908. These *Transactions,* in addition to carrying the full texts of scientific papers presented, carried edited yet remarkably frank versions of the informal discussions, often heated, which followed. Although primarily concerned with United States and Canadian radiology, the *Transactions* were also one of the means by which news of European radiological developments was circulated through North America, for Europeans visiting the United States often addressed the Society, and Americans touring European radiological centers were accustomed to report to the Society following their return.

American Quarterly of Roentgenology (1906–1913)

This useful publication was first launched, as the official organ of the American Roentgen Ray Society, in October 1906, under the editorship of Dr. Preston M. Hickey of Detroit and Ann Arbor, Michigan. It took the place of the *Transactions* for the 1906 meeting. In addition to publishing papers and discussions from the annual meetings of the Society, Dr. Hickey brought together a variety of original contributions by American radiologists and others. Many articles were abundantly illustrated despite the fact that authors were required to pay the added cost of publication of illustrations out of their own pockets. Publication was temporarily suspended after the fourth (July 1907) issue, but the *Quarterly* was revived in December 1909, and continued under the same name, with Dr. Hickey as editor, through September 1913. Together with its companion publication, the *Transactions,* the *Quarterly* constitutes the richest and fullest historic record of American radiology through most of the "gas-tube era"; Part II of this history, above, depends on these ARRS publications for much of its documentation.

American Journal of Roentgenology (November 1913 to Date)

In November 1913, the *Quarterly* blossomed out as a monthly in a new and larger format under the name *American Journal of Roentgenology,* with Dr. Hickey still as editor. It remained the official organ of the American Roentgen Ray Society. In January 1923, it became the official organ also of the American Radium Society, and its name was extended to become the *American Journal of Roentgenology and Radium Therapy.* Finally, in January 1952, the name was further stretched to *American Journal of Roentgenology, Radium Therapy, and Nuclear Medicine,* although it continued to be familiarly known to radiologists as "the *Journal.*"

The history of the *Journal* from its roots in the 1906 *Quarterly* to its esteemed position today as one of the world's great medical periodicals would require—and deserve—a volume for itself. In addition to original scientific and clinical contributions, the *Journal* publishes abstracts of radiological papers appearing in other American and foreign publications, news of the medical specialty throughout the world, book reviews, and brief but often outspoken editorials. Thus, the *Journal,* in addition to its communications function from month to month, remains a primary source of historic documentation for almost every major radiological advance since the announcement of the invention of the Coolidge tube in its second (December 1913) issue. Without the *Journal,* the present volume would have been much slimmer and not nearly so rich.

In 1916, Dr. Hickey was succeeded as editor by Dr. James T. Case of Battle Creek, Michigan. In 1918, Dr. Case was succeeded by Dr. Harry M. Imboden of New York City, and in 1924, Dr. Imboden was succeeded by Dr. Arthur C. Christie of Washington, D.C. Next in the distinguished line was Dr. Lawrence Reynolds of Detroit, who edited the *Journal* during its years of major expansion from 1930 until his death in 1961. He was succeeded by his associate and partner, Dr. Traian Leucutia of Detroit, the present editor. Many of the distinguished radiologists of the United States and Canada have served at one time or another as associate editors and as members of the editorial board. A review of the 100 volumes published from 1913 to 1968 reveals a remarkable maintenance of uniformly high editorial standards from the days of Preston Hickey through the regime of Traian Leucutia.

RADIUM (1913–1925)

Neither the *Transactions of the American Roentgen Ray Society* nor the *American Quarterly of Radiology* made more than rare casual mentions of radium or radium therapy during the years from 1902 through 1913. When Joseph M. Flannery launched the production and sale of radium in the United States in 1913 (page 271), accordingly, he needed some means of publicizing his product. His house organ, named simply *Radium,* began publication in Pittsburgh as a monthly in April 1913, under the joint editorship of Flannery's medical and physical consultants, Dr. W. H. Cameron and Dr. Charles H. Viol. The publisher was the Radium Publishing Company, affiliated with Flannery's Radium Chemical Company and Standard Chemical Company; each issue carried the advertisements of these two affiliates and of no other companies.

Through the years, however, *Radium* rendered excellent service by abstracting the major literature on the subject, both European and American, and by publishing occasional original articles of merit. It was converted from a monthly to a quarterly in 1922, when the *Journal* added *Radium Therapy* to its title and scope. In 1924, *Radium* became a semiannual, and in 1925 it ceased publication.

WESTERN ROENTGEN SOCIETY (WRS) (1915–1920)

From 1902 on, as noted above, the American Roentgen Ray Society was a vigorous, distinguished, but small organization, boasting only 155 members on May 1, 1913. The membership, moreover, was heavily concentrated in the East, due in part to the withdrawal of many Western members. More than half of the active members in 1913 resided in four states: New York (38), Pennsylvania (26), Ohio (12), and Massachusetts (10). Nine resided in Canada, only six came from Illinois, and only 16 from west of the Mississippi. Twenty-three states were not represented at all, and six states had only one member each. Thus, it was hardly surprising that a demand arose either for broader Western representation in the ARRS or for a new Western organization of radiologists. Westerners complained that admission to membership was more difficult for them, since many of them did not personally know two active ARRS members in good standing who could sponsor them. They also complained that most meetings were held in the East and that attendance was therefore costly both in money and in time away from their practice. As a result of these Western concerns, a schism developed in the organizational structure of American radiology.

The records of the ARRS from 1913 to 1916 suggest that there was a general awareness of Western dissatisfaction, and a willingness to make conscientious efforts to meet it. In November 1913, for example, the ARRS cooperated in establishing a new Chicago Roentgen Society (CRS). The CRS president, Dr. Hollis E. Potter, and the other officers were all ARRS members. The first CRS scientific meeting, held in Chicago on December 12, 1913, was announced in the ARRS publication, the *American Journal of Roentgenology,* and the proceedings were reported in that *Journal.* Clearly the new Chicago Roentgen Society had the blessings of the ARRS.

In 1915, a Pacific Coast Roentgen Society was similarly organized, with membership limited to "any graduate physician in reputable standing in his community *who can qualify for membership in the American Roentgen Ray Society.*" [7]*

Furthermore, a "Western Section" of the ARRS met at the Hotel Cadillac in Detroit on February 21, 1914, and the Annual Meeting of the ARRS itself was held in Cleveland from September 9 to 12, 1914. There was sentiment for continuing this precedent of "Western" meetings; thus, an editorial in the *American Journal of Roentgenology* for October 1914 noted, "The successful midwinter meetings which have been held both in the East and West cause one to wish that arrangements are being made for similar gatherings this year. It is to be hoped that there will be a one-day meeting for the Eastern members and a one-day meeting for the Western members."

This suggestion was adopted. In 1916, one midwinter meeting was held at the Hotel Chalfonte in Atlantic City on January 21 and 22, and another, for Western members, at the Hotel Statler in Chicago 2 weeks later. The *American Journal of Roentgenology* for February 1916 thereupon reported "sentiment" favorable to an even broader geographical decentralization through "creation of an eastern section, a middle section, and a western section." Also, no doubt as a further step to conciliate Western radiologists, the next annual meeting of the Society was scheduled for the Congress Hotel in Chicago, September 27 through 30, 1916.

Finally, modest moves were made to open the ARRS door to additional members. At the Cleveland meeting in September 1914, for example, a new class of "Associate Members" was established, open to applicants who were not physicians but rather "persons of scientific attainment who are interested in the advancement of roentgenology." The number of

---

* Italics added.

ARRS active members climbed from 155 on May 1, 1913, to 170 on October 1, 1914; new members from Illinois and from states west of the Mississippi accounted for nine of the 15 additional active memberships. But these steps, although impressive, were not sufficient to prevent the launching of a rival organization in the West.

One young physician concerned with the problem of Western representation in the ARRS was Dr. Edwin C. Ernst of St. Louis. Dr. Ernst journeyed east during the winter of 1914–1915 to take post-graduate training at the New York School of Roentgenology, recently established by five radiological leaders: Drs. Lewis Gregory Cole, Leopold Jaches, Fred M. Law, William H. Stewart, and Arthur Fenwick Holding. At the conclusion of the course he attended the midwinter meeting of the ARRS held in Atlantic City on January 29 and 30, 1915.

At the Atlantic City meeting, Dr. Ernst talked with Dr. Willis F. Manges, secretary of the ARRS, and, as he recalled nearly half a century later, he mentioned that "I understood prominent roentenologists in the West would be interested in applying for membership." Dr. Ernst cited as examples Dr. Fred O'Hara of Springfield, Illinois, and several others. After all, the society had been founded in St. Louis; why not re-open its membership to Westerners? Dr. Manges "did not appear very enthusiastic," Dr. Ernst recalled, "but promised to let me know at the close of the scientific sessions." [8]

Dr. Ernst was apparently right in suspecting Dr. Manges's lack of enthusiasm. The application of Dr. O'Hara of Springfield was one of 13 such applications pending before the Executive Committee at the time of the Atlantic City meetings.[9] Dr. O'Hara's sponsors for membership were Dr. Miles B. Titterington of St. Louis and Dr. Albert Soiland of Los Angeles. Nine of the 13 applicants were subsequently admitted, including one each from Colorado, Nebraska, and Utah—but Dr. O'Hara was not.[10] Thereafter Drs. Ernst, Titterington, and Soiland became leaders in the movement to establish rival organizations.

Dr. Ernst met Dr. Manges again at the end of the Atlantic City sessions, he later recalled, and was informed that Dr. Manges and the other members of the Executive Committee "actually didn't know much about those from the Midwest I had suggested, and would take it under advisement.... Naturally, I was disappointed.... I then offered to buy a drink at the bar in the name of the West and offered a toast looking at Dr. Manges: 'Here's to the Western Roentgen Society!'" Dr. Ernst returned home believing that "the time was ripe for the formation of an independent Central or Western Roentgen Society." [8]

An organizing meeting for the new society was held in St. Louis in 1915. Among those attending were Dr. Ernst, Dr. O'Hara of Springfield,

Dr. Titterington (who had sponsored Dr. O'Hara for ARRS membership), Dr. Gray C. Briggs of St. Louis (not an ARRS member), and Mr. George W. Brady of the George W. Brady Company, Chicago, manufacturer of *Paragon* X-ray plates and other materials. The name "Western Roentgen Society" was agreed upon for the new organization. Dr. O'Hara was chosen as temporary president and Dr. Titterington as secretary. The first annual meeting was scheduled for "our favorite hotel, the Sherman House" in Chicago, December 15 and 16, 1915. The Brady Company supplied its list of customers as potential members; so did other Midwestern X-ray manufacturers—Scheidel-Western, Kelley-Koett, and Wappler. Invitations went out from Mr. Brady's office.

By the time of the first annual meeting of the WRS in December 1915, the new Society could boast 62 paid-up charter members at $10 apiece; 30 actually attended the initial meeting in Chicago, representing 17 Western and Southern states. One charter member, Dr. Benjamin H. Orndoff, still survived in 1969. The *American Journal of Roentgenology* failed to mention this meeting, or to take any notice whatever of the organization of the Western Roentgen Society.

A further WRS meeting, including the first scientific session, was held at the Planter's Hotel in St. Louis in June 1916, at which some 40 new members were admitted; another meeting at the Hotel Sherman in Chicago in February 1917 found 76 in attendance and 20 new members; and by 1919 the Western Roentgen Society, with 472 members, was far larger—although still less prestigious—than the American Roentgen Ray Society.

Journal of Roentgenology (1918–1919)

In 1918, under the presidency of Dr. Benjamin H. Orndoff of Chicago, the Western Roentgen Society launched this official publication, a quarterly edited by Dr. Bundy Allen of Iowa City, Iowa. Only a few issues were published under this name.

AMERICAN RADIUM SOCIETY (ARS) (1916 TO DATE)

The *Transactions* of the American Roentgen Ray Society and the official *Quarterly* of the Society, as has been mentioned, carried very few references to radium from 1902 to 1913, and the *Journal* carried not a single reference during its first 2 years of publication (November 1913 through October 1915). Clearly the ARRS did not in those years consider radium within its area of interest. During the A.M.A. meetings in Detroit in June 1916, accordingly, a small group of physicians and surgeons interested in radium therapy met to discuss the formation of a new American

Radium Society. Dr. W. H. B. Aikins of Toronto was elected temporary president and Dr. R. E. Loucks of Detroit, temporary secretary. Thus, another portion of American radiology was carved out of the potential domain of the American Roentgen Ray Society.

The first annual meeting of the American Radium Society was held at the Rittenhouse Hotel in Philadelphia on October 26, 1916, with 19 active members and one associate member—Dr. Charles H. Viol, physicist of the Radium Chemical Company—in attendance. Dr. W. H. Cameron of Pittsburgh, medical consultant to Joseph M. Flannery's Radium Chemical Company, was chairman of the membership committee. Of the American radium pioneers, Dr. Robert Abbé of New York was a charter member, but Dr. Howard Kelly of Baltimore and Dr. Francis H. Williams of Boston were not. None of the 20 founding members survives.

Although initially devoted solely to radium, the ARS later extended its interests to include some aspects of X-ray therapy and the artificial radioisotopes. Its purpose, as currently stated, is "to promote the scientific study of radium *and other sources of ionizing radiation* in relation to their physical properties and their therapeutic application." † Most of its present concern is focused on cancer therapy.

To be eligible for active membership, physicians must have formal training in radiation therapy acceptable to the society plus at least 2 years of active practice after training. In lieu of formal training, 6 years of experience in the use of radiation for therapy is acceptable. In addition, a thesis or current publication pertinent to the Society's field of interest is required. Radiologists, internists, surgeons, gynecologists, and other specialists are included among its active members. Physicists, health physicists, and some others are eligible for associate membership. The current membership is approximately 500.

As noted above, the ARS has since 1923 been a co-sponsor with the American Roentgen Ray Society of the *American Journal of Roentgenology*. Its annual meetings draw a wide attendance from among members and nonmembers interested in radiation therapy and other aspects of cancer therapy; an important feature of these meetings is the annual award of the Janeway Medal and delivery of the Janeway Lecture, named in honor of Dr. Henry H. Janeway of Memorial Center in New York City.

RADIOLOGICAL SOCIETY OF NORTH AMERICA (RSNA) (1920 to Date)

Although launched as a Western organization in 1915, the Western Roentgen Society with 472 members from 38 states was by 1919 more

---

† Italics added.

nearly a nationwide organization than the American Roentgen Ray Society. In 1920, accordingly, the WRS changed its name to Radiological Society of North America. As evidence of its new national rather than merely Western scope, the RSNA invaded Boston itself, long one of the major strongholds of the ARRS, for its 1921 meeting. "With the 1921 meeting, the Society seems to have become firmly established and to have settled, more or less, into the pattern it was to follow in the future," Dr. Howard P. Doub, the RSNA's official historian, wrote in November 1964.[11]

The annual meeting of the RSNA, along with the annual meeting of the ARRS, is today among the major features of the radiological year. Scientific papers and exhibits abound, and there are extensive commercial exhibits. A notable feature of these meetings since 1938 has been the "annual refresher courses" designed to bring practicing radiologists and physicians up to date on recent developments. During the 1967 meeting, 81 such refresher courses were presented by 108 lecturers. Each year, too, the RSNA's Gold Medal is awarded to an outstanding radiologist; the first such award, appropriately enough, was made in 1919 to the co-founder of the American Roentgen Ray Society and founder of the *American X-Ray Journal,* Dr. Heber Robarts. For many years the main scientific event of the annual RSNA meeting was delivery of the Carman Lecture, named in honor of Dr. Russell D. Carman of the Mayo Clinic (see above, pages 132–135). Since 1961, an Annual Oration has taken the place of the Carman Lecture, and a different radiologist is honored each year.

Through the years, admission to the RSNA has become somewhat more selective. Today membership is open to physicians who are members of the American Medical Association or other national medical body in North America and who have devoted a major portion of their practice to radiology for 3 years prior to application. Active membership is also open to those who have practiced radiology for 1 year after completion of a residency in radiology. Radiological residents are eligible for junior membership. Currently the society has more than 4500 active members and more than 260 members in other categories. The current goals of the RSNA, as formally stated, are "to promote the study and practical application of radiology in all its aspects . . . to create a closer fellowship among radiologists and closer cooperation between radiology and other branches of medicine and allied sciences."

Journal of Radiology (1920–1925)

The quarterly *Journal of Roentgenology,* established by the Western Roentgen Society in 1918, suffered initially from the similarity of its name to that of the ARRS *American Journal of Roentgenology*. In 1920, accordingly, when the Western Roentgen Society became the Radiological Society of North America, the *Journal of Roentgenology* was renamed the *Journal of Radiology* and became a monthly.

It continued for a time under this name, with Dr. Allen of Iowa City as editor and Dr. Orndoff of Chicago as associate editor. "It was felt, however," Dr. Doub writes, "that a stronger financial background was needed, and the Radiological Publishing Company was established. Many of the officers and members [of the RSNA] subscribed to stock in this organization.

"Under the new regime the publication office was moved [from Iowa City] to Omaha, Nebraska, by its president, Dr. Albert F. Tyler. In January 1922, Dr. Tyler appointed his brother, Mr. H. S. Tyler, as business manager and assumed the duties of editor. Under these conditions it was not long before the officers and members of the Society realized that they were actually without control of their official journal. Steps were taken to change this, and after much litigation . . . dissolution of the publishing company was effected and a new journal was started." [11] The *Journal of Radiology* was discontinued with the issue of December 1925, when it merged with the *American Journal of Electrotherapy and Radiology* to become the *Archives of Physical Therapy*.

Radiology (1923 to Date)

The new RSNA publication, a monthly, was named simply *Radiology*, and was launched with the September 1923 issue under the editorship of Dr. M. J. Hubeny of Chicago. Dr. Hubeny was succeeded in 1931 by Dr. Leon J. Menville. From January 1941 until December 1965, *Radiology* thrived and prospered under Dr. Howard P. Doub of Detroit. Dr. William Eyler of Detroit succeeded Dr. Doub in 1966. Like the *American Journal of Roentgenology*, *Radiology* today holds an enviable position among the world's most respected medical journals.

AMERICAN COLLEGE OF RADIOLOGY (ACR), FIRST PHASE (1923–1934)

With the foundation of the Radiological Society of North America in 1920, it might be supposed that three flourishing national societies—the ARRS, ARS and RSNA—were enough. At least one American radiologist, however, did not think so. He was Dr. Albert Soiland of Los Angeles, a pioneer in radiation therapy on the West Coast and 1922 president of the RSNA. Dr. Soiland, it will be recalled, was one of the sponsors of Dr. Fred S. O'Hara's unsuccessful 1915 application for membership in the ARRS.

The RSNA was by 1922 much bigger than the ARRS, but it still lacked the ARRS's prestige. Dr. Soiland accordingly envisioned a new organization which would outstrip the ARRS in eminence and exclusiveness of membership just as the RSNA had outstripped the ARRS in size. The new organization would be limited to 100 outstanding Fellows "who have distinguished themselves in the science of radiology." Each Fellow must be a graduate of "a reputable institution of medicine and surgery" and must have devoted at least *10 years* to the science of radiology. Fellows were required to present an acceptable thesis at an annual meeting. Election to Fellowship required a unanimous vote of 10 Chancellors. In addition to Fellows and Chancellors, there would be an even higher class of Honorary Fellows, composed of "those whose contributions to the science of radiology warrant honorary recognition." Compared to this select organization, the once-proud ARRS might seem plebeian indeed.

Dr. Soiland initially proposed this new organization, to be known as the American College of Radiology, in a letter to prominent radiologists sent during the winter of 1922–1923. Twenty-one of these prominent radiologists, including Dr. Soiland, met in San Francisco on June 26, 1923, and the ACR was duly launched. (An American College of Surgeons had been founded in 1913 and an American College of Physicians in 1915.) Seventy radiologists initially accepted Fellowship, and the first Convocation of the College was held in Chicago on June 11, 1924, with Dr. Soiland as Executive Secretary and the following elected officers:

President . . . . Dr. George E. Pfahler, Philadelphia
President-Elect . . . . Dr. William H. Stewart, New York
Vice President . . . . Dr. Henry Schmitz, Chicago
Secretary . . . . Dr. Albert Soiland, Los Angeles
Treasurer . . . . Dr. Benjamin H. Orndoff, Chicago

The investiture ceremony at the first Convocation featured a solemn ritual: a "Charge to Candidates" delivered by the President and a five-paragraph "Fellowship Pledge" spoken in response by the candidates dressed in their academic robes.

During the 1920's, as Dr. Lowell S. Goin of Los Angeles later noted in a brief unpublished history of the ACR, "the College existed as a rather exclusive organization intended primarily to confer distinction upon its members. Lest it be thought that the foregoing constitutes a denigration of the College in its early years, it must be remembered that the decoration of a man with an order of chivalry, or the conferring upon him of an honorary doctorate, serves no purpose other than to honor the recipient and to recognize his distinction. These are, in fact, useful functions. Moreover, in these early years, the existence of the College served to emphasize the fact that Radiology had assumed its rightful place as a medical specialty, and as a peer of the other great branches of Medicine, some of which had Colleges in existence. . . ." [12]

"For a number of years after its organization," writes Dr. Arthur W. Erskine of Cedar Rapids, Iowa, "the activities of the College were limited to an annual Convocation, a dinner, and an oration. During that period many radiologists were doubtful that it was useful enough to justify its continued existence, and its death from inanition would not have been surprising." Nine Fellows, including one former president, tendered their resignations, but the College did survive, "probably because the governing body, the Board of Chancellors, carried out its task of selecting Fellows with conscientious care. Radiologists were indeed rare who could bring themselves to decline the real and implied honor of election to Fellowship." [13] Once the initial limit of 100 Fellows was reached, the ceiling was raised and then abolished altogether. Instead of requiring a unanimous vote of the Chancellors, Fellowship could be achieved despite two dissenting votes among the Chancellors and 10 dissenting votes among the Fellows.

That this almost wholly honorary organization, with its initial emphasis on exclusivity and ritual, would shortly emerge in its "second phase" as a fighting spokesman for its medical specialty (see below, page 320) is among the more curious quirks in the history of radiology.

Section on Radiology of the American Medical Association

It was at the June 1923 meeting of the American Medical Association, it will be recalled, that the little group of radiologists brought together by Dr. Albert Soiland launched the American College of Radiology. However, that was not Dr. Soiland's only organizational activity at the June 1923 A.M.A. meeting. He also pressed intensively for A.M.A. recognition of radiology as a full-fledged medical specialty.

This matter of A.M.A. recognition had long been a radiological sore spot. The annual A.M.A. meeting was potentially an excellent "showplace" where radiologists could display their prowess and progress to their fellow physicians on whom they were dependent for the referral of patients, yet as far back as the 1912 meeting of the A.M.A. in Atlantic City, radiologists had complained that "the space for Roentgen plates was confined to an out-of-the-way gallery with absolutely no conveniences provided for those who might desire to exhibit." At the next A.M.A. meeting, in Minneapolis in 1913, the radiological exhibit "was placed upon the top floor of the scientific building and it required a maximum of enthusiasm to climb the long flights of stairs." An editorial in the *American Journal of Roentgenology* for March 1913 accordingly urged that "one member of the [A.M.A.] committee of scientific exhibits ... be a man interested in roentgenology ... who would see that better accomodations were provided."

The *Journal's* proposal was accepted, and a radiologist was appointed to the A.M.A. exhibit committee for 1914. However, this did not solve the problem; the radiologists also needed a place on the program for scientific papers. Hence, Dr. Soiland urged in 1923 that the 15 official "Sections" of the A.M.A. be expanded to 16 to make room for a new "Section on Radiology." As a delegate from California to the A.M.A. House of Delegates, he presented a resolution calling attention to the fact that more than 1000 members of the A.M.A. were engaged fulltime or part-time in the practice of radiology, and he warned that various state bodies were attempting to legalize the practice of radiology by laymen. An A.M.A. Section on Radiology, he argued, would recognize radiology as an integral part of the science of medicine and surgery.

The A.M.A. House of Delegates in response made a modest bow to radiology. It recommended that each of the 15 Sections include in its program at least one paper pertaining to some other specialty such as radiology, but it refused to create a 16th Section.

Dr. Soiland was disappointed, but not discouraged. During the following year, no doubt at his behest, the A.M.A. received "numerous communications from all parts of the country requesting one or more sessions on radiology" at the next A.M.A. meeting. A resolution passed by the RSNA, and endorsed by the ARRS and ARS, called for an A.M.A. Section on Radiology. Dr. Soiland lost again in 1924, but in 1925 the A.M.A. formally approved establishment of such a Section.

The A.M.A. Section on Radiology has functioned effectively ever since, both in arranging radiological programs and exhibits at the various A.M.A. meetings and in urging upon the A.M.A. actions in the interest of radiology. The Section is represented in the A.M.A. House of Delegates by one delegate and one alternate, and it also has a representative on the A.M.A. scientific exhibit committee.

Advisory Committee on X-Ray and Radium Protection (1929–1946)

The schism in American radiology which led to the founding of the Western Roentgen Society in 1915 and of the Radiological Society of North America in 1920 continued through the following decade. This Advisory Committee arose in 1929 out of the schism.

An international congress of radiologists was scheduled to be held in Stockholm in July 1928, and prior to this international meeting several countries, including the United States, were invited to send representatives to the congress to consider establishing a new international organization concerned with radiation protection. The representatives, it was hoped, would discuss radiation protection problems and perhaps draw up tentative standards of protection. Most of the countries invited had radiological societies, and the representatives were selected by these societies or by government agencies. Since the United States had both the ARRS and the RSNA, a problem arose of how to choose a delegation. It was solved by having the ARRS and RSNA send one representative each; to keep peace between them, a young physicist recently employed by the National Bureau of Standards (NBS), Mr. (later Dr.) Lauriston S. Taylor, was taken along. The American College of Radiology was still primarily a ceremonial organization and did not send a representative.

"When attempts were made to reach agreement between the United States and other countries," Dr. Taylor recalled 30 years later, "serious difficulties arose. Each of our two radiological societies offered different recommendations, and each claimed to be the authoritative body. The NBS had no recommendations to offer and was there more by way of an observer. As a result, the recommendations ... prepared by the British protection committee were adopted as the first international recommendations. In the process, the United States delegates showed up rather poorly, in that agreement could not be reached on who authoritatively represented the views of the United States." [14]

An International X-Ray and Radium Protection Committee was established at this meeting, and, to avoid future disagreements within national delegations, it was recommended that "a single central committee be established within those countries having more than one radiological organization. . . ." Lauriston Taylor of the NBS accordingly shouldered the chore of bringing the ARRS and RSNA together. At the ARRS meeting in September 1928, he discussed the problem with the ARRS president, and in December he had a similar informal discussion with the RSNA president. "As a result of these discussions, these organizations agreed to consolidate their protection activities into a single committee," [14] with activities to be coordinated by the National Bureau of Standards.

The first meeting of the U.S. Advisory Committee on X-Ray and Radium Protection, jointly sponsored by the ARRS and RSNA, was held in September 1929, and during the years which followed it rendered notable service to radiology—not merely in representing the United States at later international meetings, but also in preparing a series of NBS *Handbooks* on X-ray protection, radium protection, and related problems. The American Radium Society as well as the ARRS and RSNA participated. These NBS *Handbooks* remained for many years the authoritative guides to radiation protection procedures and standards in American radiology, and recently revised editions remain in common use.

AMERICAN CONGRESS OF RADIOLOGY (1933)

Another step toward healing the organizational schism followed: the planning of an American Congress of Radiology in 1933.

Discussion of such a Congress, a sort of nationwide showcase for radiology to be held in connection with the Chicago Century of Progress Exposition in 1933, was initiated within the American College of Radiology in 1929 as one of its earliest nonceremonial activities. In 1931 the ARRS, ARS, and RSNA joined with the ACR in these discussions, and the Congress was successfully held in Chicago as scheduled. As part of the plan, a historical survey of radiology was prepared by 26 contributors and edited by Dr. Otto Glasser of Cleveland. This survey was published as *The Science of Radiology* in 1933, with extensive bibliographies, and it has remained an important historical resource ever since, very helpful in supplying leads for the research underlying the present volume. A successor volume, *The Science of Ionizing Radiation,* edited by Dr. Lewis E. Etter, was published in 1965.

AMERICAN BOARD OF RADIOLOGY (ABR) (1934 TO DATE)

Following the precedents of interorganizational cooperation set in establishing the Advisory Committee on X-Ray and Radium Protection and in planning the American Congress of Radiology, the major radiological organizations went on to launch jointly a far more ambitious undertaking, the American Board of Radiology. The ARRS, ARS, RSNA, ACR, and A.M.A. Section on Radiology all cooperated in this project.

The basic qualifications of a physician in the United States are in general an M.D. degree from a recognized medical school plus a license to practice issued by his state government. Prior to 1917 there was no similar requirement for recognition as a medical specialist. In that year the American Board of Ophthalmology was established to set examinations and issue certificates to fully qualified specialists in ophthalmology. In 1924, a similar American Board of Otolaryngology was established, and in 1932, two more: the American Board of Obstetrics and Gynecology, and the American Board of Dermatology and Syphilology.

In the absence of such a board, any licensed physician who so desired, regardless of his qualifications or lack of them, could limit his practice to any specialty he chose and hold himself out as a specialist in that field. Clearly a certifying board would serve a useful purpose in distinguishing fully trained and qualified specialists from others merely self-announced. Also, there was a concern in some quarters that if the various specialties did not organize their own certifying boards, the state governments might regulate entrance into the specialties by law as they already regulated entrance into the general practice of medicine. A welter of 48 or 50 different state standards of qualification for each of 15 or 20 specialties was hardly a welcome prospect to a profession which prided itself on freedom from governmental regulation.

These motives were as valid for radiology as for the other specialties, and in 1932 the five nationwide radiological organizations followed the lead of the other specialties and moved toward the organization of an American Board of Radiology. The ARRS, ARS, RSNA, ACR, and A M.A. Section on Radiology each sent three delegates to an organizing meeting to be held in connection with the 1933 A.M.A. meeting, and the American Board of Radiology was formally incorporated on January 31, 1934. The first candidates for board certification were examined in June 1934.

Through the years, control of the Board has remained in the five sponsoring organizations. Standards have been progressively raised, types of certification have multiplied, and the number of board-certified radiologists has grown. In December 1967, there were more than 8300 living diplomates.

To be eligible for certification today, medical applicants must prove good moral and ethical standing in medicine, a license to practice medicine in their state or country of residence, and completion of approved medical school, internship, and residency training. They must limit their practice to radiology. They must pass intensive examinations either in radiology as a whole or in one of its two main branches— diagnostic or therapeutic radiology.

Following World War II, the ABR expanded its field to provide for the certification of radiological physicists. To be eligible for certification a physicist must have at least a master's degree in science, membership in a professional society, and affiliation with an approved department of radiology. Candidates may be examined in radiological physics generally, or in one of its two main branches: (1) X-ray and radium physics or (2) medical nuclear physics. As of 1968, more than 100 physicists had been certified.

American College of Radiology, Second Phase (1935 to Date)

Even though it functioned during its early years primarily as an exclusive honorary society, the logic of events and the concerns of its eminent Fellows increasingly led the American College of Radiology to interest itself in the substantive problems of the specialty.

As early as 1927, for example, the ACR developed a concern with medical economics and with the economic aspects of radiological practice. A national committee on the costs of medical care had been established in Washington, and radiology needed a voice on that committee. Dr. Arthur C. Christie of Washington, D.C., was the radiologist member of the committee; he was also a Fellow of the ACR. To strengthen his role, the ACR established a Commission on Medical Economics with Dr. Christie as chairman. Thus, while the ARRS and RSNA remained the voices of American radiology in professional and scientific matters, the ACR tentatively assumed the role of spokesman on the economic front.

In 1933, as has been noted, the ACR played a central role in planning the American Congress of Radiology, and in 1934 it participated in the founding of the American Board of Radiology. In the latter year, under the presidency of Dr. Henry K. Pancoast of Philadelphia, it also launched a *Bulletin* devoted to economic and educational matters, and it held the third of a series of conferences on the future development of the specialty. In addition to the ACR Commission on Medical Economics, a Commission on Radiological Education and a Commission on Public Instruction actively functioned within the College framework. Dr. Benjamin H. Orndoff of Chicago served as executive secretary, coordinating these rapidly expanding activities.

In 1935, under the leadership of Dr. W. Edward Chamberlain of Philadelphia, the gradual transformation of the College from an honorary society to a functioning professional organization led to a drastic reorganization of the ACR structure. In place of the 1924 objective—"to create a Fellowship among men who have distinguished themselves..."—a new constitution adopted in 1935 cited "the purpose of advancing the science of radiology by means of the study of the economic aspects of radiology and the encouragement of improved educational facilities for radiologists." In addition to Fellows, Honorary Fellows, and Chancellors, the College now began to admit ordinary members. A new post of Chairman of the Board of Chancellors was established for Dr. Chamberlain, and under his vigorous leadership from 1935 to 1940 total membership rose from about 200 to more than 1,000. Beginning in 1939, all diplomates of the American Board of Radiology became eligible for membership. Ten classes of membership are now recognized, including physicists as well as radiologists. The membership at the beginning of 1968 consisted of nearly 6800 radiologists, plus 1500 in other categories.

One major reason for this thoroughgoing transformation of the ACR was the growing concern of radiologists for the economic future of their specialty. The Great Depression had affected them as it had affected other groups. The very rapid rise of Blue Cross and of other medical prepayment and insurance plans during the years of economic recovery had greatly expanded the role of the hospital on the American medical scene. "Hospitals were increasingly demanding that radiologists should be only employees of hospitals and that radiology must be considered a purely ancillary hospital service," wrote Dr. Goin in Los Angeles in his manuscript history of the ACR already cited.[12] There was also a concern among many radiologists that plans for a nationwide health insurance program then under discussion in Washington might impair their traditional fee-for-service relations with patients. In these and many other matters, radiologists needed a strong voice. The continuing rivalry between the ARRS and RSNA made it difficult for either of them to speak for radiology as a whole. Following its 1935 reorganization, the ACR increasingly stepped into this breach.

California radiologists were particularly alarmed by prospective changes in medical economics, for their state was the battleground of Upton Sinclair's EPIC (End Poverty in California) movement with its proposal to provide all medical services out of tax funds. In February 1936, accordingly, the Pacific Roentgen Society instructed one of its leaders, Dr. Goin, to propose to the ACR Board of Chancellors the formation of a new Intersociety Committee for Radiology, capable of speaking for the entire specialty on radiologist-hospital relationships, Blue Cross-Blue Shield relationships, compulsory health insurance, and other economic issues. This Western proposal was accepted, and from 1937 to 1939 the ACR, ARRS, ARS, RSNA, and A.M.A. Section on Radiology jointly supported an Intersociety Committee—yet another step toward healing the 1915 breach. A "war chest" was collected to finance the committee's activities, and an executive secretary was employed—perhaps the first full-time employee of any American radiological organization.

In 1939, this rather cumbersome interlocking-committee arrangement was superceded by an interlocking-directorate arrangement. The ARRS, ARS, and RSNA each elected one representative to the ACR board, so that the ACR became, in effect, the united voice of all of the organizations on economic issues. The ACR also took over the executive secretary of the Intersociety Committee. This arrangement continues to date, and the paid staff of the ACR continues to provide certain joint services for the other societies.

Currently the ACR engages in a very wide range of activities through its Board of Chancellors, its Council, and its Commissions and committees. Major areas of concern include standards in radiological practice, standards and protection, education, public health, health insurance, technologist affairs, and radiological units. More than 100 delegates, known as councilors, maintain a close relationship between the College and its members and their local radiological organizations, including 46 statewide ACR chapters and one in the District of Columbia. The ACR also maintains a Professional Bureau to assist residents and young radiologists in finding appointments. A Liaison Committee to Medical Care Insurance Plans represents radiology in this important field. Headquarters are maintained in Chicago. Affiliated with the ACR are the American College of Radiology Foundation and the Foundation Museum, also in Chicago.

The pomp and circumstance of Fellowship have been maintained, and election to Fellowship in the College remains a high radiological honor; indeed, the ceremonial aspects have taken on a new depth and significance against the background of the vigorous College activities in so many other fields.

Canadian Association of Radiologists—Association Canadienne des Radiologists (CAR-ACR) (1937 to Date)

As early as 1901, it will be recalled, the Roentgen Society of the United States changed its name to the Roentgen Society of America in order to welcome Canadian members, and all the leading American radiological societies ever since have welcomed Canadian radiologists, not only to membership, but to leadership roles.

In addition, Canadian radiologists formed their own association in 1937 at the invitation of Dr. G. E. Richards of Toronto General Hospital. The CAR now maintains headquarters in Montreal and has more than 800 members.

The establishment of the CAR, however, has not lessened the participation of Canadian radiologists in American organizations. The roster of society presidents and committee chairmen is liberally sprinkled with the names of eminent Canadian radiologists. The leading American societies hold their annual meetings in Canadian as well as United States cities. Thus, radiology in the United States and Canada remains an almost seamless web.

In addition, however, English-speaking and French-speaking Canadian radiologists continue to maintain close ties with British and French radiology, and with other Canadian medical organizations. To cite a relevant example, membership in the CAR is open alike to radiologists certified by the Royal College of Physicians and Surgeons of Canada, the American Board of Radiology, or the British Faculty of Radiologists.

Journal of the Canadian Association of Radiologists—Journal de l'Association Canadienne des Radiologists (1950 to Date)

This quarterly, the official organ of the CAR, publishes articles in English or French with summaries in the other language. Canadian radiologists publish reports of their work in it, but many, in addition, publish also in the British, French, and American radiological periodicals.

Following World War II, a major expansion occurred in the field of radiology. To the two conventional sources of ionizing radiation—the X-ray tube and radium—were added a host of new artificially produced radioisotopes arising out of research into the nature of atomic nuclei and out of World War II military needs. The invention of nuclear reactors and of many new kinds of particle accelerators also opened new realms for radiology. Part IV of this volume, below, is concerned with these developments.

It may here be noted, however, that the artificial radioisotopes and the particle accelerators produced significant changes in the organizational structure of American radiology, and stimulated additional periodicals. The old-line organizations—the ARRS, ARS, RSNA, ACR, and A.M.A. Section on Radiology—all developed a growing interest in the new fields, but, in addition, new organizations were founded to meet the needs of nonradiologists concerned with nuclear medicine and related topics. These organizations in turn launched new periodicals. The major examples are cited below.

National Committee on Radiological Protection and Measurements (NCRP) (1946 to 1965)

Prior to World War II, as noted above, the organization primarily concerned with radiation safeguards was the Advisory Committee on X-Ray and Radium Protection, launched jointly in 1929 by the ARRS, RSNA, and National Bureau of Standards. This relatively narrow base was clearly inadequate to face the vast new problems of radiation protection arising out of the new scientific developments and out of the many new nonmedical applications of ionizing radiation. Accordingly, the old Advisory Committee was superceded in 1946 by the National Committee on Radiation Protection and Measurements (NCRP), with 51 members representing 20 professional societies and government agencies. The National Committee became The National Council on Radiation Protection and Measurements in 1965, with nearly 150 members, under a Congressional charter as a Federal nonprofit organization. The publications of the NCRP are the authoritative guides to radiation protection in the United States today. In addition, however, a number of other government agencies have a concern with radiation safeguards, notably the National Center for Radiological Health of the U.S. Public Health Service, the National Academy of Sciences—National Research Council (NAS-NRC), and the Atomic Energy Commission (AEC). A cabinet-level Federal Radiation Council, established in 1959, coordinates Federal government activities with respect to radiation protection. These and subsequent developments are described in more detail below (pages 422–424).

SOCIETY OF NUCLEAR MEDICINE (SNM) (1954 TO DATE)

While the old-line radiological organizations provided a forum for radiologists interested in the medical uses of the newly available artificial radioisotopes, a wide range of physicians actively engaged in using isotopes for research or for diagnosis and treatment of disease were not radiologists and hence not eligible for membership in the ARRS, RSNA, and ACR. Primarily to meet the needs of these nonradiologists—though radiologists, too, were included among the founders and members—the Society of Nuclear Medicine was launched in 1954. Its growth was rapid, to 1250 members in 1959 and to more than 1700 in 1961. Major advances in nuclear medicine are reported at its annual meetings, which feature the Ernest O. Lawrence Memorial Lecture.

Journal of Nuclear Medicine (1960 to Date)

Despite the fact that the ARRS *American Journal of Roentgenology and Radiation Therapy* added *Nuclear Medicine* to its title and scope in 1952, and despite the concern of the RSNA's monthly publication, *Radiology*, with nuclear medicine, the Society of Nuclear Medicine also felt a need for a publication of its own. It established the *Journal of Nuclear Medicine* as a quarterly in 1960, under the editorship of Dr. George E. Thoma of St. Louis. This journal became a bi-monthly in 1962.

HEALTH PHYSICS SOCIETY (1955 TO DATE)

While the old-line radiological societies all admitted physicists to membership after World War II, they tended to attract primarily physicists associated with the radiological departments of universities and hospitals. The introduction of high-voltage accelerators and nuclear reactors and the growing concern with protons, neutrons, electrons, mesons, and other forms of radiation attracted a far broader group of physicists concerned with radiation and radiation protection—men employed by government agencies, by industrial firms, and by university and hospital departments outside of radiology. To meet the needs of this broader group, the Health Physics Society was established in 1955, under the leadership of Dr. Karl Z. Morgan of Oak Ridge National Laboratory. By 1957, it had attracted 900 members from the United States and other countries. In 1968, it had more than 3000 members in 39 countries; 7 local chapters were active in the United States. In 1966, the Health Physics Society became an affiliate of the International Radiation Protection Association—an organization with 16 affiliates and with individual members in more than 50 countries.

Health Physics (1958 to Date)

In 1958 the Health Physics Society established its own journal, *Health Physics,* under the editorship of Dr. Karl Z. Morgan.

AMERICAN BOARD OF HEALTH PHYSICS (1959 TO DATE)

While the American Board of Radiology certifies diplomates in radiological physics as well as in radiology, its certification is limited to physicists associated with radiological departments; its examinations are concerned primarily with the knowledge and training required for work in medical radiology. Members of the Health Physics Society, in contrast, are concerned with many other aspects of radiation protection— the control of radiation hazards associated with nuclear reactors, with isotope separation plants, with high energy accelerators, and with industrial radioisotope applications, for example. In 1960, accordingly, the Health Physics Society established the American Board of Health Physics to provide certification in this broader field. By 1968, it had certified more than 460 health physicists.[15]

The establishment of these newer groups—the Society of Nuclear Medicine, Health Physics Society, and American Board of Health Physics—did not represent a schism comparable to the earlier schism between the ARRS and RSNA, but it did raise problems of cooperation and coordination which have not as yet been fully solved.

OTHER RADIOLOGICAL AND ANCILLARY ORGANIZATIONS

In addition to national organizations, there are more than 100 local, statewide, and regional radiological organizations and groups. Among the oldest is the Philadelphia Roentgen Society, established in 1905. The large regional societies include the New England Roentgen Ray Society, the Eastern Conference of Radiologists, the Section on Radiology of the Southern Medical Association, the Southern Radiological Conference, the Rocky Mountain Radiological Society, and the Pacific Northwest Radiological Society.

Radiologists sharing a common professional interest have also, in recent years, established organizations of their own. Examples are the Association of University Radiologists (1953), the Society for Pediatric Radiology, (1958), and the American Society of Therapeutic Radiologists (1961). For dentists specially concerned with X-ray procedures there is the American Academy of Oral Roentgenology (1951).

The technicians employed by radiologists and radiological departments also have their organizations and publication. The first of these was the American Society of X-Ray Technicians, established in 1920 and now known as the American Society of Radiologic Technologists. It has more than 12,000 members and publishes the bimonthly *Radiologic Technology*. The comparable Canadian organization is the Canadian Society of Radiological Technicians.

The American Registry of Radiologic Technologists is a certifying body sponsored jointly by the American College of Radiology and the American Society of Radiologic Technologists. The 55,000 applicants who have passed its qualifying examinations are entitled to call themselves "registered technologists," and to use the initials "R.T."

REFERENCES

1. *Amer. X-Ray J., 7:* no. 6, pp. 12–13, 1900.
2. ANON., *The American Roentgen Ray Society, 1900–1950,* pp. 5–6. Charles C Thomas, Publisher, Springfield, Illinois, 1950.
3. For these and many other details below, see KRABBENHOFT, K., "History of Radiologic Journals." In BRUWER, A. J., *Classic Descriptions in Diagnostic Roentgenology,* pp. 1991–2029. Charles C Thomas, Publisher, Springfield, Illinois, 1964.
4. *Amer. X-Ray J., 7:* no. 2, p. 10, 1900.
5. *Trans. Amer. Roentgen Ray Soc.,* 1902–1908.
6. *Amer. J. Roentgen., 76:* 1–6, 1956.
7. *Amer. J. Roentgen., 3:* 105, 1916.
8. ERNST, E. C., Unpublished papers.
9. *Amer. J. Roentgen., 2:* 618, 1915.
10. *Ibid.,* p. 873.
11. *Radiology, 83:* 771–784, 1964.
12. GOIN, L. S., Personal communication.
13. *Radiology, 45:* 549–554, 1945.
14. *Health Phys., 1:* 3–10, 1958.
15. Membership figures throughout this chapter are based on personal communications from officers of radiological societies.

PART IV. RADIOLOGY IN THE NUCLEAR ERA

   The 1918 Beginnings

Three events have often been cited as marking the dawn of the nuclear age. The earliest was on December 2, 1942, when the first nuclear reactor—an "atomic pile" of uranium and graphite, designed by Enrico Fermi and his associates and erected in a squash court on the University of Chicago campus—"went critical." The second occurred on July 16, 1945, when the first atomic explosion was set off over the uninhabited desert sands at Alamogordo, New Mexico. The third event followed just 3 weeks later, on August 6, 1945, when the first atomic bomb was detonated in deadly earnest over the city of Hiroshima, Japan (population 300,000). However, in a history of radiology, the story must begin much earlier—with a classic experiment performed at the Cavendish Laboratory in Cambridge, England, by Ernest Rutherford back in 1918, while World War I was still raging.

Rutherford's experiment had a simplicity strongly reminiscent of Roentgen's pioneering discovery.[1] He placed a bit of radium in a container, filled the container with oxygen, and mounted a zinc sulfide screen nearby. Alpha particles emitted by the radium struck the zinc sulfide screen and produced on its surface pinpoints of light called *scintillations*. By watching the screen through a microscope, Rutherford could observe and even count the scintillations (Fig. 35).

Next Rutherford placed enough silver foil between the container and the zinc sulfide screen to block the alpha rays. The scintillations ceased. Finally, he substituted nitrogen for the oxygen in the container. Despite the continuing presence of the silver-foil barrier, scintillations reappeared on the zinc sulfide screen. Something different was now being emitted from the nitrogen-filled container—something capable of penetrating a barrier impervious to alpha rays.

What were these emanations, and where did they come from? They were deflected when a magnet was brought near them, proving that they were not X rays. By further studying their behavior in electrical and magnetic fields, Rutherford was able to identify them as positively charged nuclear particles—protons.

Further deductive reasoning by Rutherford and an associate, James Chadwick, reconstructed the process which must have been going on inside the container. The nitrogen nucleus, they knew, contains seven

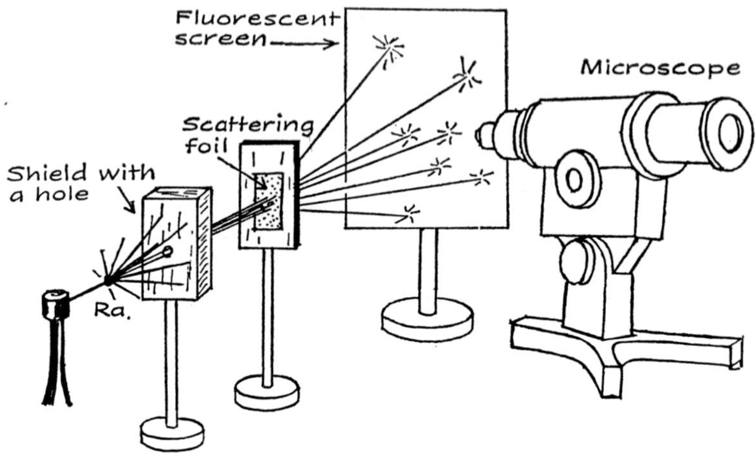

FIG. 35. From GAMOW, GEORGE, *The Atom and the Nucleus,* p. 26. Prentice-Hall, Inc., Englewood Cliffs, New Jersey, 1961.

protons, and the alpha particle emitted by the radium contains two protons. When an alpha particle struck a nitrogen nucleus in the Rutherford experiment, one proton was ejected. The remainder of the nitrogen atom and the alpha particle joined together to form a new atom with eight protons—that is, an oxygen atom. Rutherford had thus achieved the goal of the medieval alchemists: transmutation of elements. An atom of nitrogen bombarded by an alpha particle had been converted to an atom of oxygen plus a left-over proton, ejected at high energy.[2]

During the 1920's, countless variations on this basic Rutherford experiment were performed in many laboratories, and the foundations of nuclear physics were thus laid. Not only was it possible to convert one familiar element like nitrogen into another like oxygen; bombardment also produced previously unknown species of matter—*isotopes* of the familiar elements, having the same numbers of protons and electrons, but different atomic weights. The oxygen produced in Rutherford's initial experiment, for example, was not ordinary oxygen-16, with an atomic weight of 16, but rather a heavier isotope, oxygen-17. A whole new world, it seemed, might be hidden in the interior of the atom.

Unfortunately, only a few tantalizing glimpses into this new realm could be secured during the 1920's, because of the inherent limitations of radium and the other radioactive elements as sources of bombarding particles. In the first place, the alpha particles emitted by radium carry a strong positive electrical charge—twice the charge of a proton. They are therefore strongly repelled by the positive electrical field surrounding the nucleus. Moreover, the emission of an alpha particle by an atom of radium is a relatively rare event. Thus, transmutations could be produced only a few atoms at a time. A nuclear chemist, Dr. Martin D. Kamen, recalls that in the course of experiments of this kind at Yale as late as 1933, it took him "three years of constant labor to produce and analyse a few hundred proton recoils—in fact, ten man-hours per track had been required! This statistic shows how slender were the means available for researches in nuclear physics. . . ." [3] To learn more about the nucleus, and to produce the fascinating new isotopes on a useful scale, a far richer source of bombarding particles was urgently needed—a source which would yield vast quantities of high energy electrons, protons, and perhaps other particles as well for bombardment experiments.

By 1928, accordingly, laboratories in many countries were consciously engaged in a sort of scientific race to see which would be the first to develop "particle accelerators" or "atom-smashers" capable of speeding up subatomic particles to the energies required for effective nuclear bombardment. The starting point of this race was inevitably the one kind of particle accelerator already familiar to physicists: the X-ray tube itself.

Conventional X-ray tubes accelerate electrons to a speed of 93,000 miles per second—half the speed of light—when operating at energies as low as 75,000 volts. Energies of 200,000 volts were readily available from 1920 on. Early efforts of physicists were accordingly devoted to the design of X-ray tubes which would operate at even higher voltages, producing electrons of even higher speeds and energies. Chapter 23 describes how these "supervoltage" X-ray tubes were designed and built, and how radiologists soon secured access to them, or to modifications of them, for use in radiation therapy.

By the early 1930's, however, the inherent limitations of the conventional X-ray tube and its conventional power supply for nuclear research came to be recognized; hence, physicists went on to develop ingenious new devices to meet their own research needs: the electrostatic generator, the linear accelerator, the cyclotron, the betatron, and the synchrotron, to name only a few. Chapter 23 traces how these new devices, too, were one by one adapted for radiological use.

Some of the new devices were electron accelerators; they could therefore be used to produce X rays of extremely high energy. Could these new "supervoltage" X rays accomplish more than conventional X rays in the treatment or cure of disease? Chapter 23 reviews the laborious efforts, continuing for a quarter-century, to secure a reliable answer to that question.

The new devices also opened wholly new therapeutic doors. They could be used, for example, to hurl beams of high-energy electrons, protons, neutrons, and even heavier particles—atomic nuclei—*directly* into human tissue, such as cancer tissue. Chapter 24 reviews how radiologists have been exploring these new modes of therapy as well.

Finally, both the particle accelerators and the nuclear reactors have made available many hundreds of new kinds of isotopes, at first in trivial quantities, later in very large quantities at low cost. Many of these new isotopes proved to be themselves radioactive—emitting not only the familiar alpha particles, beta particles, and gamma rays emitted by radium, but also neutrons, positrons, and other particles whose very existence was unsuspected when the race for higher voltages began. Chapter 25 describes how radioisotopes have in their turn been harnessed for radiological uses, both diagnostic and therapeutic.

REFERENCES

1. *Phil. Mag. (London)*, 6th series, *37:* 537–580, 1919.
2. *Phil. Mag. (London)*, 6th series, *42:* 809–825, 1921.
3. *J. Chem. Educ., 40:* 234–242, 1963.

23 Supervoltage

THE PHYSICISTS RACE TOWARD HIGHER VOLTAGE

Scores of scientists in many countries participated in the development of high-energy particle accelerators. The early work of four Americans—W. D. Coolidge, Charles C. Lauritsen, Robert J. Van de Graaff, and Ernest O. Lawrence—will be reviewed here because of its direct relevance to the history of radiology.

W. D. Coolidge

Throughout the 1920's, as has been noted, the 200,000-volt Coolidge X-ray tube was standard equipment for "deep" radiation therapy. No doubt some radiologists would have liked X rays of even higher voltage, but these were not easy to produce. Dr. Coolidge explained why.

"Early in our work on the hot-cathode high-vacuum X-ray tube," he recalled in 1928, "we were made conscious of a certain limitation. Such a tube behaved consistently only so long as a certain applied voltage was not exceeded. When this voltage *was* exceeded, current flowed through the tube even when the cathode was not heated." [1]

This current flow is known as the "cold-cathode effect" or the "field-current effect." As Dr. Coolidge explained, it "sets a limit to the voltage which can be used on a given tube, for if one attempts to appreciably raise voltage in spite of it, he either punctures the tube, through the local heating attending bombardment of the glass, or gets a runaway arc discharge, through bombardment of the anode.

"In our earlier attempts to build experimental X-ray and cathode ray tubes for voltages appreciably in excess of 250,000, we have seemed to be continually contending with and limited by the 'cold-cathode' effect."

By 1926, however, Coolidge had developed a method to limit this effect which was subsequently used also by several of his successors. [2] Coolidge called his new tube the "cascade" tube, and it was built in sections. An electron leaving the cathode went through one of these sections and then another en route to the anode. Each section might operate at 250,000 or even 300,000 volts; thus, a three-section tube might reach 900,000 volts without the need for a potential in excess of 300,000 volts at any single point in its interior.

Dr. Coolidge described this new tube in some detail to an audience of

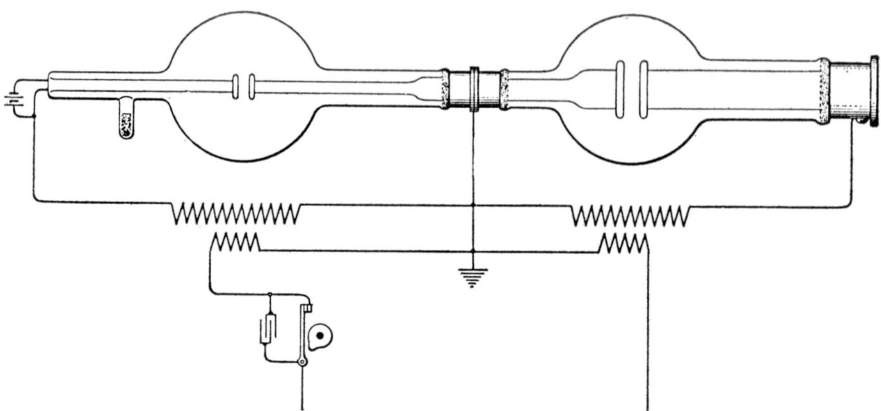

FIG. 36. From *American Journal of Roentgenology, 19:* 315, 1928.

radiologists at the Montreal meeting of the American Roentgen Ray Society in September 1927.[3] One model consisted of two cascaded sections, each operating at 300,000 volts (Fig. 36).

"As the anode of the first section is electrically connected to the cathode of the second section," Dr. Coolidge reported, "the composite tube may be considered as having three electrodes which may be referred to as a cathode, intermediate electrode, and anode. Experiment shows that the tube will stand the highest voltage when the applied potential difference is divided equally between the two sections ... by connecting the intermediate electrode to the electrical center of the high-voltage circuit."

Dr. Coolidge also showed a picture of a three-section cascade tube capable of operating at 900,000 volts. It was essentially the same except that it contained two intermediate electrodes. "... It seems reasonable to hope," he concluded, "that a cascade type of tube can be developed for as high a potential difference as can be produced, and work will be continued along this line."

At a meeting of electrical engineers a few months later, Dr. Coolidge indicated that his new high-voltage tube held promise for nuclear research as well as for radiology. It should prove easy, he declared, to produce with such a tube X rays as penetrating as the gamma rays from radium, and it might even be possible to produce electrons at 3,000,000 volts, equivalent to the beta rays from radium. Moreover, "the capacity or quantity factor would be tremendously in our favor, as with 12 milliamperes of current we would have as many high-speed electrons coming from the tube as from a *ton* of radium." [1] This, of course, was precisely what the nuclear physicists and nuclear chemists needed to speed their experiments and shorten their vigils.

However, there were difficulties in the way. Despite use of the cascade principle, Dr. Coolidge's 1927 three-section tube was nearly 11 feet long, and, even so, the glass was occasionally punctured by runaway cold-cathode currents. A very high vacuum was needed—so high that, to maintain it, a vacuum pump attached to the tube had to be kept in continuous operation while the current was on. Dr. Coolidge used an induction coil as his source of high voltage, and this made difficulties, too. The output of the coil was an alternating current, which meant that maximum voltage was achieved only at the peak of each cycle. Finally, the tube that Dr. Coolidge described in 1927 produced high-voltage electrons but not X rays; further engineering would be needed to bring the electrons into focus on a target—and to devise a target capable of withstanding bombardment by 900,000-volt electrons. Nearly 3 more years were to elapse before the first General Electric cascade tube was ready for delivery.

Charles C. Lauritsen

At the California Institute of Technology, meanwhile, Dr. Charles C. Lauritsen entered the race for higher voltages with a head start. During the early 1920's, the Southern California Edison Company had established a high-voltage laboratory at Caltech to study problems of long-distance electric power transmission; in 1925 an engineer in this laboratory, Professor R. W. Sorenson, had cascaded four 250,000-volt transformers to produce a peak potential of 1,000,000 volts.[4] Professor Sorenson and Dr. Robert A. Millikan, who headed Caltech, made this transformer array available to Dr. Lauritsen, and in 1928 he and his research assistant, R. D. Bennett, reported on its use to produce 750,000-volt X rays.[5]

"The radiation is very powerful," they declared, "and can be observed by means of a fluoroscope at a distance of 100 meters [328 feet]."

However, Dr. Lauritsen's initial equipment had shortcomings, too. The transformer array, for example, was hardly likely to whet the appetite of a practicing radiologist for a similar installation. It occupied a room 138 feet long and 64 feet wide, with a ceiling 50 feet high—and even so, one of the four transformers had to be placed in a pit "in order to get sufficient overhead clearance." The tube was made of four glass cylinders, "each 12 inches in diameter and 28 inches long, of the kind used in gasoline dispensing pumps." To support his tube, Lauritsen found it necessary to erect "a tower 14 feet high and 8 feet square at the base, constructed of redwood timber crossed and braced to give rigidity"

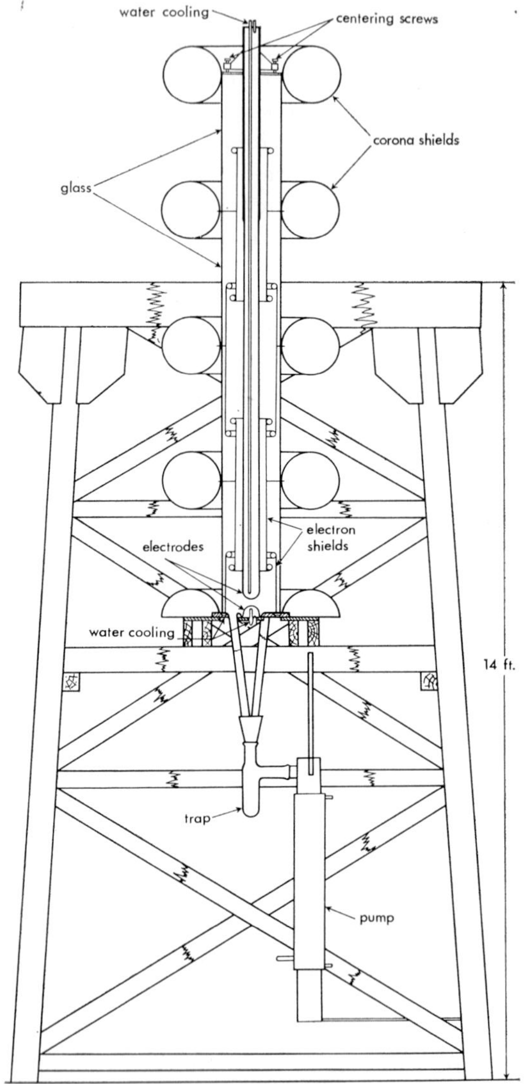

Fig. 37. From *Physical Review, 32:* 852, 1928.

(Fig. 37). Like Coolidge's tube, Lauritsen's required continuous pumping to maintain the vacuum, and it achieved maximum power only during the peak of each alternating-current cycle.

Robert J. Van de Graaff

In Europe, too, high-energy variations on conventional voltage sources and discharge tubes were being studied and tested, but the dimensions and costs involved were high and seemed likely soon to become prohibitive. Altogether new approaches were clearly needed. One of the earliest and most ingenious of these new approaches was devised by Robert J. Van de Graaff (1901–1967).

While still a Rhodes scholar studing under Ernest Rutherford at Oxford in 1927 and 1928, young Van de Graaff had become fascinated by the high-voltage problem, and on his return to Princeton as a National Research Fellow he built in 1929 a "hastily improvised" [6] little device which he had recently thought up. This device, the electrostatic generator, belonged to the same family of devices as the old "static machine" used as a source of electrical potential for X rays in 1896. When his first electrostatic generator proved successful, he built a second model which he described at the September 1931 meeting of the American Physical Society in Schenectady, New York. [7]

This second electrostatic generator, unlike Coolidge's and Lauritsen's elaborate installations, cost Van de Graaff only about $100 for parts, yet "in recent preliminary trials," he told his fellow physicists, "spark-gap measurements showed a potential of approximately 1,500,000 volts.... The generator has the basic advantage of supplying a direct steady potential, thus eliminating certain difficulties inherent in the application of non-steady [alternating-current or pulsating-current] high potentials. The machine is simple, inexpensive, and portable. An ordinary lamp socket furnishes the only power needed."

Van de Graaff's curious device consisted essentially of two hollow copper spheres, each 24 inches in diameter, mounted on two upright Pyrex pedestals 7 feet tall. A continuous silk belt, mounted on two pulleys, ran up and down each pedestal at 3500 feet per minute. These "conveyor belts" were run by a toy motor. The lower pulleys were grounded. An array of metal points (Van de Graaff used phonograph needles) sprayed electrons and other negatively charged ions onto one of the conveyor belts. The belt carried the negative ions to the top of the pedestal where another set of points picked them off for storage on the surface of the copper sphere. Simultaneously, a second set of points was spraying protons and other positively charged ions onto the second belt, and these were being simultaneously carried up and stored on the second sphere. Since each sphere could be charged to 750,000 volts, a potential of 1,500,000 volts could be built up between them. [6] It was fortunate that Van de Graaff was able to assemble his gadget with $100 worth of parts, for it hardly seems likely that any responsible agency would have financed so implausible a device at the behest of an unknown young inventor.

Once the device was demonstrated, however, its advantages were obvious. Among those present at the Schenectady meeting where Van de

Graaff described his model was President Karl T. Compton of the Massachusetts Institute of Technology,[8] who had known and encouraged Van de Graaff at Princeton. Dr. Compton hired Van de Graaff for M.I.T. without delay, and the next report on the Van de Graaff generator, completed in 1932, was signed by an M.I.T. team composed of Van de Graaff, Compton, and L. C. Van Atta.

However, electrostatic generators, like their predecessors, were soon plagued by growing size and rising costs. A model described in 1933, for example, was too big to be built at M.I.T. in Cambridge; Compton therefore arranged to have it constructed in the largest unused structure he could find—an airship hangar 140 feet long, 75 feet wide, and 75 feet high, located on the estate of Colonel E. H. R. Green at Round Hill, Massachusetts. The 24-inch spheres of the earlier model were superseded by spheres of aluminum alloy 15 feet in diameter, with walls $\frac{1}{4}$ inch thick. Multiple belts instead of only two carried ions up to the spheres. The inside of one sphere was a laboratory provided with a floor and containing accessory apparatus. At one time it was contemplated that an X-ray tube would be mounted between the spheres, and that radiologists would treat their patients inside one of them. The generator was "mobile" in a sense, for it was mounted on very wide railroad trucks, and a quarter of a mile of track with rails 14 feet apart, donated by the New Haven Railroad, was laid into the hangar so that the device could be wheeled in and out on the trucks.

This generator was completed in 1934 and achieved a potential of 7,000,000 volts, but additional time was needed to create an X-ray tube capable of handling that much energy.

Ernest O. Lawrence

While Van de Graaff was still at Princeton designing his first preliminary model, another brilliant young American physicist, Dr. Ernest Orlando Lawrence (1901–1958) of the University of California at Berkeley, was pondering several even more revolutionary solutions to the high-voltage problem.

During the summer of 1929, Lawrence was browsing casually through some physics journals in the university library[9] when he came upon a paper by a European physicist, Rolf Wideröe,[10] which described how a 25,000-volt potential could be used twice to produce 50,000-volt particles in a discharge tube. The trick was a simple one. Like Coolidge, Wideröe divided his tube into sections, but he did not connect his intermediate electrode to the middle tap of his power supply. Instead, he applied the whole voltage twice—once as the particle was moving through the gap between electrodes in the first section, and again as it was moving through the gap in the second section. A high-frequency alternating potential was used, and the circuits were arranged so that the electrical potential changed polarity in just the time that it took the particle to pass from gap to gap. Thus, the two "pushes" received by the particle were in the same direction.

Lawrence's fertile mind promptly developed variations on Wideröe's promising technique, and he set his graduate students to work on several of them. One student, David H. Sloan, was soon accelerating particles through a series of 10 cylindrical electrodes mounted in line inside a discharge tube, and in December 1930, Sloan and Lawrence reported on a linear accelerator of this kind which accelerated particles by means of 30 successive electrodes.[11] Positive ions rather than electrons were accelerated in these devices. Such an ion, when it reached the gap between the first and second electrodes, was in effect leaving a positive electrode and approaching a negative one; it was therefore accelerated as it crossed the gap just as an electron would be accelerated in a conventional X-ray tube. By the time it reached the next gap, the polarity had changed, and it was again leaving a positive electrode for a negative one. Hence, it was accelerated again. To keep the particle in phase with an alternating potential as its speed increased, the length of the successive tube sections had to be increased. Subsequent linear accelerators were developed for electrons as well as positive ions, and enormous energies have been reached (see pages 353–354).

Lawrence's next contribution to the solution of the high-voltage problem was the *cyclotron,* the first of the circular accelerators.[12, 13] It was built between the pole faces of a powerful electromagnet. The pole faces in most models were circular and parallel to one another. In the space between them a hollow vacuum chamber or "can" was lodged, and in the vacuum chamber were two D-shaped electrodes, familiarly known as "dees," separated by a narrow gap.

The operation of the cyclotron had an esthetic beauty as impressive as the device's utility. Positively charged particles were introduced into the circular vacuum chamber near its axis. The magnetic field caused the particles to begin circling the axis through the two dees. When a particle reached the first gap between the dees, it found itself leaving a positively charged electrode and approaching a negatively charged electrode, just as in the linear accelerator. It was therefore accelerated. Halfway round the circle it reached the next gap. By then the potential had been reversed, as in the linear accelerator, and the particle was accelerated again. The faster it went, the larger the diameter of the path it followed and hence the longer the path. However—and this was the heart of the matter—the longer path did not force the particle out of step with the alternating potential, for, as Lawrence had correctly for-seen, the laws of motion kept the length of the path directly propor-tional to the velocity of the particle, so that particles circling relatively slowly and particles circling rapidly all took exactly the same time to get from one gap to the next.

Eventually the particles, spiralling outward, reached the periphery of the vacuum chamber at maximum energy and were led out through a window or harvested in other ways. Some took many rounds to reach the periphery, others achieved maximum energy in fewer rounds, but all of the particles reached the periphery at substantially the same energy. Thus, the emerging beam was "monoenergetic."

Lawrence's ingenious cyclotron accelerated protons and other posi-tively charged ions rather than electrons, and it therefore could not be used directly for the generation of X rays, yet it was to have a profound effect on the history of radiology. By 1932, a model which Lawrence built with his student, M. Stanley Livingston, proved capable of accel-erating protons to an energy of 1,000,000 volts.

Livingston later recalled Lawrence's "sparkling eyes and dramatic gestures . . . when the small cyclotron at the University of California produced million-volt protons for the first time in scientific history." [9] However, in a formal sense, Lawrence lost the race for a successful "atom-smasher." Just a few months earlier two English researchers, J. D. Cockcroft and E. T. S. Walton at the Cavendish laboratory in Cam-bridge, had reached the goal. Using equipment of their own design, they beamed protons accelerated in a discharge tube at a lithium target. The lithium nucleus, which contains three protons, captured a fourth from the beam to become a beryllium nucleus; this beryllium nucleus then split into two helium nuclei containing two protons each. For the first time, in the language of the day, "the atom had been split" by bombardment with laboratory-accelerated particles. Lawrence and Liv-ingston had to be content to confirm and extend the English findings with their cyclotron.[9]

Far from putting an end to the race, of course, the Cockcroft-Walton achievement injected new vigor into it. Nuclear physics, a relatively unstylish field during the 1920's, quickly rose to the pre-eminence that it still enjoys. Further nuclear discoveries followed in rapid succession. These discoveries made nuclear physicists increasingly eager to build particle accelerators of even greater capabilities. Thus, even today, when accelerators have been built which reach tens of billions of volts, the race for higher energies and improved devices continues toward the hundreds of billions of volts (see page 354).

One of Lawrence's initial goals, voiced in 1931, was to accelerate particles "with quite modest laboratory equipment" [14] rather than with giant machines like Lauritsen's transformer array. Initially he succeeded; his first cyclotron had magnets with pole faces only 4 inches in diameter, and his million-volt protons were produced in a magnet with pole faces only 11 inches in diameter. But soon Lawrence's cyclotron, too, was afflicted by the elephantiasis of its predecessors. Within a few years Lawrence was constructing a cyclotron with a magnet weighing 200 tons and pole faces 60 inches in diameter; far larger and heavier devices followed.

PUTTING SUPERVOLTAGE TO USE

Soiland in Los Angeles

What would happen if "supervoltage" X rays made possible by the new physical apparatus were beamed into human tissues—tumors, for example? Until October 1930, no one knew. No doubt hundreds of radiologists would eagerly have welcomed the first opportunity to find out. The radiologist given the first opportunity was Dr. Albert Soiland of the Soiland Clinic in Los Angeles (now the Los Angeles Tumor Clinic).

When any new form of therapy such as a new mode of radiation first becomes available, effects may be studied initially on physical dummies or "phantoms," then on biological objects such as plant seeds and insect eggs, then on laboratory animals, and ultimately, after these possibilities have been fully explored, cautious human trials may be begun. The approach used by Caltech and Dr. Soiland, however, was much more direct.

"During the summer of 1930," Dr. Soiland told a meeting of the Radiological Society of North America in 1932, "I was invited by Dr. R. A. Millikan and Dr. C. C. Lauritsen of the California Institute of Technology to inspect the high-voltage X-ray tube installation at the Institute. Dr. Lauritsen . . . had succeeded in building a large X-ray tube of glass through which 5 milliamperes of current operated successfully at 750,000 volts. This equipment, which was designed for physical research purposes only, had been in successful operation for many months. It occurred to Dr. Lauritsen that the radiation produced by this tube might have some biological effect which could be utilized in the treatment of disease." [15]

Dr. Soiland reacted to his first look at the Caltech apparatus as Dr. Millikan and Dr. Lauritsen had no doubt expected him to. He requested permission to make use of the tube, and "Dr. Millikan and Dr. Lauritsen agreed, with the consent of the Board of Trustees of the California Institute of Technology, that we be allowed to bring some of our own patients to the Institute for experimental clinical tests.

"The experimental treatment schedule was begun in October 1930. The first patient treated was a middle-aged man with an inoperable adenocarcinoma of the rectum, a patient of Dr. C. Edgerton Carter. The electrical factors for this first experimental treatment were: voltage, 600,000; milliamperes on the tube, 4; filters, 6 mm. of steel and 1 cm. of felt; skin-target distance, 50 centimeters. Those present at the dedication of the Lauritsen tube were Dr. Millikan, Dr. Lauritsen, Dr. Carter, and Dr. Soiland."

Two years after the first treatment, Dr. Soiland was able to report that the patient "has gained 20 pounds in weight, has no pain, and attends his daily duties. The proctologist who has examined him recently says there is but a vestige of the old lesion present." Additional patients followed. "To the clinical radiologist," Dr. Soiland predicted, "the outcome of this research work will be of momentous importance."

Dr. Soiland made no revolutionary claims for the new 600,000-volt therapy, but he did call attention to its potential effects on the practice of radiology. "The cost of equipment and accessories," he pointed out in 1932, at the pit of the great depression, " . . . would vary from $30,000 to $50,000. . . . Such a formidable installation would, in the writer's opinion, be prohibitive for the average radiologist even to consider. It would be more feasible for centralized institutions, geographically selected to serve their respective communities—preferably the larger hospitals having suitable clinical and physical facilities." [15]

While these early clinical trials were going on, W. K. Kellogg, the "breakfast-food king," visited Caltech. The first therapeutic use of 200,-000-volt X rays (see page 290) had taken place at his brother Dr. John Kellogg's Battle Creek Sanitarium in Michigan; Kellogg now gave the money for a W. K. Kellogg Laboratory at Caltech where further supervoltage therapy could be undertaken. By June 1933, patients were being treated in the Kellogg laboratory at 750,000 volts, and by August at 1,000,000 volts. The new Lauritsen tube used was 30 feet long and was made of porcelain instead of glass. It had four ports through which four patients could be treated simultaneously.

The new laboratory was under the direction of Dr. Seeley G. Mudd of Caltech. At the American Congress of Radiology in September 1933, Dr. Mudd and three associates, Dr. Clyde K. Emery of Caltech and Drs. Orville M. Meland and William E. Costolow of the Soiland Clinic, reported on their first 285 patients treated with supervoltage. Patients with inoperable neoplasms of the bladder, prostate, rectum, esophagus, pharynx, and larynx were included.

Skin reactions, the Caltech group reported, were similar to those seen after conventional radiation therapy, although higher doses could be delivered before these reactions made their appearance. It was still too early, they stated, to evaluate clinical results.

Failla in New York

While this work was under way, General Electric in June 1931 installed a Coolidge two-section cascade tube and associated supervoltage power supply at Memorial Hospital in New York City.[16] The Memorial approach was very different from Dr. Soiland's. Exhaustive tests of the new equipment were immediately launched by the director of Memorial's Biophysical Laboratory, Dr. Gioacchino Failla. These tests were designed not only to determine the characteristics of the 700,000-volt X-ray beam from the new apparatus, but also to compare this beam with the beam from the conventional 200,000-volt X-ray apparatus and with the gamma-ray beam from a 44-gram pack of radium.[17]

The first fruits of this research program were presented by Dr. Failla, Dr. Edith H. Quimby, and a dozen other members of the Memorial staff at the September 1932 meeting of the American Roentgen Ray Society. At the conclusion of their presentation, Dr. Henry Schmitz of Chicago declared that it presented "a turning point in cancer radiation therapy." After a third of a century, this accolade requires no modification—but, as described below, it was in some respects a distressing turning point.

Dr. Failla, Dr. Quimby, and their associates described first their efforts to *measure in roentgens* the three kinds of radiation. For this purpose they used half a dozen ionization chambers of various kinds— three made of aluminum, copper, and lead, and three of Celluloid. To their amazement, the results were utterly inconsistent. The number of roentgens varied with the size of the chamber and the material of which it was made.

Next, depth doses were determined in a water "phantom" having approximately the radiation-absorbing characteristics of human tissue. The results left little doubt that 700,000-volt radiation delivered a higher dose to deeper layers as compared with the surface dose than did 200,000-volt radiation, but the phenomenon proved to be quite complex, and subject to a number of variables.

With scrupulous care and much labor, the Memorial group next compared the effects of the three kinds of radiation on five different radiation-sensitive chemical solutions and on photographic films with and without intensifying screens. The results could only be described as capricious. " . . . It is evident," the Memorial group concluded, "that the *apparent* radiation emission . . . varies with the chemicals and reactions which are used to determine it."

Biological measures of relative effectiveness were also studied. Fruit-fly eggs, wheat seedlings, mouse tails, and rabbit ears were all irradiated under comparable conditions by the three kinds of rays. Here the results were on the whole consistent. It was possible to conclude that the relative biological effectiveness of 700,000-volt radiation on these test objects fell somewhere between the effectiveness of 200,000-volt radiation and of gamma radiation from radium.

Now tests were made on human skin. The forearms of patients were irradiated under standardized conditions with the three kinds of rays. Here again, consistent results were secured—but the comparisons made on human skin proved quite inconsistent with the comparisons made on fruit-fly eggs, wheat seedlings, and mouse tails.

Finally, clinical observations based on actual therapeutic trials were reported. These trials had begun in October 1931. During the early months, patients with osteogenic sarcoma and with carcinoma of the lung, breast, stomach, and rectum were irradiated. Small doses were used initially, and these were gradually increased. Skin reactions could be readily evaluated, but with these tumors the reaction of the tumor itself could for the time being only be guessed.

Beginning in March 1932, therefore, trials were run on visible carcinomas of the larynx, pharynx, hypopharynx, and tonsil. The Memorial team concluded that with 700,000-volt X rays given in divided doses, as compared with 200,000-volt X rays given in the same way, "the present indications are that at least the same results can be obtained *using a dosage which causes considerably less discomfort to the patient locally and generally."* *

Here was the first clear indication that supervoltage might have an advantage in actual clinical practice. It was therefore of great historic significance in encouraging further trials of supervoltage. However, it was subject to two obvious limitations. The evaluation of "discomfort to the patient" was at best a clinical impression. Also, the tumors were relatively superficial; the effects on deep tumors remained undetermined.

In summarizing the Memorial findings, Dr. Failla came directly to the point.[17] The question is not, he stressed, whether one kind of ray is more effective than another in killing cancer cells. That is almost immaterial. The therapeutic question is whether a *wider margin of difference* between the effect on cancer cells and on surrounding tissue can be secured at one voltage than at another. The Memorial findings indicated that the margin of difference might or might not be the same. A wider margin was at least possible, and this was good news. However, the findings also indicated that the task of determining the margin at various voltages

* Italics added.

would be far slower and far more laborious than anyone could have anticipated.

Thus, far from leading radiation therapy into the promised land, the preliminary Memorial findings in a sense made it seem even more distant. Before the Memorial results were announced, radiologists dealt with what they thought was a complex art, requiring considerations of dose measurement, dose fractionation, filtration, skin-target distance, multiple portals, and other variables (see Chapter 20). However, the variables were at least *measurable,* and radiologists believed that they had one rock on which to stand: the roentgen. To paraphrase Gertrude Stein, "a roentgen was a roentgen was a roentgen"—until 1932. Now the rock had turned to quicksand. The effect of a 1-roentgen dose delivered to fruit-fly eggs was not the same as one delivered to human skin. A 1-roentgen dose delivered at 700,000 volts differed from one delivered at 200,000 volts. Indeed, a roentgen was seen not to be a measure of dosage at all. Worst of all, a roentgen measured with one device was not the same as a roentgen measured with another. The already complex art of radiation therapy had suddenly become vastly *more* complex. More than a quarter-century was to be required to re-establish firm physical and biological foundations for the art of radiation therapy.

The Memorial Hospital installation nevertheless evoked, as might be expected, a considerable demand for high-voltage X-ray units from other medical centers. Custom-built units rated at from 500,000 to 1,000,000 volts were placed in operation at Lincoln Hospital in Lincoln, Nebraska, in April 1933, at Harper Hospital in Detroit in September 1933, at Mercy Hospital—Loyola University Clinics in Chicago in October 1933, at Swedish Hospital in Seattle in January 1934, and at the University of California School of Medicine in San Francisco in May 1934. In 1935 General Electric introduced a 400,000-volt stock model; by 1936 Dr. Otto Glasser of the Cleveland Clinic could describe 10 such units, some made by GE and some by other companies, installed in hospitals and medical centers within a few hundred miles of Cleveland.[18]

Leucutia in Detroit

The Harper Hospital unit in Detroit and the University of California School of Medicine unit in San Francisco merit further description. The former was assembled by the Kelley-Koett Manufacturing Company for Dr. Traian Leucutia in 1932 and was similar in conception to the device with which Cockroft and Walton had first "split the atom" that same year. Six transformers, each with its own rectifier array, were cascaded to produce a 900,000-volt direct-current supply with very little "ripple" or irregularity. This current was fed into an anode-grounded Lauritsen-type porcelain tube 13 feet long, having a capacity of 650,000 volts. Because the current was direct and steady, however, the X rays emitted were on the average much "harder" than a 650,000-volt beam from an alternating-current tube. During the years after 1932, a series of scholarly papers by Dr. Leucutia and his Harper Hospital physicists, Dr. Kenneth E. Corrigan and Dr. Benedict Cassen, not only reported on findings made with this apparatus but also comprehensively reviewed supervoltage developments elsewhere.[19] Many of the details in this chapter are drawn from the Leucutia-Corrigan-Cassen papers.

Stone in San Francisco

The other unusual installation was a high-frequency device designed by David H. Sloan of the University of California Radiation Laboratory—Lawrence's laboratory—as part of the UCRL drive for high-voltage particle accelerators (see page 341).[20] Lawrence's cyclotron proved superior for nuclear research, but the Sloan high-frequency system had obvious practical advantages for radiology. It consisted essentially of a cylindrical vacuum tank only 40 inches high and 42 inches in diameter, in which were lodged both the high-energy source and the X-ray generator (Fig. 38). Indeed, the tank itself functioned as the X-ray tube. No high voltage existed anywhere outside the tank—a major safety factor.

Electrons emitted by a tungsten filament in the tank were beamed at a target connected directly to one end of the high-frequency secondary coil. This coil had a diameter of 15 inches; it consisted of 12 to 15 turns of 1-inch copper piping with water circulating through the piping to cool it. The primary consisted of a single turn of copper piping, also water-cooled. The source of power was in effect a radio transmitter lodged in the tank, delivering power to the primary coil much as it would to a radio antenna. It operated at a frequency of 6,000,000 cycles per second, producing a potential of 1,000,000 volts at the tip of the secondary coil where the X-ray target was mounted. An ingenious grid mounted between the filament and the target allowed electrons to reach the target only during the $\frac{1}{30000000}$ second in each radio-frequency cycle when the positive potential on the target was highest. Because of this grid, and because the potential was alternating so rapidly, Sloan reported, "the X-ray output can be made to simulate that from constant-potential direct current." M. Stanley Livingston and Milton A. Chaffee installed the device for Dr. Robert S. Stone at the University of California Medical School in 1934; Dr. Stone used it in fruitful therapeutic research for many years thereafter.[20]

"The apparatus is rugged to an extreme, with its welded steel vacuum tank serving both as an X-ray tube and a high-voltage insulator for the

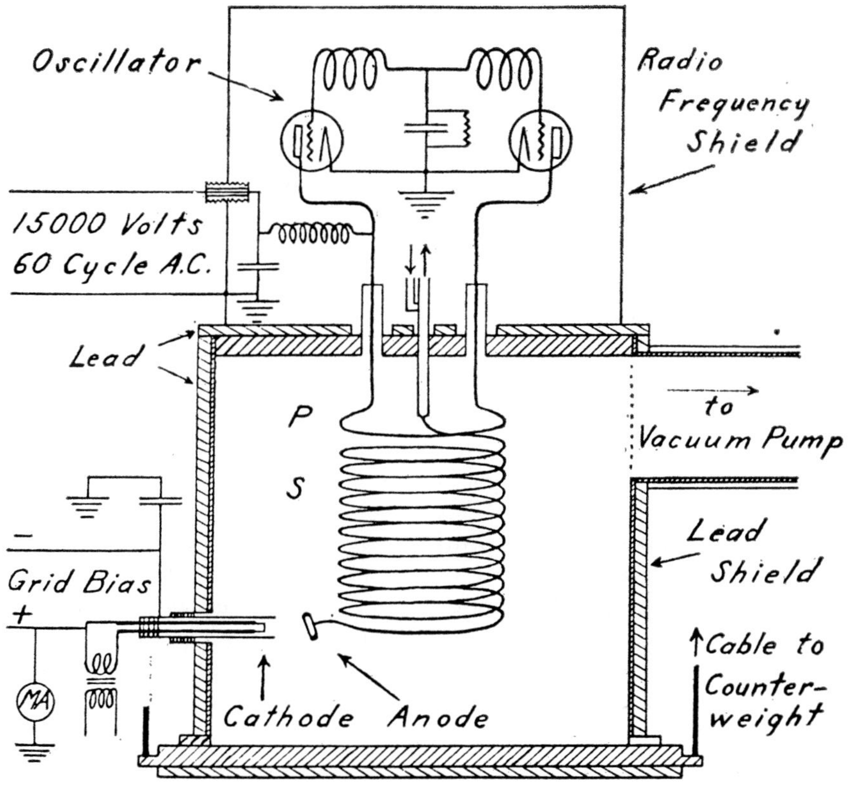

Fig. 38. From *Radiology, 24:* 153, 1935.

transformer," Dr. Stone told a meeting of the Radiological Society of North America in December 1934. "Punctures such as occur in glass or porcelain X-ray tubes are impossible. High-voltage discharges, which are certain to occur when increasing the voltage applied to any apparatus, are confined in a metal chamber where no damage can result. Whenever a discharge takes place, the inherent characteristics of the circuit are such that the voltage in the coil drops to nearly zero.... Far from causing damage, the high-voltage discharges merely clean the all-metal surfaces so that even greater voltages may be applied. Because of the absence of any exposed high-voltage conductors, the installation can be made in a room of ordinary size, instead of requiring a large building to surround it." [21]

It was with this device that Dr. Stone treated the mother of Drs. Ernest and John Lawrence for a malignant growth in 1937; "the treatment was so successful," Sir Mark Oliphant later wrote, "that it reinforced the faith of the brothers in the possibility of developing still more effective uses of radiation in the treatment of cancer." [22]

Dresser in Boston

Meanwhile, the Van de Graaff group at M.I.T. was also making progress. The monstrous spheres of the 7,000,000-volt generator in the airship hangar at Round Hill had attracted the attention of Dr. Richard Dresser, chief radiologist of the Huntington Memorial Hospital in Boston, who was seeking a supervoltage installation of his own.

"One sunny afternoon in the spring of 1935," one of Van de Graaff's young associates, Dr. John G. Trump, later recalled, "a radiologist called at my laboratory. He had heard our assertions regarding the Van de Graaff belt generator, and wondered if it could power a 400,000-volt therapy tube. My parting remark to Dr. Richard Dresser now seems rather brash. 'Make it a million volts,' I said as he left, 'and we *might* be interested.' " [23]

Dr. Dresser soon returned to M.I.T. with a bulbous glass 200,000-volt X-ray tube, which Dr. Trump attached to his own 700,000-volt Van de Graff generator. "As the generator voltage was raised in the darkened laboratory, the hissing of corona could be heard. Then came ominous crackling sounds. Suddenly a bright discharge flashed from one end of the tube to the other. This threat to the tube and a dull glow from the anode terminated the demonstration."

A makeshift tube of higher capacity was next rigged up inside a steel vacuum chamber, and a further demonstration was held for Dr. Vannevar Bush and other scientific notables. "On that beautiful Sunday morning," Dr. Trump continued, "the inadequate radiation shielding was hastily reinforced by some lead bricks near the target. Removing ourselves as far as possible from the radiation source, several measurements of X-ray output were then attempted." The meter readings were high, and the beam penetrated ½ inch of lead. "Everyone was convinced that we were witnessing an unprecedentedly high and penetrating output and that we had better stop while we were still intact." On the basis of this demonstration, the Godfrey M. Hyams Trust gave the Harvard Medical School a $25,000 grant; with this modest sum Dr. Dresser was able to secure for Huntington Memorial Hospital not only a Van de Graaff machine and a tube but also an extension to the hospital needed to house them.[24]

The Van de Graaff machine in this installation was improved in several respects. It required only one sphere instead of two, and the sphere was no longer a sphere but a tubular "high voltage body" (Fig. 39). A

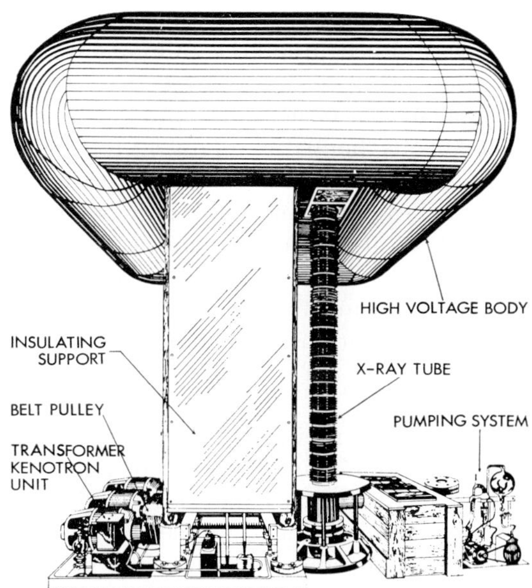

FIG. 39. From *American Journal of Roentgenology, 91:* 24, January 1964.

belt conveyor carried negative ions up to this electrical storehouse as in earlier models, but, in addition, positive ions were carried down on the return trip, thus doubling the efficiency of the belt. Mounted next to the pedestal which held up the charge-storing body was a vertical porcelain tube 16 feet long, divided into 20 sections by metal diaphragms. The whole apparatus was installed in a room only 25 by 23 feet with a ceiling 20 feet high; the target end of the tube projected into the treatment room below. The X rays generated were rated at a steady 1,000,000 volts.

NEW SOURCES OF SUPERVOLTAGE

Until 1939, all of the 1,000,000-volt devices except the Sloan UCRL radio-frequency X-ray generator were big, clumsy, and expensive to install. In 1939, E. E. Charlton and his General Electric associates borrowed a tip from the Sloan device and "miniaturized" the GE 1,000,000-volt unit by enclosing it in a tank like Sloan's. They gained even more compact insulation by filling the tank with a gas—usually Freon—under pressure.[25] The first of these pressurized 1,000,000-volt units, only 7½ feet long and 4 feet in diameter, was installed at Memorial Hospital in New York City; subsequent units went to St. John's Hospital in Cleveland and Roswell Park Memorial Institute in Buffalo, New York. The M.I.T.

group, too, mounted their Van de Graaff generators in pressurized tanks, and the X-ray tube was placed inside the column supporting the charge-storing body.[26] By the spring of 1940, M.I.T. had supplied Dr. George Holmes at the Massachusetts General Hospital with a unit capable of operating at 1,250,000 volts, housed in a tank 13 feet high and 4½ feet in diameter. Still smaller tank sizes were later made available—2,000,000-volt Van de Graaff units, for example, in a tank only 5½ feet high and 3 feet in diameter.[27] More than 40 such units were in use by hospitals in 1965 for cancer therapy.

Lawrence's cyclotron, meanwhile, had been revolutionizing nuclear physics and making contributions to radiology which are described in subsequent chapters. It could not be used efficiently for the acceleration of electrons or the generation of X-rays, however, for a reason which to laymen may seem curious. Einstein's special theory of relativity decreed that nothing can move faster than the speed of light, 186,000 miles per second, and that as objects approach the speed of light, they increase in mass. An electron accelerated in a 5,000,000-volt field reaches 99.5 per cent of the speed of light, and increases in weight by 1100 per cent. The weight increase of an electron accelerated in a cyclotron would almost immediately cause it to get out of step with the alternating potential impressed on the dees (see page 341). A cyclotron can be used to accelerate protons and other heavy ions because their relativistic weight increase is negligible until a much higher voltage is reached.

In 1940, another step forward in high-voltage technology was taken when Dr. D. W. Kerst of the University of Illinois completed the first betatron.[28] Like the cyclotron, Kerst's compact device accelerated particles in circular orbits between the poles of an electromagnet, but in other respects it was quite different. Its main advantage for radiology was that it could accelerate electrons up to tens of millions of volts despite their relativistic weight increase.

The heart of the betatron was an evacuated "doughnut" in which electrons, guided by a carefully shaped, *pulsating* magnetic field, were accelerated in circular orbits *as if they were traveling through the secondary coil of a transformer.* Since there was no physical transformer, there were no problems of insulation or heating, nor was it necessary first to achieve a high potential and then apply it to the electrons; the high potential was generated in the circling electrons directly. Dr. Kerst described a 20,000,000-volt model designed for radiation therapy in *Radiology* for February 1943; many betatrons are now used throughout the world for radiation therapy and other purposes.

World War II stalled the climb toward higher X-ray energies, but after the war three very different developments affected radiology.

One was initiated by Dr. Robert S. Stone at the University of California Hospital in 1949. His 1,000,000-volt Sloan apparatus installed in 1934 was by then obsolete, and a decision to replace it was made. What should his laboratory acquire?

Four-million-volt linear accelerators, Dr. Stone knew, were already undergoing clinical trials in England in 1949. At least two 24,000,000-volt betatrons were already in clinical use and three more were in the planning stage. In Europe a 31,000,000-volt betatron was being used to treat patients, and two more were on order. In England, two 31,000,000-volt machines of a new design were being installed in hospitals. "It seemed as if the field of energies up to 30,000,000 volts was likely to be well investigated," Dr. Stone concluded.[29]

A betatron of higher voltage could be secured, of course, but Dr. Stone's attention was attracted to a new device, which resembled the betatron, known as the *synchrotron*. The synchrotron principle had been conceived in the U.S.S.R. in 1944 by a Russian physicist, V. Veksler,[30] and independently a little later by E. M. McMillan at the Los Alamos Laboratory in New Mexico.[31] The chief advantage of the synchrotron was lesser size and weight; a 70,000,000-volt electron synchrotron would weigh no more and take up no more space than a 50,000,000-volt betatron. The two 31,000,000-volt installations being readied in England in 1949 while Dr. Stone was reaching his decision were both synchrotrons. Dr. Stone decided that what he wanted was a 70,000,000-volt synchrotron which would make possible "the investigation of a range so far not examined." [29]

"The General Electric Company had made a synchrotron of this capacity," Dr. Stone later recalled, "and said it was willing to make such an instrument for clinical use. The order was given for such a machine and it was installed in 1951. It took from then until July 1956 to put it in proper shape to treat patients."

Most earlier installations of this magnitude had been supported either by educational institutions and medical centers, or by wealthy donors like W. K. Kellogg, or by foundations. A few were aided by the U.S. Public Health Service. Several were WPA projects, aided by the Works Progress Administration. World War II added another major sponsor: Dr. Stone's 70,000,000-volt synchrotron and the building which housed it, like many of the post-war medical-physical undertakings, were financed by the U.S. Atomic Energy Commission. Most of the operating funds also came from the AEC.

A second important development following World War II was renewed interest in *linear* accelerators. At Stanford University and elsewhere these devices were notably improved under contracts with the

AEC, the Office of Naval Research, and the Office of Air Research; compact electron-accelerating models suitable for generating X rays were developed at Stanford, with technical assistance from General Electric and Varian Associates and with financial support from the American Cancer Society and the U.S. Public Health Service.[32] It proved possible to generate X rays at voltages up to 10,000,000 volts in an accelerating "pipe" only 6 feet long. One such device, designed by Edward L. Ginzton and Kenneth B. Mallory of Stanford to operate at 5,000,000 volts, was installed in 1955 at the Stanford University School of Medicine in San Francisco for the use of Dr. Henry S. Kaplan.[33] A 50,000,000-volt linear accelerator for electron-beam therapy (see Chapter 25) is in operation at the Argonne Cancer Research Hospital, University of Chicago.

The largest linear accelerator, placed in operation at Stanford in 1966, is 2 miles long, cost $114 million, and accelerates electrons to energies as high as 20 *billion* volts for physical research. It was surpassed in 1967 by the Soviet Union's synchrotron at Serpukhov, near Moscow, capable of accelerating protons to an energy of 76 billion volts.[34] Still in the planning stage in 1968 was an accelerator to be erected at the National Accelerator Laboratory near Weston, Illinois. It will cost an estimated $300 million and will accelerate protons to at least 200 billion and perhaps 400 billion volts.[35] There are no current plans, however, for the medical use of these monsters.

The third important development following World War II was the introduction of *radioisotopes,* particularly cobalt-60, as sources of powerful gamma-ray beams for radiation therapy. Cobalt-60 emits gamma rays at two specific energy levels, 1,170,000 volts and 1,350,000 volts, but because the beam from a cobalt-60 radiation therapy unit lacks the "softer" rays present in beams from X-ray tubes, a cobalt-60 beam is roughly equivalent in hardness to the filtered beam from a 2,000,000- or even 3,000,000-volt X-ray tube.[36] Another radioisotope, cesium-137, was also in use in therapy units. During the 1950's and 1960's, these isotope-powered units became by far the most popular sources of supervoltage radiation for therapy; they were installed in hospitals of moderate size and even in radiologists' offices as well as in large medical centers. Out of 704 supervoltage units in use for radiation therapy in the United States and Canada, according to a survey published in 1968 by the International Atomic Energy Agency, 623 were cobalt-60 units and 37 were cesium-137 units—as compared with 35 linear accelerators, 27 betatrons, 13 Van de Graaff units, and 6 resonant transformers of the Lawrence-Sloan type first used by Dr. Stone.

The availability of cobalt-60 equipment, says Dr. William T. Moss of Wesley Memorial Hosital in Chicago, proved "a major stimulus to radiation therapy. For the first time we had a readily available beam with good percentage depth dose, good skin and bone sparing. No longer were intense skin irritations a prerequisite to the adequate irradiation of many of the deeply situated cancers. Thus the reaction was less for the patient and the technique of treating the patient was easier for the radiologist." [37]

Thus, during the 1960's radiation therapists had available compact, convenient sources of X rays covering the range from 1,000,000 to 30,000,000 volts, a custom model generating rays at 70,000,000 volts; and gamma rays from cobalt-60. A vast clinical experience was being accumulated, on the basis of which it became possible to give at least tentative answers to the question of the practical therapeutic superiority of supervoltage that Dr. Failla had raised in 1932.

What Has Supervoltage Accomplished?

The radiologists who had access to supervoltage devices, beginning with Dr. Soiland in October 1930, were initially cautious in reporting the merits of the new equipment. They made only modest claims for the superiority of higher voltages over conventional 200,000-volt therapy, but even these modest claims were challenged.

At a meeting of the Section on Radiology, Illinois State Medical Society, in May 1934, for example, Dr. Roswell T. Pettit stated with considerable eloquence the case *against* supervoltage, and particularly against the recently introduced 400,000-volt models, from the point of view of the practicing radiologist.

"It is not my purpose to belittle the efforts now being made by the several research institutes," he told the Illinois radiologists, " ... but to warn against too hasty conclusions drawn from insufficient experimental and clinical evidence, to warn against the too hasty expenditure of large sums of your own and other people's money, and to point out that many of the advantages of supervoltage can be procured at practically no cost." [38]

Dr. Pettit conceded that the higher-voltage X rays made possible a larger "depth dose"—that is, a higher dose delivered to a deep-lying tumor as compared with the dose delivered to the skin—but he pointed out that this valuable advantage could also be achieved by moving the patient farther away from the conventional X-ray tube and increasing the filter. A 400,000-volt machine costing more than $10,000, he declared, would improve by only 3 per cent the depth dose he could achieve at 200,000 volts with a Thoraeus filter which then cost only $4. Radiologists should acquire a Thoraeus filter "before succumbing to the pressure exerted by super-high voltage representatives of X-ray manufacturers looking for ten, twenty, and fifty thousand dollar orders...." [38]

Through the succeeding years, Dr. Leucutia, Dr. Stone, Dr. Failla, Dr. Edith Quimby, and many others contributed notably to the evaluation of supervoltage therapy. However, as experience with the new machines accumulated, it became increasingly clear that no simple evaluation was possible.

In the first place, clinical results as well as laboratory investigations showed that "supervoltage" was not a single entity. Effects at 500,000 volts, as might be expected, were not like those at 1,000,000 or 70,000,000 volts. Thus, separate answers would have to be found for each voltage range explored.

Again, the "quality" of the beam from two machines operating at what purported to be the same voltage is not necessarily identical. A machine operating on alternating current produces rays of maximum voltage only at the peak of each cycle, and even a machine operating on direct current with steady input generates X rays at all voltages up to the voltage of the electrons striking the target. Thus, the beams from an X-ray machine cannot be compared volt-for-volt with the relatively homogenous gamma rays from radium, cobalt-60, or other radioisotopes. The "softer" rays mixed in with rays of higher voltage from an X-ray machine, however, can be filtered out; thus, quality also depends on the composition and thickness of the filters used. Years of experiment and of clinical experience were required before data sufficient to correlate quality of beam with biological effects could be accumulated.

Next, what tumor sites are we talking about? For skin cancer in some circumstances, supervoltage therapy may in fact be seriously inferior. The problem in some cases may be to irradiate the skin with a *minimum* dose to the underlying tissues. For deep therapy, higher voltages have an apparent advantage—but how deep, and at how high a voltage? Obese patients may benefit from voltages unnecessary in ordinary practice.

The type of tumor is also relevant. Thus, before the therapeutic questions could be answered, it was necessary to accumulate experience at various voltages for tumors of each type and at each site and for their metastases.

Moreover, how were doses to be compared? The r, or roentgen unit, adopted as an international standard in 1928, was merely a physical measurement based on the amount of ionization produced in air. It proved to be wholly inadequate for supervoltage evaluations, since at such voltages substantial amounts of radiation might pass right through a tissue with negligible ionizing effect. Hence, it was necessary to introduce a new unit, the *rad*, defined in terms of the energy *absorbed* by a gram of tissue from a given beam of radiation.

Rad for rad, do X rays at higher voltages have greater biological effects? The answer, laboriously secured through countless experiments in many laboratories, proved to be no, for most practical purposes. Indeed, multi-million-volt X rays turned out to have a slightly *lesser* biological effect than lower voltages in some tissues. Thus, it was necessary to introduce a new concept: "relative biological effectiveness," or RBE, for each type of radiation. Alas, RBE turned out to be itself a variable concept. The RBE of one beam might be higher than the RBE of another when measured in wheat seeds, but lower when measured in insect eggs, human skin, human fat, human muscle, or human bone. Soon another new unit for comparing radiation effects emerged: the *rem*, defined as the dose in rads multiplied by the RBE for man.

The *rate* at which the dose was delivered proved to be important, too, for comparisons. A beam delivered at 100 r per minute for 1 minute does not have the same effect as a beam delivered at 1 r per minute for 100 minutes. Also, *fractionation* of the dose over a period of days or weeks made a major difference; 200 r per day, delivered 6 days a week for 4 weeks, add up to 4800 r, but the effect is not the same as 4800 r delivered in daily doses for 2 weeks or 4800 r delivered in doses every other day for 4 weeks.

Working with 200,000-volt X rays, radiologists had learned to gauge the deeper effects by observing the appearance of reddening, tanning, and other skin effects. So long as the skin was not severely damaged, no irreparable damage to underlying tissues need be anticipated. Supervoltage, however, has a "skin-sparing" effect; thus, it was slowly learned that serious damage to mucous membrane, nerve cells, intestinal lining, and other deep tissues might make their appearance without prior warning from the skin reaction.

This and other discoveries led, in turn, to further variations on the themes discussed in an earlier chapter—the use of multiple fields and of rotational therapy. Fields and "isodose curves" had to be carefully coordinated, and doses had to be prescribed which would irradiate a tumor as heavily as necessary and as uniformly as possible without delivering too heavy a dose to sensitive neighboring structures. Ingenious methods had to be worked out to fit the geometry of each patient and of each tumor or metastasis within each patient.

With earlier forms of therapy, the radiologist walked a tightrope stretched between "too little" and "too much." Low doses meant a low cure rate; high doses meant damage to normal tissue. With supervoltage the tightrope became a slackrope, on which it was even more difficult to maintain a balance.

Supervoltage, moreover, brought into question afresh the *ultimate* aims of cancer therapy. To cure is the highest goal, but what if the odds are heavily weighted against cure? Should not doses be moderated in such cases in order to achieve a good palliative effect with minimum discomfort for the patient—even at the sacrifice of a 1-in-100 chance to cure? Few would dispute the desirability of such a sacrifice, but should a 1-in-50 chance of cure be similarly sacrificed for comfort—or a 1-in-5 chance? To achieve how much benefit in patient comfort? How should the chances be calculated, for each patient, and each tumor, and each type of radiation?

Answers inevitably came slowly. We quote only a few.

Back in 1934, Dr. Leucutia could already point to specific technical advantages such as increased depth dose and skin sparing, for super-voltage beams. However, he hastened to add that "as great as these advantages are from the point of view of the biological action of the rays and the clinical response of the individual tumor, the group of neoplasms as a whole continues to be governed by the same general laws of radiosensitivity as formerly. Highly sensitive tumors respond readily whereas the recalcitrant tumors, although they may show some degree of improvement in their response, in the main continue to remain intractable also at the higher voltages." Metastases outside the radiation field would, of course, not be affected at any voltage. Thus, "super-high roentgen therapy, while it may be expected to lead to decided improvement in the end results...will not prove a panacea for the cancer problem as a whole." [39]

In May 1937, Dr. Robert S. Stone summed up his own experience with supervoltage over a 3-year period in an address to the Minnesota State Medical Society.

"There is a common belief, held by both the medical profession and the laity," he began, "that higher and higher voltages are synonymous with better and better treatments, and more and more cures of cancer. This popular feeling is stampeding radiologists into procuring apparatus capable of producing higher and higher voltages." Did the evidence warrant this trend? The University of California clinical trials were relevant to this problem. "In adjacent rooms we have machines capable of producing 200,000-volt and 1,000,000-volt radiations and we have endeavored to compare the physical and clinical observations on the various voltages as accurately as possible.... The same technique, except for voltage, has been used on the 200,000-volt and 1,000,000-volt machines." [40]

The proportion of patients cured with the 1,000,000-volt beam, Dr. Stone reported, was no higher than at 200,000 volts. However, he added, cure statistics do not tell the whole story. "A great many patients who come in suffering severely from cancer can be relieved of a large part of their suffering. Their tumors can be reduced in size, and an attitude of depression changed to one of hope. The older textbooks are filled with pictures of emaciated, suffering patients in advanced stages of cancer. By our radiation methods we are able to keep many such patients comfortable until they die of *internal* metastases, such as those to the liver, and their deaths are much less painful." He summarized what 3 years of supervoltage had accomplished in his concluding sentence: "Many of the patients treated were made much more comfortable and their remaining years of life more enjoyable." [40]

By 1950, additional advantages of supervoltage had been established, but the over-all outlook was not much different. "From the physicist's point of view," wrote Dr. Milford D. Schulz of the Massachusetts General Hospital in *Radiology* for July 1950, "there are a considerable number of advantages in treating malignant tumors with X rays generated at supervoltage levels. From the patient's point of view, supervoltage has the advantage of sparing him to a limited degree some of the undesirable effects of radiation. From the clinician's point of view, supervoltage radiation offers another tool with which he can attack malignant neoplasms with a little greater nicety than before, but probably with no remarkable increase in success.... *From the point of view of the tumor,* there is little to indicate that in the range of therapeutic X rays commonly available it cares greatly at which potential the X ray that falls upon it is generated." †

During the 1950's, as more data became available, somewhat improved 5-year survival rates were reported from several centers. However, many changes had occurred as the years went by; it was difficult indeed to gauge how much of the statistical improvement reflected higher-voltage therapy and how much reflected improved techniques of use, earlier diagnosis, the greater frequency with which patients with curable cancer were being referred for radiation therapy instead of surgery, and other factors.

At the December 1955 meeting of the Radiological Society of North America, a symposium was held with the title: "Supervoltage: Should We Junk 250,000 Volts?" [41] Four participants summed up a quarter of a century of experience with supervoltage in these terms:

> *Dr. Simeon T. Cantril, Tumor Institute of the Swedish Hospital, Seattle:* "If one takes the whole cabinet of patients who are candidates for irradiation . . . because one has the full compliment of apparatus available, from superficial X ray to supervoltage up to 2,000,000 volts, I would say, from our experience, that the actual percentage increase in survival is something of the order of 15 percent."

---

† Italics added.

Dr. Milton Friedman, New York University College of Medicine: "How is the patient load divided? For malignant neoplasms, 15 percent 250,000 volts and 85 percent supervoltage radiation. But that is chiefly because we are still, after 13 years, in an exploratory phase, trying to find special indications for supervoltage irradiation."

Dr. Ruth R. Guttman, Francis Delafield Hospital, New York City: "I believe that a supervoltage unit should be present in any well-equipped radiotherapeutic department of large hospital, but I do not think that we should try to do without the 300,000 or 250,000-volt unit."

Dr. T. A. Watson, Director of Cancer Service, Province of Saskatchewan, Canada: "In regard to the question of survival, I imagine that the survival rate would be very little improved by supervoltage therapy. However, there are many other factors which enter into consideration, such as less discomfort to the patient, both constitutional and local."

In July 1956, a symposium on supervoltage was held at the Oak Ridge Institute of Nuclear Studies (ORINS) in Oak Ridge, Tennessee. The conclusions of this symposium were summarized by Dr. Marshall Brucer of ORINS and Dr. Milton Friedman of the New York University College of Medicine. With respect to relative cure rates in general, they concluded that "a complete answer will not be available for many years." However, answers could be given with respect to particular tumors. "In a few tumors, such as cancer of the testes, osteogenic sarcoma, and possibly some advanced cancers of the cervix, supervoltage irradiation has demonstrably increased the cure rate. In others, such as cancer of the lung, esophagus, anterior two-thirds of the tongue, and the parotid, it has been disappointing.

"The reason for the disappointment with supervoltage irradiation lies in the 60–30–10 law. This restatement of a well-known principle is as follows: The value of the factors that influence irradiation cures are 60 percent for the nature and extent of the tumor, 30 percent for the skill and experience of the therapist, and 10 percent for the modality used. Thus supervoltage may potentially increase the cure rate for cancer only about 10 percent." [42]

In 1957, Dr. Henry S. Kaplan of the Stanford Medical School summarized the latest physical understanding of supervoltage advantages in terms which may be paraphrased as follows[32]:

1. X rays entering a tissue begin immediately to liberate electrons which are emitted in all directions. With X rays of conventional voltage, this electron liberation and other ionization effects are at a maximum at or very close to the surface of entry. With supervoltage, in contrast, "the skin is spared because ionization equilibrium occurs below the surface; the actual equilibrium depth may range from several mil-

limeters to several centimeters." The higher the voltage, the greater the depth of tissue spared.

2. There is a pronounced increase in depth dose as compared with skin dose, "which greatly simplifies the problem of delivering tumoricidal doses to deep-seated neoplasms."

3. At conventional voltages, the depth dose increases with the *size* of the field, so that fields larger than the size of a deep-lying tumor must often be irradiated to get an adequate dose to it. With supervoltage, "depth dose is relatively independent of field size, making it possible to confine fields to the actual dimensions of the tumor...." This, in turn, cuts the total dosage to the patient; "systemic reactions and injury to normal tissues can thus be minimized."

4. At conventional voltages, X rays have a greater effect on heavy atoms such as those found in bone than on the lighter atoms of soft tissue. Thus, the rays may kill bone cells in or near the beam, producing a condition known as osteoradionecrosis. Electrons emitted by the heavy atoms in irradiated bone cells, moreover, may enter nearby tissues and increase the dose that *they* receive. However, the "selective absorption in bone disappears at energies above 1,000,000 to 2,000,000 volts; the hazard of osteoradionecrosis is thus materially reduced, and inhomogeneities of dosage in tissues adjacent to bone are eliminated."

The net clinical effect of these physical advantages, Dr. Kaplan continued, is three-fold:

> (a) "Curative" therapy is made possible for *some* cancers which are treatable only with great difficulty, if at all, with 200,000 volts.
> (b) Greater precision and homogeneity may be attained in the treatment of *all* deep tumors.
> (c) Palliative therapy for such tumors may be offered without exacting an excessive price in terms of radiation sickness and cutaneous reaction.

Dr. Kaplan went on to emphasize, however, that "these advantages are purely physical; there are no qualitative differences, and only slight quantitative differences," in the biological effectiveness of 200,000-volt as compared with supervoltage X rays.[32]

Beginnings have also been made in evaluating objectively the *palliative* advantages of supervoltage radiation, from the point of view of patient comfort.

Dr. Justin J. Stein and his associates of the Cancer Research Institute, University of California at Los Angeles, for example, compared the effects of cobalt-60 beams (roughly equivalent to X rays at 3,000,000 volts) and conventional X-ray therapy on patients with inoperable lung cancer.[43] "Considerably better palliation was obtained in the cobalt-60 treated group," Dr. Stein told the September 1961 meeting of the American Roentgen Ray Society, "in that the patients felt better for longer periods of time than when treated with conventional roentgen therapy, and there was better control of hemoptysis, . . . severe cough, pain, and dyspnea. The patients tolerated the therapy much better, and there were no appreciable skin reactions even with tumor doses in excess of 6,000 r." Most patients were treated without being hospitalized during therapy.

"If the next ten years are as productive as the last decade," Dr. Stein concluded, "then certainly we have much to hope for in the ceaseless struggle against cancer."

REFERENCES

1. *J. Amer. Inst. Electrical Engineers, 47:* 212–213, 1928.
2. *J. Franklin Inst., 202:* 693–721, 1926.
3. *Amer. J. Roentgen., 19:* 313–321, 1928.
4. *J. Amer. Inst. Electrical Engineers, 44:* 373, 1925.
5. *Phys. Rev., 32:* 850–857, 1928.
6. *Phys. Rev., 43:* 153–154, 1933.
7. *Phys. Rev., 38:* 1919, 1931.
8. *Ibid.,* p. 1915.
9. LIVINGSTON, M. S. AND BLEWETT, J. P., *Particle Accelerators.* McGraw-Hill Book Company, New York, 1962.
10. *Arch. Elektrotech., 21:* 387, 1929.
11. *Phys. Rev., 38:* 586, 1931.
12. *Ibid.,* p. 834.
13. *Phys. Rev., 40:* 19–35, 1932.
14. *Phys. Rev., 38:* 2021–2032, 1931.
15. *Radiology, 20:* 99–101, 1933.
16. *Amer. J. Roentgen., 27:* 405–414, 1932.
17. *Amer. J. Roentgen., 29:* 293–367, 1933.
18. *Amer. J. Roentgen., 38:* 769–772, 1937.
19. *Amer. J. Roentgen., 31:* 628–662, 1934; *34:* 664–677, 1935; *38:* 762–768, 1937.
20. *Phys. Rev., 43:* 213, 1933; *47:* 62, 1935.
21. *Radiology, 24:* 153–159, 1935.
22. *Phys. To-day, 19:* 43, 1966.
23. *Amer. J. Roentgen., 38:* 758–761, 1937.
24. *Amer. J. Roentgen. 91:* 21–30, 1964.
25. BUSCHKE, F., CANTRIL, S. T., AND PARKER, H. M., *Supervoltage Roentgen Therapy.* Charles C Thomas, Publisher, Springfield, Illinois, 1950.
26. *Amer. J. Roentgen., 49:* 531–535, 1943.
27. GLASSER, O. (ED.), *Medical Physics,* Vol. 2, pp. 905–910. Year Book Publishers, Inc., Chicago, 1950.
28. *Phys. Rev., 58:* 841, 1940.
29. University of California at San Francisco Radiological Laboratory Semi-Annual Report. June 30, 1958.
30. *C. R. Acad. Sci. U.R.S.S., 43:* 444, 1944.
31. *Phys. Rev., 68:* 143, 1945.
32. *Stanford Med. Bull., 15:* 123–140, 1957.
33. *Ibid.* pp. 145–151.
34. *Science, 161:* 11–19, 1968.
35. *Univ. Wisconsin U.I.R. Newsletter, 3:* 3–4, 1968.
36. *Amer. J. Roentgen., 87:* 593–599, 1962.

37. *Your Radiologist, 2:* 9–10, 1968.
38. *Illinois Med. J. 66:* 283–288, 1934.
39. *Amer. J. Roentgen., 31:* 628–662, 1934.
40. *Minnesota Med., 21:* 79–85, 1938.
41. *Radiology, 67:* 481–515, 1956.
42. U.S. Atomic Energy Commission, *Roentgens, Rads, and Riddles.* U.S. Government
    Printing Office, Washington, 1959.
43. *Amer. J. Roentgen., 89:* 191–199, 1963.

24 Particles in Therapy

While supervoltage X rays for therapy were the first radiological fruits of the physicists' race for higher voltages, other fruits were soon ripening for harvest. Ernest O. Lawrence's cyclotrons, for example, yielded high-energy neutrons which could be beamed into patients. The story of their use and abandonment constitutes one of the sadder chapters in the history of radiology.

Neutrons, as we have seen, became available for physical experiments in 1932, and the question of their therapeutic possibilities was raised not long thereafter. Lawrence himself discussed the question at the 1936 meeting of the Radiological Society of North America.[1]

"Neutron rays," he explained, "have the remarkable property of being more readily absorbed in light substances rich in hydrogen such as biological tissues than in denser substances like iron or lead. If you should use a fluoroscope and look through the body with neutron rays, you would find that the bones would appear relatively transparent and the flesh would look darker. Neutron rays also are unique in the manner in which they produce ionization. X rays produce ionization by liberating high-speed electrons from atoms, while neutrons, being tiny dense particles of neutral matter, pass right through the electron clouds of atoms and ionize only by making intimate collisions with the correspondingly dense atomic nuclei."

An X ray, Dr. Lawrence continued, travels a long distance through tissue, but the electrons that it liberates along the way produce only a few ions per centimeter along their course. The neutron, in contrast, produces no ions until it strikes an atomic nucleus. Then a proton in the nucleus "recoils" from the collision with an energy of more than 1,000,000 volts. Such recoil protons travel only a short distance, but they produce ionization 100 times more dense than that produced by X-ray-liberated electrons. "So we see," Dr. Lawrence added, "that neutron ionization, in comparison with X-ray ionization, is very much more localized and very much more intense where it occurs." To the radiologists in his audience, this news from the frontier of nuclear physics must have been exciting indeed. What they needed for therapy was precisely what Dr. Lawrence was describing: more intense ionization in a more narrowly circumscribed region of tissue. Dr. Lawrence gently underlined the point. "In view of this great difference in the physical behavior of neutrons and X rays," he declared, "one is led to wonder whether the two forms of radiation are also very different in their biological action." [1]

At the Lawrence laboratory in Berkeley, this possible difference in biological action was of great practical interest from the moment the first neutron beam emerged from the first cyclotron. Animal experiments were therefore launched almost at once. "... These experiments were originally undertaken for the immediate practical purpose of obtaining information for the protection of workers in our laboratory," Dr. Lawrence explained. "We did not want to repeat the unfortunate experiences of many of the early roentgenologists. It was fortunate that my brother, Dr. John H. Lawrence of the Yale University School of Medicine, was visiting me the summer before last [1935] and took the occasion to look into this vital question."

Dr. John Lawrence's initial experiment with the cyclotron was quite simple. "First of all he placed some rats near the source of neutrons," Dr. Ernest O. Lawrence reported, "and found immediately that the neutron rays are indeed very lethal and that they kill a rat by a few minutes' exposure. When I say kill, I mean that the rats died in about two or three days' time after exposure." [1]

A quarter-century later, while in a reminiscent mood, Dr. John Lawrence added a whimsical detail. "You will be interested to know," he told a conference of scientists held in Mexico City on November 24, 1961, "that we had one fortunate experience. We placed the first mouse to be exposed to this combined beam ... within a small chamber with an air intake and outlet for ventilation. After a five-minute exposure of the mouse we crawled in between the dees of the cyclotron to examine it. The mouse was dead! This produced a very healthy fear of these new radiations which I think was fortunate, because thereafter no one was careless about exposure. Later we discovered that the animal had died from suffocation and not from radiation, but we did not widely advertise this among our physicist colleagues." [2]

Further biological experiments with neutron beams in the Lawrence laboratory were performed in 1935 and 1936 by the Lawrence brothers themselves and by Paul C. Aebersold, Dr. E. R. Dempster, and Dr. R. E. Zirkle, the latter a visitor from the University of Pennsylvania. Fruit-fly eggs, fern spores, wheat seedlings, and mice were all irradiated with varying doses of X rays and neutrons. Dr. Ernest Lawrence summarized the results to the assembled radiologists in 1936.

It was found, he reported, that "about 87 r of neutrons kills about one-half of the flies' eggs, while for X rays...it takes about 190 r to produce the same effect.... In other words, it was found that...the neutrons were about twice as effective as X rays. In the case of the fern spore, Dr. Zirkle and Mr. Aebersold found that the neutrons are about 2.5 times as effective as X rays. Thirdly, they found, that in inhibiting the growth of wheat seedlings, the neutrons are about five times as effective as the X rays." In their ability to kill mice, neutrons proved to be about 3.8 times as potent as X rays. The experiments as a whole made it clear not only that neutrons are more potent than X rays but also—and of greater practical importance—that the effect of neutrons on one tissue was no guide to their effect on another tissue.[1]

"I think we can say," Dr. Lawrence told the radiologists, "that these experiments established quite definitely that neutron rays and X rays do not parallel each other in their biological action. The selective action of neutron rays on tissue is in general different from that of X rays."

Many radiological heads in the audience must have risen at that remark. If neutrons affect some tissues more than others, radiologists must have been asking themselves, how do they affect cancer tissues? Dr. Lawrence told them.

Tumor cells from a mammary carcinoma, he reported, were wrapped in filter paper, moistened, and placed in a plugged wood block to ensure that they would receive approximately the same quality of radiation as they would receive inside a living body. More than 1000 tumor samples were thus exposed, some to neutrons and some to X rays. It took an X ray dose of about 4500 r to kill all of the tumor cells; the same effect was produced by only 1000 r of neutrons. Similarly, to inactivate the tumor cells in half of the capsules required 3600 r of X rays but only 700 r of neutrons. "Dividing 3,600 by 700," Dr. Lawrence concluded, "we see that the neutrons are about 5.1 times more lethal."

However, these figures, although impressive, still left the essential question unanswered. The radiation therapist is not greatly interested in how large a dose of radiation it takes to kill a cancer. Even with relatively primitive equipment, he could deliver as large a dose as he pleased if there were no other effects to be considered. His problem is to deliver a killing dose to the cancer without also killing or severely damaging normal tissues in the vicinity. What the radiologists in Dr. Lawrence's 1936 audience wanted to know was whether the *therapeutic margin* between effects on cancer cells and on normal tissues was wider for neutrons than for X rays. Dr. Lawrence presented evidence suggesting that it might in fact be wider.

"In therapy," he reminded the radiologists, "one is interested in the effect on the tumor relative to the effect on the host, the mouse in these experiments. The ratio of the 50-percent tumor dose to the perceptible killing mouse dosage for X rays is 3,600 divided by 400, a ratio which is 9. In other words, the mouse can tolerate over its whole body only one-ninth the dose of X rays required to kill 50 percent of the tumor particles *in vitro*. With neutrons the ratio is 700 divided by 120, that is, 5.8. Instead of only one-ninth of the tumor dose, the mouse can stand about one-sixth of the 50-percent tumor-killing dose and so we see that the experiments indicate that a more effective dose on the tumor using neutrons can be given without killing the mouse.

"If these indications of a greater selective action of the neutron rays on tumor tissue prove to be true for carcinomas *in vivo,* it is a very important matter." [1]

For the assembled radiologists, Dr. Lawrence's report must have raised many hopes, but it must also have evoked some concern. Suppose that neutron rays from a cyclotron did prove to be a treatment of choice for cancer. Small hospitals and radiologists in private practice could hardly to be expected to secure cyclotrons of their own for clinical use. On this point, however, Dr. Lawrence was reassuring. "The view of the cyclotron which I have shown in the illustrations perhaps gives you the impression that the apparatus is extremely large and costly, but it is not so bad as it seems at first sight. At the present time I am of the opinion that a cyclotron can be engineered and developed in a way which will make it entirely practical for the purposes of medicine." [1]

Which radiologist would be afforded the first opportunity to try out a neutron beam on human patients? The choice fell on Dr. Robert S. Stone of the University of California Medical School, in association with Dr. Ernest O. Lawrence's radiologist brother, Dr. John H. Lawrence. Dr. Stone, Dr. John Lawrence, and Dr. Paul C. Aebersold, a UCRL physicist, made their first clinical report on the new therapy at the December 1939 meeting of the Radiological Society of North America[3]; Dr. Stone and Dr. John C. Larkin, Jr., made a second report before the same organization in December 1941[4]; and Dr. Stone gave his final report—one of the classics of investigational radiology—before the America Radium Society in June 1947.[5] The account which follows is drawn from all three of these reports.

Work began in 1938, Dr. Stone explained, with the UCRL 37-inch cyclotron used to accelerate deuterons (heavy-hydrogen nuclei composed of one proton linked to one neutron). When beamed at a beryllium traget, the 8,000,000-volt deuterons caused the beryllium atoms to emit neutrons at energies up to 12,000,000 volts. In December 1939, this device was succeeded by the first "medical cyclotron," which was set up in the new Crocker Radiation Laboratory, close to the UCRL on the Berkeley campus, and which produced an intense yield of neutrons at energies up to 21,000,000 volts.

How should dosages be determined? As Dr. Ernest O. Lawrence had reported in 1936, numerous preliminary studies had been made to determine the relative biological effectiveness of neutrons as compared with X rays. After reviewing all of these studies, Dr. Stone and his associates decided to adopt a four-to-one ratio, and to give one-fourth as many neutron units as they would have used X-ray units in comparable situations.

"The first patient," Dr. Stone reported, "was a man with a carcinoma of the upper alveolar ridge (gum) invading the maxilla. On September 26, 1938, he was given 180 n [neutron units].... The dose of 180 n produced much the same effect as we would have expected from 900 roentgens of 200,000-volt X rays." [3]

From September 1938 to February 1943, when neutron radiation was abandoned, 249 patients were treated with the new medical cyclotron. Many of them were chosen by physicians of the Visible Tumor Clinic. "They were patients who, in the opinion of that group of doctors, could not be cured by surgical or X-ray treatment. It was felt that neutron therapy must show decided effects in *advanced* cancer, as represented in these patients, before its use for the treatment of small localized lesions could be justified." With a single exception, every one of the patients treated was "considered incurable by any known means." [4]

The initial results on the first 24 patients, reported in 1939, were moderately promising. "In every case there was some decrease in the size of both the primary lesions and the metastases." Early skin damage and general reactions to the radiation were much like those which would have been expected from X rays. "Most of the patients presented one or more of the following symptoms: weakness, anorexia, nausea, and vomiting." [3]

By the time of the 1941 report, additional lessons had been learned. Skin reactions, it was found, depended very much on *the dose given per day* as well as on the total dose. A given degree of skin reaction might be caused by as few as 675 or as many as 1025 neutron units, depending on rate of application. When "crossfiring" was used, the exit skin dose from one beam had to be added to the entering dose from the other. When two fields overlapped even slightly, severe reactions were noted. The estimated four-to-one ratio for the relative biological effectiveness of neutrons as compared to X rays was increased to a six-to-one estimate so far as minimal skin reactions were concerned. While the statistical survival rates of the patients were described as "discouraging," the effect of the neutrons on particular tumors was sufficiently impressive "to encourage further study in selected cases. It was demonstrated, both clinically and pathologically, that some cancers disappeared as a result of neutron therapy." [4]

Much happened between the time of that second report and Dr. Stone's final report in June 1947. World War II had intervened. Additional patients subjected to neutron therapy had died, and those who survived had developed late and severe reactions. Neutron therapy itself had been discontinued. Dr. Stone might quietly have moved on to other matters. However, he chose to lay the facts on the table, both in a personal appearance before his fellow radiologists and in the pages of the *American Journal of Roentgenology and Radium Therapy. He* must have approached the preparation of this final report with a heavy heart.

He began with an important point: "The theoretical reasons for testing the biological effects of neutrons were sound." [5]

The tests, however, had run into a phenomenon that was unprecedented, that had not been anticipated, and that could not have been anticipated. *Early effects on the skin and other normal tissues proved to be an unreliable guide to subsequent effects.* Thus, patients who had benefitted from therapy and whose cancers had disappeared, with seemingly only minor effects on the irradiated skin, began 2 or 3 or even 4 years later to show changes altogether out of proportion to what had been expected.

An example was the one patient, a 58-year-old salesman, who was accepted despite the fact that his tumor might have been curable by X rays or surgery—the only exception to the rule limiting neutron therapy to patients with incurable cancer. This patient had carcinoma of the larynx and had requested to be treated by neutrons. His immediate reaction to neutron radiation was just about what would have been expected with X rays, and all seemed to be proceeding on schedule. "The skin healed well—but before a year had passed it became very blotchy in appearance and the subcutaneous tissues became indurated. Gradually the skin became more atrophic. Telangiectatic vessels appeared after the third year.... He now has fixation of the skin and subcutaneous tissues in the larynx—the whole area feeling very hard and containing numerous telangiectatic vessels."

There were compensations. "The lesion promptly disappeared and has not recurred. The patient is content because he has his voice and has lived without evidence of his cancer for more than six years. *We* are not content because we believe that if roentgen rays had been used he might have been 'cured' with less damage to the normal tissues." [5]

Other cases told the same story. Far from widening the "therapeutic margin" between the effect on cancer cells and the effect on surrounding tissue, when neutrons were used the margin appeared to be almost non-existent. "Eighteen patients have been kept alive," Dr. Stone wrote, "but none of them is free from distressing side effects." He recommended: "Neutron therapy as administered by us has resulted in such bad sequelae in proportion to the few good results that it should not be continued."

Dr. Stone's final report on neutron therapy thus stands as a monument of clear-eyed objectivity and blunt truth. It was well received by his fellow radiologists.

Dr. Stone made one final point which can serve to introduce the sections which follow. "The late results from the use of neutrons," he declared, "should serve as a warning to those proposing to use protons, multimillion volt beta rays [electrons], and multimillion volt roentgen rays in the treatment of human cancer.... [They] should study the relative biological effectiveness...by late reactions as well as by acute early ones." [5]

Electron Beams for Therapy

When an X-ray beam enters living tissue, it liberates electrons from atoms and these electrons, in turn, may liberate additional electrons from additional atoms. Indeed, most of the biological effect of an X-ray beam is in fact the effect of electrons. Thus, the question was raised at least as early as the 1920's: Why bother with X rays at all? Why not beam electrons themselves into tissues?

Among the pioneers to whom this notion must have appealed was Dr. W. D. Coolidge. Indeed, his development of the cascade tube during the 1920's (see page 335) did not arise solely out of X-ray considerations but also out of an effort to produce an electron beam of sufficient voltage to have biological usefulness.

Dr. Coolidge reported on a cathode-ray tube—that is, a tube for emitting electrons—at the October 1926 meeting of the Franklin Institute in Philadelphia.[6] His tube, like the Lenard tube which had given Roentgen his clue in 1895, had an extremely thin metal window through which electrons could escape. It was designed to emit electrons at voltages up to 250,000 volts. In an accompanying paper,[7] Dr. Coolidge and his associate, C. N. Moore, described the effects of the electrons emerging from this tube when beamed at diamonds, at other crystals, at various chemical compounds, and at such biological targets as bacteria, fruit flies, snails, cockroaches, rubber-plant leaves, and rabbit ears. "Cockroaches seemed badly injured when rayed for a quarter of a second and one was killed by being rayed for one-half second," Coolidge and Moore noted. The effects on rabbit ears were similar to X-ray effects, varying "from a slight tanning of the skin to complete destruction of the tissues throughout the entire thickness of the ear, depending upon the time of the exposure and the amount of current used." Although they did not mention tumor irradiation, it was clearly in their minds. They concluded: "The effect of cathode rays on animal tissues would seem to offer a very promising subject for medical research." [7]

Their suggestion, however, was premature, for subsequent studies showed that, at voltages under 1,000,000 volts, electrons did not penetrate deeply enough to be of much practical value. Interest did not revive until higher-voltage electrons became available.

Two German investigators, A. Brasch and F. Lange, tried electron-beam therapy in 1934,[8] and in 1940 the M.I.T. electrostatic-generator group—Trump, Van de Graaff, and R. W. Cloud—suggested the use of their device in this way.[9] Although medical use of electron beams had not as yet been tried in the United States, they indicated, the opportunities were now ripe. Electrons accelerated to 1,500,000-volt energies could readily be extracted from a Van de Graaff machine in enormous quantities; indeed, an important problem was the reduction of the beam to a manageable intensity. At 1,500,000 volts, the electrons would penetrate in tumoricidal quantities to a depth of several millimeters—deep enough to be "of medical interest in the treatment of certain types of very superficial malignant conditions." A major advantage that they anticipated would be the rapid falloff of intensity beyond this depth, thus sparing the deeper tissues below the tumor from radiation damage. They also called attention to the fact that electrons accelerated in a Van de Graaff machine were for all practical purposes "monoenergetic"; that is, they all carried approximately the same energy and would therefore produce ionization at approximately the same depth.[9]

For 10 years this suggestion lay dormant. Then in 1951 Drs. Hugh Hare and Magnus Smedal of the Lahey Clinic consulted the M.I.T. physicists concerning a 76-year-old patient with a rare skin disease, lymphoma cutis.[10] For years the Lahey Clinic radiologists had kept this man's malignant skin condition controlled by means of X-ray therapy, but the skin's tolerance for X rays had by now been exceeded, and the disease was rampant over the entire surface of his body. A beam of electrons from a Van de Graaff generator at M.I.T. was delivered over the patient's entire skin surface, and the disease was thereby held in control for an additional 4 years. Thereafter many additional patients with shallow but widely disseminated skin diseases were successfully treated with electron beams of relatively low energy (1,500,000 to 3,800,000 volts) by the M.I.T.-Lahey Clinic group.

Electrons of higher voltage were also put to good use. The invention of the betatron by Dr. Donald Kerst in 1940 and the design of a convenient way of harvesting betatron electrons by Lester S. Skaggs and Kerst in 1946 made available electron beams of far higher energies —up to 30,000,000 volts or even more—which penetrated considerably deeper into human tissue. The therapeutic use of 6,000,000-volt electrons from betatrons was explored in Germany beginning about 1948, and at the Second National Cancer Conference in March 1952, a group from the University of Illinois College of Medicine, Chicago, reported on the use of betatron electrons at energies up to 22,000,000 volts to treat head and neck cancer. At the October 1953 meeting of the American Roentgen Ray Society, this group gave a fuller report on their first 13 patients.[11]

The number was small, they explained, no doubt recalling Dr. Stone's experience with neutrons, because "we did not want to treat a large number of patients only to discover years later that our methods were wrong."

On the basis of physical characteristics alone, the University of Illinois group—which included Drs. Lewis L. Haas, Roger A. Harvey, and John S. Laughlin—reported,

> we could assume that the high-energy electron beam might result in the following advantages over conventional roentgen rays:
> 1. Homogeneous dosage in all layers of a lesion.
> 2. Insignificant exit dose beneath the lesion in healthy tissue.
> 3. Faster and better recovery [from] radiation reactions.
> 4. Low volume dose per tumor dose.
> 5. Less damage of tumor bed.
> 6. Fewer general symptoms.
> 7. Less bone and cartilage damage.
> The actual application of these advantages has been confirmed.[11]

During the years immediately following 1953, however, electron-beam therapy remained a procedure under study at only a few centers, and few reports were published.

At the December 1960 meeting of the Radiological Society of North America, a group from the Stanford University School of Medicine—Drs. L. M. Zatz, C. F. von Essen, and Henry S. Kaplan—reported on their clinical experiences with 10,000,000- to 40,000,000-volt electrons from the Stanford Mark IV linear accelerator.[12] Their clinical program ran from May 1958 to April 1960, when the accelerator was commandeered for nonmedical purposes. During this period 42 patients were irradiated.

The Stanford group reported that the beam appeared to be useful for shallow lesions lying within 8 centimeters of the surface, but skin reactions were "brisk." When efforts were made to treat deeper tissues by crossfiring at the tumor from two directions, difficulties were encountered which suggested that there was little advantage in electrons over supervoltage X rays for depth therapy.

A physicist and a radiologist, Drs. J. E. Morgan and Andrew H. Dowdy of the U.C.L.A. Medical Center in Los Angeles, reported in 1963 on electron therapy with 6,000,000-volt electrons from a linear accelerator.[13] They found considerable difficulty in shielding the eyes and genitals of patients from stray electrons, and they recalled a remark by Dr. Failla that electrons can "sneak around behind a shield and hit you in the back." They described, however, ingenious methods of dealing with this problem.

At the International Congress of Radiology in Montreal in August 1962, a group from Memorial Hospital in New York City—Drs. Florence C. H. Chu and Lourdes Nisce, radiologists, and Dr. John S. Laughlin, physicist—reported on 218 patients with carcinoma of the breast treated since 1955 with electrons of up to 24,000,000 volts from the Memorial Hospital betatron.[14] Several difficulties were encountered, and some of these were overcome.

"Advantages of electron irradiation," the Memorial group concluded, "include easy manipulation, convenient adjustment of the depth of penetration of radiation, absence of increased bone dose, and satisfactory dose distribution in most cases." Disadvantages included limitation of field size to 24 by 24 centimeters and problems in setting up multiple fields without "hot spots," "cold spots," and overlapping. "The advantages, however, appear to us to outweigh the disadvantages. Electrons of the energies available to the authors have proved to be worthwhile, convenient, and effective in the treatment of tumors situated close to the body surface, such as breast cancer."

Rather similar results were reported at the November 1963 meetings of the Radiological Society of North America by Drs. Norah duV. Tapley and Gilbert H. Fletcher of the M. D. Anderson Hospital and Tumor Institute, University of Texas, Houston. They irradiated 92 patients with head or neck cancer and 21 with breast cancer, using electron beams at an energy of from 6,000,000 to 20,000,000 volts. "After using the electron beam in the treatment of more than 100 patients," they concluded, "we have the impression that this therapeutic modality can be of particular value for lesions no deeper than 5 centimeters from the skin surface. [15]

Perhaps the most interesting of the recent work with electron-beam therapy has been reported from the Argonne Cancer Research Hospital, University of Chicago.[16] A linear accelerator there makes available electron beams at voltages as high as 50,000,000 volts. The pencil of electrons emerging from this accelerator, as at other installations, is far too intense and covers far too small a field (½ centimeter in diameter) to be directly used. At other institutions, the electrons are therefore first scattered by projection through a foil in order to achieve a useful field size, and are then collimated into a parallel beam again by passage through a diaphragm. The Argonne beam instead is used "raw." The pencil of electrons is deflected in accordance with a planned pattern by a magnetic scanning system, similar to that in a television tube. At any one instant, only a ½-centimeter cylinder of tissue is irradiated, but the beam-scanning system systematically moves the beam to provide essentially uniform radiation over a field of any size and shape up to 20 by 20 centimeters. The beam is not continuous; on the contrary, it delivers 2856 successive "bunches" of electrons in each *millionth* of a second, and 60 "pulses" of electrons, each composed of many thousands of "bunches," are delivered every second. The *instantaneous* dose rate can only be described as fabulous—as high as 500,000,000 rads per second during the small fraction of a millionth of a second when a "bunch" of electrons hits a cell.

The first cancer patient was treated with this beam on June 16, 1959; at the October 1962 meeting of the American Roentgen Ray Society, Drs. J. W. J. Carpender and M. L. Griem, radiologists, and Drs. Lester S. Skaggs and L. H. Lanzl, physicists, made their preliminary report on the treatment of the first 97 patients, 51 of them with malignancies of the head or neck.

The most significant finding was a considerably lesser skin reaction than most earlier workers with electron-beam therapy had reported. The Argonne group offered a number of possible explanations for this apparent skin-sparing effect. It might be due to the scanning system, which irradiates only a small area at any given instant. It might be due to the absence of a beam-scattering foil. It might be due to the enormous instantaneous dosage—or it might be due to the pulsed nature of the beam.

A similar skin-sparing effect and other advantages of 10,000,000- to 22,000,000-volt electron-beam therapy was reported for 150 tumors of the head and neck by Dr. Herbert E. Brizel, University of Louisville, at the March 1968 meeting of the Canadian Association of Radiologists.

While no proof had yet been secured that survival rates are improved, Dr. Brizel concluded, "the *quality* of survival certainly appears to be markedly improved, even in our own limited series." [17]

Electron-beam therapy had thus come a long way, both in terms of engineering and in terms of usefulness, since Coolidge made his first suggestion in 1926. However, it had still not established itself as a standard technique of radiology.

THERAPY WITH PROTONS, DEUTERONS, ALPHA PARTICLES, AND OTHER HEAVY IONS

The disappointing results with neutron beam therapy (reviewed earlier in this chapter) made clinical trials with protons and other heavy particles comparatively uninviting; in any event, protons at a voltage sufficient to penetrate deep tissues were not available until after 1946. In that year, however, Dr. Robert R. Wilson of Harvard's Research Laboratory of Physics called the attention of radiologists to some interesting future possibilities.[18]

Particle accelerators then under construction, Dr. Wilson pointed out, would soon be able to accelerate protons to any energy up to 400,000,000 volts—high enough to pass right through the human body. To project protons to any desired depth in tissue, a radiologist need only use protons of the right voltage. There would be very little scatter of the protons en route to their target and relatively little ionization of the tissues along the way, but, as the protons approached the end of their range and slowed down, they would produce intensive ionization in a restricted region deep in the tissue—a phenomenon known as the "Bragg effect."

Similar or even more selective effects might be secured, Dr. Wilson continued, with deuterons and alpha particles, and perhaps with even heavier particles such as carbon nuclei. Thus, the door might at last be opened to a widening of the therapeutic margin between the effects of radiation on a lesion and the effects on surrounding tissue. A deep-lying tumor might be heavily irradiated with only limited ionization in the tissue ahead of it, beyond it, and surrounding it.

The first experimental trials of heavy-ion beams confirmed these predictions. They were reported in 1952 by Dr. John H. Lawrence of the Donner Laboratory in Berkeley and two associates, Drs. C. A. Tobias and Hal O. Anger. Protons were accelerated in the new Berkeley 184-inch synchrocyclotron (a device which combines the principles of the cyclotron and the synchrotron) and were then channeled from the device to an adjoining treatment room.[19]

To an even greater degree than Wilson had predicted, it proved possible with such a beam to limit the ionizing effects to a cylindrical volume of tissue beginning well below the skin and ending before the skin was reached again. "In small animals," the Lawrence-Tobias-Anger group reported, "cylindrical lesions one millimeter in diameter are easily produced." The longitudinal boundary of this cyclinder of damaged tissue, they added, was "microscopically sharp." No such precise localization had ever been achieved with any other type of radiation.

"High energy protons, deuterons, and alpha particles," the group pointed out, "have great advantages over other radiations in producing *localized* radiation damage in a deep region in tissue.... The particles, when focused, travel in a straight beam with little divergence and may be directed to any portion of the body. A suitable aperture, made of brass or other metal, is used to decide the shape and size of the beam. As the particles penetrate tissue, their scattering is very small compared with electrons, and for practical purposes negligible amounts of radiation fall outside the main beam. The background radiation can be kept to less than one-tenth of 1 percent of the beam."

How could these characteristics of the synchrocyclotron beam be put to clinical use? One possibility immediately suggested itself. In late cancer of the breast and a number of other conditions, clinical benefits had been reported from removal of the pituitary gland or suppression of its function. Surgical excision of this gland is difficult. Why not destroy it *in situ* with a heavy-particle beam—a sort of "radiation surgery"?

Following several years of biological tests and animal experimentation, the first human patients were treated in 1954; in 1963, Dr. Lawrence and his associates reported on 159 patients with breast cancer, diabetic retinopathy, chromophobe adenoma, malignant exophthalmos, acromegaly, Cushing's syndrome, and other conditions whose pituitaries had been ablated with heavy-ion beams. Dr. Lawrence, on the basis of this experience, was now advising against pituitary irradiation for breast cancer because "the remissions are temporary and responses are not predictable." However, for other conditions trials were continuing.

Proton and alpha-particle beams have also been used for the direct irradiation of tumors at the University of California in Berkeley, at Harvard, and in Europe. Dr. Lawrence's first case was a 43-year-old woman with disseminated cancer of the breast. A metastasis in the right deltoid muscle was treated beginning in January 1960. "The beam was modified so that the maximum dose was delivered under the skin and almost no dose went further than 2.2 centimeters beneath the skin, a point still about $\frac{1}{2}$ centimeter from the surface of the bone. The skin dose was about one-third the tumor dose, the major part of the dose going to the tumor itself. Therapy was well tolerated and three months later there was only a depressed, slightly indurated area that was non-tender and showed no definite mass. There had been no skin reaction." Dr. Lawrence reported this case, and three cases of brain tumor irradiated with alpha particles, at a meeting of the American Medical Association in June 1962.[20]

Dr. R. N. Kjellberg and his Harvard associates also reported in 1962 on the therapeutic use of heavy ions; they delivered from 4,000 to 10,000 rads of 160,000,000-volt protons from the Harvard cyclotron to brain tumors in four patients.[21]

Currently available at the UCRL in Berkeley are beams of high-energy particles of far greater mass than protons, deuterons, or alpha particles—for example, ions of lithium-7, boron-11, carbon-14, oxygen-16, neon-20, and even argon-40. These particles can be accelerated to enormous energies in the Berkeley HILAC (heavy-ion linear accelerator). Their use for therapy remains a problem for the future, but in Berkeley, at least, hopes are high.

"A new era in teletherapy," Dr. John Lawrence declared in 1961, "seems to be opened up by these investigations [of heavy ions] during the past ten years." [22]

REFERENCES

1. *Radiology, 29:* 313–322, 1937.
2. *Symposium on the Use of Radioisotopes in Animal Biology and Medicine,* pp. 1–21. Academic Press, London and New York, 1963.
3. *Radiology, 35:* 322–327, 1940.
4. *Radiology, 39:* 608–620, 1942.
5. *Amer. J. Roentgen., 59:* 771–785, 1948.
6. *J. Franklin Inst., 202:* 693–721, 1926.
7. *Ibid.,* pp. 722–736.
8. *Strahlentherapie, 51:* 119, 1934.
9. *Amer. J. Roentgen., 43:* 728–734, 1940.
10. *Amer. J. Roentgen., 88:* 215–228, 1962.
11. *Amer. J. Roentgen., 72:* 250–259, 1954.
12. *Radiology, 77:* 928–939, 1961.
13. *Radiology, 81:* 317–319, 1963.
14. *Ibid.,* pp. 871–879.
15. *Radiology, 82:* 327–328, 1964.
16. *Amer. J. Roentgen., 90:* 231–239, 1963.
17. Canadian Association of Radiologists. Press release, March 7, 1968.
18. *Radiology, 47:* 487–491, 1946.
19. *Amer. J. Roentgen., 67:* 1–27, 1952.
20. *JAMA, 186:* 236–245, 1963.
21. *Trans. Amer. Neurol. Ass., 87:* 216–218, 1962.
22. *J. Neurosurg., 19:* 717–722, 1962.

25   The Radioisotopes (Radionuclides)

To the major sources of ionizing radiation with which this history has so far been concerned—X-ray tubes, radium and other naturally occurring radioactive elements, and the various particle accelerators— one more very important group of radiation emitters must now be added: the artificially produced radioactive isotopes. **Known as radio-isotopes** during most of the period with which this chapter is concerned, they have in recent years become known also as radionuclides. They have earned for themselves a major role in all branches of **biological research** and a limited but significant use in therapy. Many additional uses, it seems likely, have yet to be found.

Artificial radioactivity was discovered in Europe, and the new artificial radioisotopes were first put to use there. It is therefore necessary once again—as at a number of earlier turning points in radiological history—to transgress geographical boundaries and consider European origins.

The 1934 Discovery

While American physicists from 1928 on were inventing Van de Graaff machines, linear accelerators, cyclotrons, and other complex devices for nuclear research, many physicists in European countries as well as in the United States and Canada continued to work with nature's own atom-smashers—the alpha particles emitted by radium, polonium, and other naturally occurring sources of ionizing radiation. Their techniques were essentially the same as those Rutherford had used in 1918 to transmute nitrogen into an isotope of oxygen. They simply brought a radioactive source close to a target of some element, and studied what happened when alpha particles emitted by the source struck the nuclei of the target substance.

The discovery of two new subatomic particles—the neutron in 1932 and the positron or positively charged electron in 1933—re-invigorated this type of experiment. At the Radium Institute in Paris, for example, a series of Rutherford-type experiments was conducted in 1933 by Irène Curie, the daughter of Pierre and Marie Curie, and her husband, Frédéric Joliot. Their methods differed from Rutherford's of 15 years earlier in only one substantial respect. They were looking for positrons as well as for alpha particles, beta rays, and gamma rays emitted during nuclear bombardment. "The apparatus they were using...could be built at a cost of only a few dollars in any university physics laboratory," Dr. Jacob Sacks of the far more lavishly equipped Brookhaven National Laboratory on Long Island afterward remarked, perhaps with envy.[1]

The Joliot-Curies soon discovered that a number of light elements emitted positrons when bombarded by alpha particles from their radioactive source, a modest supply of polonium; they reported their findings in 1933. However, on further study, the bombardment of three elements—aluminum, boron, and magnesium—was found to produce a far more curious effect. *The emission of positrons continued even after the polonium source had been taken away from the target!* There was only one plausible explanation, and the Joliot-Curies announced it in a brief paper published in *Nature* for Feburary 10, 1934: "The transmutation of boron, magnesium, and aluminum by alpha particles has given birth to new radioelements [radioactive isotopes]...."

The details of the transmutations were soon worked out. The aluminum nucleus, for example, contains 13 protons and 14 neutrons; the alpha particle contains two protons and two neutrons. When they collide, one neutron is emitted as radiation; the remaining 15 protons and 15 neutrons join together to form a new nucleus, phosphorus-30. This isotope of phosphorus, however, is itself unstable. After a time one of the neutrons in its nucleus emits a positron, and the phosphorus-30 is thereby transmuted into a stable nucleus of silicon-30.

The Joliot-Curie announcement set physicists throughout the world off on a search for additional radioactive isotopes, and within 1 year nearly 100 were discovered by European and American researchers.

Hevesy's Radioisotope Tracers

To a Hungarian-born physicist working in Denmark, Dr. George Hevesy, the news of artificial radioactivity carried a special significance. He *needed* the new radioisotopes to bring to fruition a promising research technique that he had invented more than a decade earlier.

Hevesy's technique can best be illustrated by a story that he himself once told.[2] While living in a boarding house in 1923, he had become suspicious of the cuisine. He therefore brought to the table with him a speck of one of the naturally occurring radioisotopes and deposited it on a scrap of meat which he left on his plate. Next day he brought a radiation detector—an electroscope—to the dinner table; sure enough, when the hash was served the electroscope revealed that it was radioactive. Hevesy had thus used a naturally occurring radioisotope as a *tracer* to follow the course of the meat scrap from his plate to the kitchen, through the meat chopper, through the hash pot, and back to the table again.

In a more typical 1923 experiment, Hevesy had grown bean plants in a solution containing a known amount of radioactive lead (thorium B). At intervals he had picked some of the plants, reduced their tissues—roots, stalks, leaves, beans—to ash, and measured the radioactivity in each tissue; thus, he could trace the course of the lead through the plants.

The early Hevesy experiments established a number of principles underlying the use of radioisotopes as tracers today. First and foremost, an isotope of an element appeared to participate in biochemical and physiological processes in precisely the same way as does the element itself. Thus, by tracing the course of an isotope through a living cell or a complex organism, the course of the stable element is also revealed.

Again, Hevesy's bean experiments established the principle of *selective uptake*. When he grew his beans in a solution containing only trivial amounts of lead, for example, as much as 60 per cent of the lead might be taken up by the roots. When more substantial quantities of lead were placed in the nutrient solution, as little as 0.3 per cent of it entered the bean plants. The maximum uptake of a substance is determined, in short, by the organism and its state at the moment, rather than by the amount of the substance available. This principle holds in animal and human as well as plant physiology.

Furthermore, Hevesy's early experiments revealed the principle of *metabolic turnover*. When a lead atom enters a living tissue such as a bean leaf, he was able to show, it does not stay there indefinitely. Rather, it is displaced in due course by another atom of lead subsequently picked up by the roots and carried to the leaf. Thus, the concept of the living organism as the scene of an unceasing dynamic interchange was established, and the characteristic turnover rate could be clocked. This rate can be expressed in terms of "biological half-life"—the time it takes for one-half of a dose of some substance administered to a living organism to leave the organism again.[3]

During the years after 1923, Hevesy continued his work with radioactive lead, radioactive bismuth, and other naturally occurring radioactive substances, but progress was disappointing, for lead and bismuth were of little biological importance.

In 1926, three physicians at Boston City Hospital and the department of medicine, Harvard Medical School—Drs. Herrmann L. Blumgart, Soma Weiss, and Otto C. Yens—used a similar radioisotope technique in human clinical research. They injected minute amounts of radium

C into a vein in a patient's right arm, then measured the time it took for the radium C to affect a Wilson cloud chamber held close to the patient's left arm. Blood circulation time, thus measured, ranged from 14 to 24 seconds in patients with normal circulation but rose to 71 seconds in a patient with cardiac decompensation. Circulation time proved quite stable when repeated measurements were made on the same patient, and time was little affected by the amount of radium C injected for the test.[4]

In 1932, Professor Harold C. Urey of Columbia University discovered a stable isotope of hydrogen—heavy hydrogen or deuterium—which was not radioactive but which could be distinguished from ordinary hydrogen because each atom weighed twice as much. When combined with oxygen, heavy hydrogen produced "heavy water"; in 1934, Hevesy and an associate performed the first tracer experiment with this fluid by drinking small amounts of it themselves, monitoring its excretion in their urine, and thus establishing its biological half-life.[5]

An important new technique was developed in this study. The heavy water that the two scientists drank was, of course, diluted by large quantities of ordinary water already in their bodies. By measuring the ratio of heavy water to ordinary water in the urine excreted, they were able to determine the total volume of body water with which the heavy water had been diluted. This *isotope dilution principle* has several clinical applications today; it is used, for example, to determine total blood volume in a human patient.

Still, Hevesy was handicapped. What he urgently needed to exploit his brilliant tracer technique fully was something that nature had failed to supply—radioactive isotopes of such biologically important elements as phosphorus, sodium, and carbon. It is reported that Hevesy and his associates sometimes speculated on how much *might* be accomplished if these elements could by some unexpected miracle be rendered radioactive. The Joliot-Curie discovery of 1934 brought that miracle within reach.

Problems remained, however. One was the rapidity with which the Joliot-Curie radioisotopes lost their radioactivity. Their phosphorus-30, for example, had a half-life of only 3¼ minutes, which meant that after 6½ minutes only one-quarter of the original activity remained, after 13 minutes only one-sixteenth, and after 3 hours less than 1 per cent—too little to measure. Also, the maximum quantity of a radioisotope that could be produced using the Joliot-Curie polonium source was exceedingly limited—only about 100,000 atoms of phosphorus-30 at a time, for example. After that ceiling was reached, the phosphorus-30 decayed to silicon as rapidly as their polonium source could manufacture new phosphorus-30.

Enrico Fermi in Rome took the next step toward supplying physiologically significant radioisotopes in quantities sufficient to be useful to researchers like Hevesy. Fermi prepared a mixture of radium and beryllium. When the alpha particles from the radium bombarded the beryllium nuclei, neutrons were emitted, and the emerging neutrons could be used in their turn to bombard other nuclei. Fermi discovered many new radioisotopes with this source, including phosphorus-32, with a half-life of 14.3 days instead of only $3\frac{1}{4}$ minutes as in the case of the Joliot-Curie phosphorus-30. With this relatively long half-life, and with a radium-beryllium source of substantial strength, it was possible to build up a considerable supply of phosphorus-32 before the decay rate caught up with the rate of manufacture.[6]

Fermi promptly informed Niels Bohr of the University of Copenhagen of his phosphorus-32 discovery, and Bohr dedicated his own radium-beryllium source—given to him by friends as a present on his 50th birthday—to the manufacture of phosphorus-32 for his colleague Hevesy on weekends and at other times when he did not need it for his own research. The manufacturing process was simple. Bohr merely hung his source inside a flask containing carbon disulfide; the neutrons from the source transmuted the sulfur atoms into phosphorus-32.

Hevesy and his associate D. Chiewitz reported their first tracer experiments with the new radioisotope in a letter to the editor of *Nature* published November 9, 1935. Thus, the man who had invented the tracer technique with a naturally radioactive isotope in 1923, and who had performed the first human experiments with a stable isotope in 1934, was also afforded the honor of performing the first biological experiments with one of the new artificial radioisotopes in 1935. Niels Bohr, a physicist with an eye for poetic justice as well as for scientific merit, had seen to that.

"Recent progress in the production of radioisotopes by neutron bombardment makes the radioisotope of phosphorus-32 easily accessible," Hevesy and Chiewitz began their letter to the editor of *Nature*. "This isotope ... can be used as an indicator of inactive phosphorus in the same way that the radioactive isotopes of lead, bismuth, and so on were formerly used as indicators of those elements." The method, moreover, was incredibly sensitive. "If, for example, we add active phosphorus-32 to 1 milligram of inactive phosphorus in such quantity that the Geiger counter registers 1,000 impulses per minute, carry out with the phosphorus activated in this way any sort of chemical or biochemical reaction, and then find out that the product obtained gives one impulse per minute, we may conclude that 1/1000th of a milligram of the phosphorus originally introduced is present in the product investigated."

Hevesy and Chiewitz treated their phosphorus-32 with nitric acid to secure phosphoric acid. They then treated a sodium compound with this radioactive phosphoric acid to secure *labeled* sodium phosphate—that is, molecules of sodium phosphate which behaved chemically and physiologically like ordinary sodium phosphate, but whose fate in living organisms could be traced by detecting the radiation emitted when a phosphorus atom in one of the molecules of the labeled compound decayed. Much of the progress in radiochemistry, the biological sciences, and medical research during subsequent years arose out of precisely this technique of labeling; with sufficient ingenuity, almost any substance can now be radioactively labeled by incorporating into each molecule one or more radioactive atoms.

Hevesy and Chiewitz fed their precious initial supply of labeled sodium phosphate to laboratory rats, and made careful daily determinations of the amount of radioactivity excreted in the urine and feces. They were able to show that, many days after a rat had eaten the radioactive phosphorus and had excreted the portion not absorbed by its tissues, it continued to excrete small additional amounts. "We have obviously to deal," the investigators concluded, "with the excretion of phosphorus which has already been deposited for a while in the skeleton, the muscles, or other organs, and which has been displaced again. From our experiment it follows that the average time which a phosphorus atom thus spends in the organism of a normally fed rat is about two months. This is also supported by the fact that rats killed about a month after the intake of phosphorus contain only about half the active phosphorus found in those killed after a week's time. The result strongly supports the view that the formation of the bones is a dynamic process, the bone continuously taking up phosphorus atoms which are partly or wholly lost again, and are displaced by other phosphorus atoms."

At autopsy, moreover, Hevesy and Chiewitz found that more than half of the phosphorus remaining in the rat after 20 days was lodged in its bones, a third was contained in the muscles and fat, and the modest remainder was distributed through the liver and other organs. This *selective localization* of particular radioisotopes in particular tissues was another finding which was to have far-reaching consequences in subsequent research.

Finally, and quite by accident, Hevesy and Chiewitz learned something of the transport of phosphorus through the placenta to the unborn rat fetus. "During one of the experiments," they reported, "the rat produced six offspring on the seventh day [after the phosphorus-32 meal], of which five were eaten by the mother; this caused a large increase in the active phosphorus content of the [mother's] excreta in the following three days." The surviving offspring was then sacrificed and its tissues were analyzed. Two per cent of the total radioactivity was found in its body, suggesting that 12 per cent of the original dose of phosphorus-32 had passed through the placenta and had been retained by the six fetuses.

All this was learned with only a few hundredths of a microgram of phosphorus-32.

RADIOISOTOPES FROM THE CYCLOTRON

In the United States, the news of the Joliot-Curie discovery of artificial radioactivity opened new vistas for Ernest O. Lawrence and his associates at the University of California Radiation Laboratory. The Lawrence cyclotron was capable of producing beams of high-energy protons, deuterons, and other particles vastly more intense than the radiation from the modest polonium source used by the Joliot-Curies or the radium-beryllium sources used by Fermi and Bohr. Thus, Lawrence could manufacture the new radioisotopes in far greater quantity, and he could also create new radioisotopes not achievable with the more primitive techniques. By the end of 1936, at least 18 radioisotopes of biologically significant elements were being manufactured in the Lawrence cyclotron. Most of them, however, had so short a half-life that their utility was quite limited, as the following table, prepared by Dr. Lawrence at the time, suggests[7]:

Oxygen-15	2 minutes	6 seconds
Nitrogen-23	10 minutes	23 seconds
Magnesium-27	10 minutes	25 seconds
Iodine-128	25 minutes	
Chlorine-34	40 minutes	
Barium-139	1 hour	20 minutes
Manganese-56	2 hours	30 minutes
Calcium-45	4 hours	
Copper-64	12 hours	48 minutes
Sodium-24	14 hours	48 minutes
Potassium-12	16 hours	
Arsenic	27 hours	
Bromine	35 hours	
Mercury	40 hours	
Iron-59	72 hours	
Phosphorus-32	14 days	7 hours
Sulfur-35	2 months	
Sodium-22	6 months	

"In those days," Dr. Glenn T. Seaborg—then a young associate of Lawrence's, later chairman of the U.S. Atomic Energy Commission—has recalled, "we were able to find a new radioisotope every month or two." Also, as skill with the procedures developed, it even became possible to search for, find, and manufacture new radioisotopes to meet specific needs.[8] Dr. Seaborg has reported two examples of this kind of "tailoring."

"Dr. Joseph G. Hamilton . . . mentioned to me," Dr. Seaborg later told the Society of Nuclear Medicine,[9] "the difficulties he was having with radioactive iodine tracer in his experiments. At that time he was using the iodine-128 isotope, which has a half-life of only 25 minutes. He inquired as to the possibility of finding another iodine isotope with a longer half-life, which led me to ask him what value would be best for his work. He replied, 'Oh, about a week.' You may recall that soon after that we synthesized and identified iodine-131, with a half-life of eight days.

"Similar requests from other specialists in nuclear medicine led to the identification of several other applicable isotopes in our laboratory at Berkeley. Dr. George H. Wipple, the Nobel pathologist at the University of Rochester, needed an iron isotope with a half-life of several weeks for his studies of hemoglobin formation in blood. For this use we provided iron-59, with a half-life of 45 days. I cannot claim that we in the physical sciences always fulfill the needs of our colleagues so precisely, but these examples do serve to illustrate the importance of a close tie between the sciences."

Isotopes for Blood Diseases

Among the radioisotopes which could be manufactured in the cyclotron in 1936 was sodium-24. Ernest Lawrence made some for two of his associates, Drs. Joseph G. Hamilton and Robert S. Stone. What should they do with it?

One obvious possibility was to administer the sodium-24 to animals or to human volunteers and then, using the Hevesy technique, to trace the course of the sodium through the living organism as Hevesy had done with phosphorus in rats. A more significant possibility, however, captured the interest of Drs. Hamilton and Stone.

In preliminary animal experiments, small amounts of a sodium-24 solution had been injected into white mice.[7] No ill effects were noted except that the number of white cells in the blood of the mice fell after moderate doses. This result was not surprising. For many years patients with chronic leukemia—a disease characterized by too many white cells in the blood—had been treated with X rays to lower their white-cell count. The X rays depressed the activity of the bone marrow where the white blood cells are manufactured. Apparently the radiation from sodium-24, given internally to mice, produced the same effect; the possibility was thus suggested that sodium-24, if given internally to leukemia patients, might similarly lower their white-cell counts and improve their clinical condition.

No therapeutic trial of an artificial radioisotope administered to human patients had ever been reported. Before launching a human trial, accordingly, Drs. Hamilton and Stone reviewed the earlier literature on the intravenous injection of naturally radioactive substances. As early as 1913, they learned, Dr. Frederick Proescher and Dr. B. R. Almquest had injected radium chloride into the veins of more than 20 patients suffering from various diseases, including a patient with chronic leukemia.[10] Numerous other investigators (including Dr. Stone himself) had also given radium internally to patients, either orally or by injection. Some preliminary reports on these treatments were favorable, but Drs. Hamilton and Stone found few follow-up reports on the long-range after-effects. Instead, they found numerous reports of radium poisoning, bone tumors following radium ingestion or injection, and other major hazards (see page 417). It was hardly surprising that the internal use of radium had gone out of style. "The amount which would be sufficient to be clinically effective," Drs. Hamilton and Stone noted, "probably would be fatal within a few years, due to the tendency of the radioactive elements to be deposited in the bones."[11]

With sodium-24, however, there appeared to be no comparable hazard. "It was felt," Drs. Hamilton and Stone reported at the December 1936 meeting of the Radiological Society of North America, "that many of the disadvantages of internal radium therapy could be avoided by the use of radiosodium, inasmuch as this latter substance does not become fixed in the body tissues, and the duration of its effect is limited by the short half-life of only 14.8 hours." Accordingly, a cautious clinical trial of sodium-24 on a patient with chronic leukemia was decided upon. A double advantage could thus be secured from the limited supply of the radioisotope, for, even if no therapeutic effect was demonstrated, the course of the sodium through the patient's body—its uptake, distribution, storage, and excretion—could be traced.

The selection of patients was easy. Since sodium-24 had a half-life of only 14.8 hours, it was administered to "the only patients with leukemia available at such times as the radiosodium could be obtained."

The first patient was a 29-year-old male who had developed symptoms of chronic leukemia in February 1935. He had been given an intensive course of deep X-ray therapy which produced considerable improvement. In March 1936, however, he returned to the hospital in relapse and "after consultation, it was decided to make this patient the recipient of the first intravenous administration of radiosodium. On March 23, 1936, he was given ... radiosodium by vein, and four days later he received ... more in the same manner." No improvement was noted, nor were there any signs of toxic effects.

In September 1936, another patient was given a sodium-24 injection, and a few days later a second dose was administered to this patient by stomach tube. Again there was neither clinical improvement nor toxic effects. The course of the sodium through his body was traced, however. "Further investigations with the use of larger amounts [of sodium-24] in other patients are essential before any estimation of its therapeutic value can be made," Drs. Hamilton and Stone concluded. "A similar line of investigation can be followed, using other artificially prepared radioactive elements."

The most hopeful of the other known radioisotopes for use in chronic leukemia was phosphorus-32. Hevesy's initial experiment with phosphorus-32 had shown that it accumulated selectively in the bones. Drs. K. G. Scott and S. F. Cook had given some phosphorus-32 to chickens, in May 1936, and reported a selective effect on their white blood cells. Dr. John Lawrence, accordingly, decided to test the effect of phosphorus-32 on leukemic patients, and Drs. Hamilton and Stone thereupon discontinued their work with sodium-24. Dr. Lawrence administered the first dose of phosphorus-32 to a patient with chronic leukemia on Christmas Eve, 1936; in 1956 that patient, aged 74, was still alive and well. By early 1939, Dr. Lawrence was able to report on half a dozen leukemia patients given the treatment.

The results could be described as mildly promising. "When the larger doses are given to patients with leukemia," Dr. Lawrence declared, "decrease in the number of white blood cells can be produced similar to that following roentgen radiation. The greater deposition of phosphorus in bone marrow and in bone than in other human tissues (as shown by experiments on leukemic mice) suggests that this offers a method of giving selective radiation in leukemia. Since at present there is no completely satisfactory method for the treatment of this disease, it seems justifiable to use this material cautiously in therapeutic attempts, in addition to its use as a tracer of the metabolism of phosphorus in this disease." [12]

Dr. Lawrence's most sensational finding, however, followed later in 1939. Polycythemia vera is a disease characterized by an excess of red blood cells rather than white blood cells. Dr. Lawrence tried his phosphorus-32 on two women patients with polycythemia vera, and at the

December 1939 meeting of the Radiological Society of North America he was able to report that both of them experienced a fall in their red cell count and a marked clinical improvement without objectionable side-effects.

This proved to be the first clear-cut success for radioisotope therapy. By October 1946, despite the limited availability of the isotope, nearly 300 patients with polycythemia vera had been treated with phosphorus-32 by Dr. Lawrence and Dr. L. A. Erf at the University of California, by Dr. Bryon E. Hall and Dr. Charles H. Watkins at the Mayo Clinic, and by others at other medical centers.[13]

"Radioactive phosphorus possesses distinct advantages over other methods in the treatment of polycythemia," Dr. Bruce K. Wiseman of the Ohio State University College of Medicine could report in 1951, "as judged by almost ten years' experience. The method is hematologically sound, effective, convenient for the physician and patient, inexpensive, and, with proper safeguards, presents less treatment hazard to the patient than other methods of therapy currently employed." [14] Other radioisotopes have also been used for the treatment of polycythemia vera, notably yttrium-90.

Ruben, Kamen, and Carbon-14

Much of the most interesting early work with radioisotopes concerned neither human patients nor laboratory animals, but primitive organisms such as bacteria, yeasts, and algae. The reasons were twofold. First, the basic biochemical processes common to all living cells could be conveniently traced in these organisms; second, complex compounds of great physiological interest such as amino acids, proteins, enzymes, and vitamins could be *labeled* with the help of these organisms. If radioactive carbon were combined with oxygen to form carbon dioxide, for example, and if one-celled plants were then incubated in an atmosphere containing the radioactive carbon dioxide, the plants took up the gas and incorporated its radioactive carbon atoms into the far more complex metabolic compounds, such as proteins and enzymes, which they were manufacturing. By extracting these products of the plant's metabolism and purifying them, it was hoped, labeled compounds might be secured which could then be used for further biochemical and physiological tracer experiments in higher organisms. However, in practice there were many obstacles. In 1937, for example, a group of scientists at Ernest Lawrence's laboratory was trying to extract from algae metabolic products labeled with carbon-11, a radioactive isotope having a half-life of only 21 minutes.

Dr. Martin D. Kamen, the nuclear chemist assigned to the group, has published in *Science* for May 10, 1963, a dramatic reminiscence of what life was like while such experiments were being performed in Lawrence's laboratory during the years 1937 to 1940.

In one experiment recalled by Kamen, 23-year-old Dr. Samuel Ruben and others proposed to grow algae in a carbon-dioxide atmosphere labeled with carbon-11 and then use an ultracentrifuge to separate the metabolic products into which the algae had incorporated the carbon-11 atoms. However, the nearest available ultracentrifuge was at Stanford University in Palo Alto, 50 miles away through heavy California traffic. In 1937 there was no throughway from Berkeley to Palo Alto. Ruben and Kamen calculated that they would have time to secure the carbon-11 from the Berkeley cyclotron, incorporate it in carbon dioxide, incubate the algae in the carbon dioxide, and extract the metabolic products from the algae. By the time the products were driven to Stanford and centrifuged, however, there would not be enough carbon-11 left to measure. "We considered a number of possible courses of action," Kamen recalled, "such as arranging a police escort for the motor trip to Stanford.... One night a brilliant solution occurred to Sam Ruben; he woke me by phone at 2 a.m. to suggest carrier pigeons!" [15]

The best solution, of course, would be to produce a longer-lived isotope of carbon, and Kamen considered carbon-14 the likeliest possibility. Traces of carbon-14 had appeared in a few earlier experiments, but only a few atoms at a time, so that its half-life was still in doubt. If carbon-14 could be produced in a cyclotron at all, which seemed unlikely at the time, it would presumably require long exposure of some target substance in the beam of the device—and Lawrence's cyclotrons were much too busy to be used for long periods on so speculative a project.

"It was with some amazement, therefore," Kamen recorded, "that I found myself... being told by Lawrence that both cyclotrons must be diverted forthwith to a full-time effort to determine definitely whether long-lived isotopes of hydrogen, carbon, nitrogen, and oxygen did or did not exist. The reason for this was soon evident. During Lawrence's most recent efforts to achieve increased and continued subsidies for cyclotron development, some question had been raised as to the real value of radioactive isotopes in biological research." Indeed, *stable* isotopes of hydrogen, carbon, nitrogen, and oxygen were at that time proving more useful as tracers than cyclotron-produced radioisotopes, because they did not vanish while a biological experiment was under way. If the cyclotrons were to repay the many millions of dollars Lawrence hoped to raise and expend on them, they would have to produce something less evanescent than oxygen-15 (half-life 2.1 minutes) and nitrogen-13 (half-life 10 minutes, 23 seconds). As Lawrence himself explained in a 1937 letter to Ernest Rutherford, "In this country medical research receives generous support, and it was the possible medical applications of the artificial radioactive substances and neutron radiation that made it possible for me to obtain adequate financial support." [16]

Several further experiments designed to produce carbon-14 were accordingly launched. One of them involved storing two 5-gallon bottles of ammonium nitrate solution in an area not far from the cyclotron, near the beam-deflector controls. Measurements had shown that a considerable flux of neutrons leaked into this area, and it was barely possible that if the bottles were stored there long enough the leaking neutrons which would otherwise be wasted might bombard the solution in the bottles and produce carbon-14. A more hopeful experiment involved inserting a copper probe coated with a paste of graphite directly into the cyclotron; it was possible that the intensive bombardment of the graphite by the direct beam of circling deuterons might transmute it to carbon-14. The probe could only be inserted into the cyclotron at night, in order not to interfere with Dr. Stone's neutron-beam therapy (see page 367) and many other daytime activities. Kamen recalled:

> I undertook the night bombardments, aided occasionally by others. . . . The probe target was not designed to withstand intense bombardment. I had merely smeared colloidal graphite on the water-cooled copper surface, and had counted on replacing, during frequent inspections, whatever graphite was found to be blasted off. . . .
>
> This experiment . . . was performed in a spirit of mixed desperation and resignation, and it involved a considerable bit of hazard from radiation exposure, as it was necesssary to examine the intensely radioactive probe nightly to insure that some graphite still clung to the target surface. Occasionally I found the irradiated graphite almost on the verge of flaking off and had to cement it back on with more graphite.
>
> On February 15 [1940], during a particularly violent storm, I terminated this bombardment. . . . Shortly before dawn I left the graphite, which looked like bits of gravel, in a weighing bottle on Ruben's desk. On the way home to get some sleep for the first time in several days I must have presented a sorry spectacle—unshaven, red-eyed, and dazed—for I was intercepted and questioned by police looking for an escaped convict. Fortunately I failed to pass muster and was released, to continue stumbling homeward toward sleep.[15]

Two weeks of work with the sample persuaded Ruben and Kamen that they had indeed produced a small amount of carbon-14, "and on Wednesday evening we motored to Lawrence's home to acquaint him with the result. Lawrence was resting in an attempt to banish a cold before his appearance the next night, February 29, to receive the Nobel prize in physics. His pleasure was unbounded. . . ."

Additional graphite probes were now placed in the cyclotron, and additional laboratory study revealed that the carbon-14 had an enormously long half-life—measurable in thousands of years, longer even than the half-life of radium. A method of producing carbon-14 had indeed been discovered, although hardly a practical method. Then fate took a hand.

While the work with the graphite probe had been under way, the two 5-gallon bottles of ammonium nitrate solution, contained in a wooden box, were standing half-forgotten near the deflector controls of the cyclotron, soaking up stray neutrons. One day an "angry deputation" of cyclotron technicians paid Dr. Kamen a visit and demanded that he remove his property. The box got in the way every time the deflector controls needed adjustment, and the crew "was weary of the constant pushing and pulling required to move the box"—especially since one of the bottles had sprung a leak and the box was thus wet with acid.

"So with no great enthusiasm," Kamen recounted, "I went over to the 60-inch cyclotron with a cart and moved the box to Ruben's laboratory in the ramshackle hut affectionately known as the 'Rat House.'" There Ruben and Kamen tested a precipitate from one of the bottles. "To our astonishment, we found that a small fraction of this precipitate was so active it completely paralyzed the screen wall counter! In a short time we ascertained that we had several microcuries [millionths of a curie] of carbon-14—a quantity greater by two or three orders of magnitude than any we had seen from the probe bombardments. Needless to say, our interest in the [probes] vanished, never to return."

Carbon-14, with a half-life of 5700 years, is today among the most useful of radioisotopes in biological tracer experiments, and many labeled biochemical compounds are routinely produced by growing microorganisms in labeled carbon dioxide and extracting the metabolic products.

RADIOISOTOPES FROM NUCLEAR REACTORS

While these and numerous other projects for the manufacture and use of radioisotopes were under way in the United States, a remarkable new idea which was to revolutionize life on our planet was conceived in Europe.

In December 1938 two physicists in Nazi Germany, Otto Hahn and Fritz Strassmann, bombarded uranium with slow neutrons and discovered some barium among the reaction products. This was amazing, for barium has an atomic weight about half the weight of uranium. How could the bombardment of uranium produce barium?

Even before publishing the findings, Hahn wrote news of the discovery to Dr. Lise Meitner, a close associate of his who had recently escaped to Sweden. Dr. Otto R. Frisch, than an associate of Niels Bohr in Denmark, has recently described the sequel.[17]

"Lise Meitner was lonely in Sweden," he wrote, "and, as her faithful nephew, I went to visit her at Christmas. There, in a small hotel in Kungälv near Göteberg I found her at breakfast brooding over a letter from Hahn. I was skeptical about the contents—that barium was formed from uranium by neutrons—but she kept on with it. We walked up and down in the snow, I on skis and she on foot...and gradually the idea took shape that this was no chipping or cracking of the nucleus...." Instead, Drs. Meitner and Frisch concluded, it must be nuclear *fission*—the actual splitting of the uranium nucleus into two approximately equal fragments, one of which was barium. In the process of splitting, moreover, a tiny portion of the mass of the uranium atom would be released as energy.

There was nothing very remarkable about this energy release; energy is similarly released in most other atomic transmutations. However, Drs. Meitner and Frisch went one long step further. They calculated that the two atomic fragments would be hurled apart with an energy of 200,000,000 electron volts—and that the total amount of energy released from even a small amount of fissioning uranium would be enormous.

Only about $\frac{1}{10}$ per cent of the mass of each fissioning uranium atom would be converted to energy, it is true, but, in accordance with Einstein's most famous theorem, $E = mc^2$, the mass (m) converted to energy (E) in such a reaction must be multiplied by the square of the speed of light (c^2)—an enormous factor. Thus, the mass in 1 pound of uranium, if completely converted, would yield as much energy as the explosion of 20 billion pounds of TNT, and even though only $\frac{1}{10}$ per cent of the mass of the uranium were to be converted, a few pounds would be enough to destroy a city.

Dr. Frisch spent only 2 or 3 days with his aunt that Christmas. "Then I went back to Copenhagen," he recalls, "and just managed to tell Bohr about the idea as he was catching [a] boat to the U.S. I remember how he struck his head after I had barely started to speak and said: 'Oh, what fools we have been! We ought to have seen that before.' But he had not—nobody had."

Bohr was met at the pier when he landed in New York by Enrico Fermi and Dr. John A. Wheeler of Princeton. He passed the news of fission to them, and later to others. Scientists at Princeton, Columbia, and other American centers tested the fission hypothesis in the laboratory, as did Frisch in Copenhagen and Joliot-Curie in Paris. By March 1939, nuclear fission was an accepted fact, and a further fact was unearthed.

When a neutron produced the fissioning of a uranium nucleus, additional neutrons were emitted, which in turn could produce fission in additional uranium nuclei, with the emission of still more neutrons ... and so on in a self-perpetuating *chain reaction*. Thus, the physicists were well on the road toward nuclear power and nuclear disaster.

The story of the atomic bomb from then until Hiroshima and Nagasaki lies outside the scope of a history of radiology. By 1946, however, the nuclear reactor which had been built for military use at Oak Ridge, Tennessee, was converted to the production of radioisotopes for civilian research. Although it could not manufacture as many different kinds of isotopes as the cyclotron, it could produce many kinds in far larger quantities at far lower cost. Public announcement of the availability of reactor-produced radioisotopes was made in *Science* for June 14, 1946; the first publicly announced shipment—a small amount of carbon-14, addressed to the Barnard Cancer Hospital in St. Louis—was dispatched from Oak Ridge on August 2, 1946, just 1 year after Hiroshima.

During the years since 1946, radioisotopes produced in nuclear reactors as well as some still produced by means of particle accelerators have become tools of enormous value in every branch of the biological sciences. More than 1000 radioisotopes are currently known, and thousands of isotope-tagged chemical compounds are for sale, conveniently packaged, as ordinary products of commerce.

By 1955, more than 1200 medical institutions were licensed by the U.S. Atomic Energy Commission to use reactor-produced radioisotopes, and by 1962 the number of medical radioisotope licensees had risen to nearly 3000. Dr. Marshall Brucer reported that there were 1,582 known species of radioisotopes in 1961, of which 300 might prove medically useful—and the numbers were still increasing. One radiologist specializing in nuclear medicine estimated in 1968 that 4,000 users of radioisotopes in 3,000 hospitals were performing 3,000,000 clinical studies with radioisotopes annually.[18]

The vast scope of these developments can hardly be covered here. Rather, the pages which follow review a few typical examples—some already routine but others still in the investigational stage—of how radioisotopes are currently being put to use by radiologists and other physicians.

RADIOISOTOPE TRACERS TODAY

Iodine-Uptake Tests

The pioneers in tracer studies—that is, the men who worked with radioisotopes from 1935 to 1946—quickly discovered that the isotopes of iodine were among the most fascinating and most useful.

Iodine follows a complex course through the human body.[19] After a dose is swallowed it is absorbed through the intestinal walls, converted to iodide, and carried in the blood plasma to the thyroid gland in the neck. The thyroid gland has an amazing ability to take up and store the iodide; indeed, it may extract additional iodide from the blood stream even though the iodide concentration inside the gland is already 100 times the concentration of the substance in the blood. The gland then combines the iodide with various proteins to form hormones and hormone-like substances, and, in response to stimulation by the thyroid-stimulating hormone (TSH) which is secreted by the pituitary gland, the thyroid gland releases these substances into the blood stream again. They circulate all through the body, regulating the metabolic rate of other organs and tissues.

Some of this was known before 1936, but many of the details were worked out through tracer studies; the researchers then went on to develop standard clinical tests to study each of the stages in the complex iodine cycle.

The simplest of these standard radioisotope diagnostic tests, and the one most commonly used by physicians, is based squarely on Hevesy's principle of selective uptake. An oral dose of a solution containing one of the radioactive iodine isotopes is given to the patient. After a time a Geiger-Müller counter or some other device for detecting radioactivity is held close to the patient's neck to determine how much of the dose has been taken up by the gland. The gland of a patient suffering from hyperthyroidism—overactivity of the gland—takes up much more of the dose than does a normal gland.[19]

A variation on this technique consists of giving an oral dose of iodine-131, measuring the iodine-131 excreted in the urine, and thus deducing the amount taken up by the gland.

A third diagnostic test determines the quantity of iodine "cleared" from the blood as it passes through the thyroid gland. Patients with hyperthyroidism may clear all of the iodine from the blood as it passes through the gland the first time; a normal gland, in contrast, may take up only one-fifth or less of the iodine contained in the blood passing through it.

Still another simple test is to administer iodine-131 orally and then use two external radiation counters, such as Geiger-Müller counters, to measure simultaneously the radioactivity emerging from the neck and from some other part of the body such as the thigh. In patients with normal thyroids, the radiation from the neck is generally less than 7 times as intense as the radiation from the thigh; higher ratios mean that the thyroid gland has picked up more than the normal amount of iodine from the blood and is therefore probably hyperactive.

Two further tests are based on the fact that normal thyroid glands and hyperactive or diseased glands react differently to thyroid extract and to the thyroid-stimulating hormone secreted by the pituitary. In one of these tests, thyroid extract is given to the patient, and one of the standard uptake tests is administered a little later. The thyroid extract suppresses iodine uptake altogether in a normal gland but not in a hyperactive gland. The other test, based on TSH, is used in the diagnosis of hypothyroidism or myxedema—a condition in which the gland is underactive. The test distinguishes between two varieties of this disease: primary myxedema, due to a defect in the thyroid gland itself, and secondary myxedema, due to lack of TSH from the pituitary. To make the distinction, a standard uptake test is first performed. TSH is then given and another uptake test is performed. If the amount of iodine taken up by the gland is increased in the second test, secondary myxedema due to a pituitary defect is indicated.

In addition to these uptake tests, all based on the quantity of iodine picked up by the thyroid gland, another series of tests is concerned with the processing of the iodine by the gland. The simplest of these tests merely determines the amount of radioactive protein-bound iodine (PBI) circulating in the blood a few days after the radioisotope is given. A variation on this test determines the ratio of the amount of iodine-131 circulating in the form of PBI to the amount still retained in the gland.

Several tests for thyroid function do not require the administration of a radioisotope to the *patient* at all. Red blood cells drawn from the patient are incubated in a test tube with various metabolic products labeled with iodine-131, and the uptake of the labeled product by the cells is determined. Cells from patients with normal thyroid glands take up more of the labeled substances than cells from patients with myxedema, but less than cells from patients with hyperthyroidism.[19]

Other Diagnostic Tests

Various gastrointestinal functions can be tested in similar ways. One of the most interesting of these tests is used to distinguish pernicious anemia from other kinds of anemia such as iron-deficiency anemia. In pernicious anemia there may be enough iron available, but the bone marrow cannot use the iron to manufacture red blood cells because vitamin B-12 is missing. Oral doses of vitamin B-12 will not help, because a defect in the gastrointestinal tract of patients with pernicious anemia prevents the uptake of vitamin B-12 from the small bowel. To check for the presence of such a defect, a dose of vitamin B-12 labeled with a radioisotope is administered. If the labeled vitamin is excreted instead of appearing in the blood stream, pernicious anemia is indicated.[19]

Liver function, kidney function, heart output, the rate of manufacture of red blood cells, the longevity of the cells, and blood volume can all be studied by means of radioisotope tests. In one simple blood-volume procedure, a small amount of albumin, labeled with a radioisotope, is injected into the blood stream. After a time a blood sample is drawn. The more blood there is circulating through the body, the more the labeled albumin is diluted, and hence the less radioactivity appears in the second sample; this is a direct application of Hevesy's dilution principle. More sophisticated blood-volume tests are commonly used to determine the volume of red blood cells and of blood plasma separately.

Very few such tests, it is true, establish a firm diagnosis when considered in isolation. Rather, their value lies in the fact that they supply significant data which, when combined with information from the patient's medical history, the physical examination, X-ray films, and other diagnostic procedures, enable the physician to make a diagnosis more confidently than would otherwise be possible.

Finally, mention should be made of the use of radioisotopes as a source of radiation for *diagnostic roentgenology*. Instead of using radiation from a conventional X-ray tube to produce an image on a diagnostic film, a beam of rays from an isotope source can be substituted. Several devices incorporate a radioisotope pellet instead of an X-ray tube as a source of diagnostic radiation. No electric power supply is required, and the device is so small and so light that it is readily portable. The convenience of such a machine for military medicine and for emergencies in remote areas is obvious. "The technique has reached the stage of clinical diagnostic usefulness," Drs. Kenneth L. Krabbenhoft and Farno L. Green of Harper Hospital in Detroit reported in 1963, but it was not yet ready to "compete with conventional roentgenography in fixed installations with adequate electrical power." [20]

Scintiscan and Photoscan

Much of the success of radioisotope research depended on the discovery of new isotopes having suitable half-lives and giving off radiation of suitable type, quality, and quantity. Much depended, too, on the convenient availability of these radioisotopes, and of compounds labeled with them, in adequate quantity, at a reasonable price. Equally important was the development of subtle, ingenious, and incredibly sensitive devices for detecting the radiations emitted by the radioisotopes. The *scintillation scanner* or *scintiscan,* developed by Dr. Benedict Cassen and his University of California at Los Angeles associates, is one very useful example.[21]

Ionizing radiation, it will be recalled, can be detected by the pinpoints of light—scintillations—which certain crystals emit when rays strike them. In 1949, Dr. Cassen mounted some crystals of calcium tungstate—the crystals that Edison had used similarly in 1896—in front of a photomultiplier tube, so that each time a scintillation appeared on the crystals the tube would emit a surge of electrical current. This scintillation counter proved to be extremely sensitive, and the electrical surges that it emitted could be "read out" in many ways. Two years later Dr. Cassen mounted one of his scintillation counters on a motorized scanning frame which moved the counter back and forth, counting as it moved, and dropping down a line at each sweep like a television scanning beam. He coupled the output of the counter to an automatic pen which moved synchronously with the counter, making a mark on a sheet of paper whenever a scintillation or a specified number of scintillations appeared on the crystals. Thus, as a radioactive area was scanned by the crystals, a *map* of the area appeared on the sheet of paper. Sub-regions emitting large amounts of radiation appeared quite dark on the map because the pen made many marks close together; sub-regions emitting little or no radiation appeared as only lightly shaded or white areas on the map.

If the area being scanned by the scintillation counter is the neck of a patient who has received iodine-131, a portrayal of the patient's thyroid gland appears on the map or scintiscan. If the gland contains a cyst or tumor which does not take up iodine-131, that sub-region appears as a "cold spot." If the gland includes a nodule which concentrates a radioisotope excessively, a "hot spot" appears on the scan.

Numerous improvements on the scintiscan have since been made. One large transparent crystal specifically "grown" for the purpose is usually used instead of many small crystals, for example. The electronic circuits may be arranged so that the scan records only radiations in a particular energy range. Thus, if a patient who has been given iodine-131 is being scanned, the device can be set to remain "blind" to all radiation except gamma rays of the voltage emitted by iodine-131. Under suitable circumstances, the presence of a radioisotope can be detected and its spatial distribution mapped even though there are billions of stable atoms for each radioactive atom.[21]

A variation on the scintiscan is the photoscan.[22] Instead of using an automatic pen and sheet of paper for recording, this device feeds the output from the multiplier tube to a moving beam of light; the brightness of the light at each moment is proportional to the number of scintillations on the face of the crystal at that moment. If a sheet of photographic paper or an X-ray film is exposed to the moving light, it records point for point the amount of radioactivity emerging from the area scanned.

The scanning of the human thyroid to determine the size of the gland and to locate hot spots and cold spots was the first clinical use to which the scintiscan was put in 1951. Many other uses have been developed since. One example is "whole-body scanning," in which a patient with thryoid cancer is given a dose of radioactive iodine and his entire body is scanned in a search for metastases. This is not always successful, since many thyroid cancer metastases do not take up radioactive iodine, but metastases anywhere in the body which do take up the radioisotope can be located in this way.

Other bodily organs, too, can be scanned in much the same way. To scan the liver, for example, a dye known as rose Bengal, which concentrates in that organ, is labeled with a radioisotope and administered to the patient. A scintiscan or photoscan made while the labeled rose Bengal is in the liver shows the boundaries of the organ and many details of clinical importance. Cysts, abscesses, fistulas, and tumors within the liver may reveal their presence by localized decreases in radioactivity shown on the scintiscan—cold spots. Patients with multiple liver metastases show multiple areas of decreased radioactivity. A diffuse decrease in activity throughout an enlarged area of activity suggests an enlarged, poorly functioning organ—perhaps cirrhosis of the liver. Liver malfunctioning can be distinguished from obstruction of the liver outflow; if the scintiscan shows activity in the intestinal area, it can be concluded that the outflow is not completely blocked. Light can also be thrown on other disease processes in the liver region.[23, 24]

Bone cancers and bone-cancer metastases can in some cases be localized by means of a scintiscan following administration of radioactive calcium, radioactive phosphorus, or some other radioisotope which is preferentially taken up by these tumors, or which is *more promptly* taken up by a tumor than by neighboring tissues. The kidneys and several other organs can be mapped by this means with the scintiscan.

No substance is known which localizes preferentially in the spleen, but an ingenious method for making a scintiscan of the spleen has nevertheless been devised. One function of this organ is to remove damaged red cells from the blood stream. Accordingly, a small sample of blood is drawn from a patient suspected of having a malfunctioning spleen. The red cells in the sample are labeled with a radioisotope, damaged by heat, and reinjected into the patient. The spleen promptly removes the tagged and damaged cells from the circulation, whereupon a scintiscan maps the regions of the organ which are performing their function properly and the regions which are not.

Still another ingenious application of the scintiscan procedure is the technique of "coincidence counting." A number of chemical compounds are taken up more promptly by certain kinds of brain tumor than by normal brain tissue, but the difference in uptake is slight. If a compound were labeled with iodine-131 in the usual way, the radiation emitted from the brain tumor would be masked by radiation from surrounding tissues. Accordingly, the compound is labeled with a radioisotope which emits *positrons*.

The positrons themselves cannot possibly be detected. A positron travels only a few millionths of a centimeter through tissue before it captures an electron; when that happens, the two annihilate one another. In the process of annihilation, however, two gamma rays are emitted at a specific voltage, and they leave the scene of annihilation in opposite directions. Hence, in coincidence counting, two scintiscan devices are stationed on opposite sides of the patient's head and the labeled compound is administered. The devices are arranged in a circuit which records radiation only when *both* devices are activated simultaneously by two gamma rays of the right energy emerging from the same positron annihilation. The background radiation or "noise" which would otherwise ruin the scan is ignored altogether.

Radioisotope Therapy

As contrasted with their widespread use in medical diagnosis, radioisotopes are being used today in the treatment of disease on a relatively limited scale. Within these limits, however, they can be remarkably effective.

The use of phosphorus-32 in the treatment of polycythemia vera and of some forms of chronic leukemia has already been noted (page 386). Much more common, however, is the use of therapeutic doses of iodine-131 in the treatment of hyperthyroidism and certain other diseases.

The procedure, which replaces surgery, is remarkably simple. After hyperthyroidism has been diagnosed with the help of an extremely small dose of radioactive iodine, a larger dose is given—indeed, a dose so large that the radiation from it damages or destroys a portion of the thyroid gland. Enough of the gland is left functioning to maintain the desired thyroid balance.

A second use of this procedure is in patients with heart disease so severe that they cannot hope to survive at their normal level of metabolic activity. To lower their metabolic rate, the thyroid gland is partially destroyed with a therapeutic dose of iodine-131, and they are thus able to live on at a lowered metabolic rate.

Great popular excitement was engendered in 1946 when it was suggested that iodine-131 could similarly be administered to patients with thyroid cancer in doses large enough to kill the cancer cells. The cure for thyroid cancer, it was alleged, could be drunk before dinner in the form of an iodine-131 "cocktail," and it was even suggested that other isotopes or compounds would soon be found which would similarly concentrate in other kinds of cancer cells and destroy them. Popular disappointment soon followed, for only a small proportion of thyroid cancers, it was found, concentrate iodine sufficiently to make this procedure helpful. In those few cases, iodine-131 is today administered with considerable success.

Radioisotopes are therapeutically useful in other respects as well.[19] In one simple approach, the old radium applicators familiar for a half-century are loaded with a suitable artificial radioisotope instead of with radium or radon, and the applicator is then used in the ordinary way. The Ernst cervical applicator, for example (above, page 289), is now used with artificial radioisotopes as well as with radium. However, many changes have been rung on this principle. Radioisotopes have been fabricated in the form of threads or wires which can be threaded through a tumor. They have been packaged in glass or ceramic "microspheres" as small as red blood cells which can be injected into a tumor's blood supply, and they have been plated on the surface of such microspheres. Radioactive colloids have been prepared—fluids laden with very finely divided radioactive particles—which can be injected directly into tumor tissues or into body cavities. Blotting paper has been soaked in a radioisotope solution and used to irradiate skin cancers.

Finally, as noted in Chapter 23, cobalt-60 and other radioisotopes have been used instead of X-ray tubes to beam gamma rays at cancer cells from a distance, and have become by far the most popular sources of supervoltage beams for cancer therapy.

This brief review is far from an exhaustive enumeration of either the diagnostic or the therapeutic applications of the artificial radioisotopes in modern medicine, nor is it possible to review here the many investigations under way which are likely to lead to new isotope uses in the years ahead. Enough has perhaps been said, however, to indicate how far the radioisotope sciences have progressed since George Hevesy dropped that radioactive speck on a meat scrap, and grew beans in a radioactive lead solution, back in 1923.

REFERENCES

1. Sacks, J., *The Atom at Work*, p. 88. The Ronald Press Company, New York, 1951.
2. *Presentation of the Second Atoms for Peace Award to George Charles Hevesy.* Rockefeller Institute, New York, Jan. 29, 1959.
3. *Biochem. J., 23:* 439–445, 1923.
4. *J. Clin. Invest., 4:* 1–31, 1927.
5. *Nature (London), 134:* 879, 1934.
6. *Nature (London), 133:* 757, 1934.
7. *Yale J. Biol. Med., 9:* 429–435, 1937.
8. U.S. Atomic Energy Commission. News release S-12-64, June 5, 1964.
9. *Yale J. Biol. Med., 9:* 429–435, 1937.
10. *Radium, 6:* 85–96, 1916.
11. *Radiology, 28:* 178–188, $$$.
12. *Int. Clin., 3:* 33–58, 1939.
13. *Med. Clin. N. Amer., 31:* 810–840, 1947.
14. *Ann. Intern. Med., 34:* 311–330, 1951.
15. *Science, 140:* 584–590, 1963.
16. *Phys. To-day, 19:* 42, 1966.
17. *Phys. To-day, 20:* 43–52, Nov. 1967.
18. *Your Radiologist, 11:* 12–17, Winter 1968.
19. Silver, S., *Radioactive Isotopes in Medicine and Biology,* Ed. 2. Lea & Febiger, Philadelphia, 1962.
20. *Amer. J. Roentgen., 90:* 1123–1142, 1963.
21. *Nucleonics, 6:* 78–80, Feb. 1950; *Amer. J. Roentgen., 68:* 963–970, 1952.
22. *Nature (London), 170:* 200–201, 1952.
23. *Radiology, 78:* 338, 1962.
24. *Arch. Intern. Med., 107:* 324–334, 1961.

26 Radiation Hazards and Safeguards in the Nuclear Era

The supervoltage X rays and the man-made radioisotopes described in the preceding chapters are the nuclear era's best-known contributions to medical radiology. However, a third radiological advance of at least equal importance also arose directly out of nuclear developments: the enormous progress made since 1942 in safeguarding radiologists themselves, their tens of millions of patients, and the public generally from the potentially deleterious effects of ionizing radiation.

Consider, for example, a patient whose head, chest, or abdomen was X-rayed for diagnostic purposes in 1942 and again in 1966. In a high proportion of cases, the radiation exposure received in 1966 would be less than one-fifth, and in many cases less than one-tenth, of the exposure commonly received during a comparable procedure in 1942.

For patients in need of fluoroscopy, the dosage reduction was even more impressive. In more than 1000 hospitals and radiological offices, patients in 1966 could benefit from new types of image-intensification equipment and new procedures capable of reducing the radiation exposure to $\frac{1}{20}$th or even $\frac{1}{100}$th of the exposure common in 1942.

Dosage to the ovaries and testes during the X-raying of other parts of the body was reduced in countless cases by an even larger factor— often to $\frac{1}{200}$th or $\frac{1}{400}$th of the gonadal dose frequently administered in 1942. Far from requiring a sacrifice of diagnostic quality, moreover, these startling reductions of dose were in a high proportion of cases accompanied by an actual improvement in quality of the X-ray films.

The ways in which these and other reductions in dosage were achieved constitute the theme of this chapter.

ATOM BOMBS AND SAFETY

The story properly begins behind the locked and guarded doors of the University of Chicago's Metallurgical Laboratory during the summer of 1942.[1] There Enrico Fermi and a picked group of associates, convinced by prior experiments at Columbia University and elsewhere that a nuclear "chain reaction" could be initiated and sustained (see page 393), were at work designing the world's first nuclear reactor or "atomic pile." In this pile, if it proved successful, the bombardment of uranium by neutrons might produce a new radioactive element, plutonium, out of which bombs of an unprecedented destructive power might be fashioned. Alternatively, atomic bombs might be made by uranium-235, a naturally occurring radioisotope found in very small quantities in uranium ores.[2] In charge of the Metallurgical Laboratory, and later of the Plutonium Project into which it blossomed, was one of America's foremost physicists, Professor Arthur Holly Compton of the University of Chicago, 1927 winner of the Nobel Prize.

Dr. Compton and his associates faced many complex problems during that summer and fall; prominent among them was the problem of radiological safeguards. Foresight was needed to prevent a catastrophic debacle such as might follow an explosion of the pile and the release of its radioactive debris over the surrounding acres or square miles. Foresight was also needed to forestall the more insidious type of damage which might result from chronic daily exposure of atomic workers to pile-emitted radiations during routine operations.

The Metallurgical Laboratory scientists, as a 1945 report recalled, realized from the very beginning "the enormity of the hazards such a unit would create. Some of them had friends and acquaintances who had been injured in experimental work with X rays and with radium, and many were aware of the harmful effects suffered by some of the workers in the radium dial industry." At this early stage, it is true, "the exact nature and extent of the hazards to be encountered was not known," but it was realized that even the first small chain-reacting pile would emit radiation "far greater...than could have been dreamed possible in earlier periods." [2]

Far larger piles, moreover, were already being planned for immediate construction, as well as plants for the separation of uranium-235 from uranium-238. Because of the radiation hazards involved in these operations, some Metallurgical Laboratory scientists "doubted whether the program could or should be prosecuted." [2]

Faced with these ominous concerns, Dr. Compton in July and August 1942 took two administrative steps which were to have far-reaching consequences. To the Chemistry, Physics, and Technical Divisions of the Metallurgical Laboratory he added a Health Division, fully equal in status to the other three, and to head the new Division he summoned to Chicago a radiologist peculiarly qualified by prior experience for the awesome responsibilities entailed: Dr. Robert S. Stone of the University of California.

Three major types of radiation hazard were anticipated during the routine operation of the piles and other atomic installations.

From the moment that a nuclear chain reaction was established,

Fermi's pile would begin to emit vast quantities of gamma rays—super-voltage X rays. Dr. Stone, it will be recalled, had been among the pioneers in the study of supervoltage effects; he had begun work with his 1,000,000-volt equipment back in 1934.

The pile would also emit vast quantities of neutrons, and Dr. Stone had had more experience with the effects of this type of radiation on human tissue than any man alive. He and Dr. John C. Larkin, Jr., had already completed their second report on the usefulness and hazards of neutron-beam therapy in the treatment of human cancer, and in 1942 they were learning through their follow-up of patients that the late effects of neutron radiation were considerably more severe than had been anticipated (see page 369).

Finally, it was known that more than 30 radioisotopes would be generated within the pile as fission products, plus countless additional radioisotopes as "daughters" and as byproducts. Periodically these "hot" materials would have to be removed from the piles and processed in complex ways. It was probable that atomic workers would be exposed to some of these substances in solid, liquid, or gaseous forms. Nothing whatever was known of the responses of the human body to most of these substances. and very little was known about the others—but whatever was known in 1942, Dr. Stone already knew. He had been a charter member of the group of California researchers who since 1936 had been conducting both animal experiments and human studies with the new radioisotopes emerging from Ernest O. Lawrence's cyclotrons. Thus, by a remarkable concatenation of circumstances, Dr. Stone could bring to the Metallurgical Laboratory precisely the three funds of experience that the new health post there demanded.

Dr. Stone entered on his new duties on August 6, 1942, nearly 4 months before the first Fermi pile "went critical," but a pressing practical problem already awaited him. Fermi and his fellow physicists had calculated how much radiation of various kinds would emerge from the piles of various sizes and designs, and they knew at least approximately how thick a shield of lead, concrete, or other materials would be needed in each instance to reduce this radiation to any desired level. Before the shielding could be designed, however, one more parameter would have to be explored: the level of ionizing radiation which could prudently be permitted in the working areas around the pile. This was a policy decision, and Dr. Stone's Health Division was responsible for making it.

One easy answer was already at hand. In 1934, the International X-Ray and Radium Protection Commission (see page 318) had recommended $\frac{1}{5}$ roentgen per working day (0.2 r) as the "tolerance dose" for radiological workers—that is, the daily dose to which workers could be exposed year after year without damage; in 1936 the U.S. Advisory Committee on X-Ray and Radium Protection had cut the tolerance dose to 0.1 r per day. These levels were quite generally accepted in 1942, and a less cautious man than Dr. Stone might have adopted them for the Metallurgical Laboratory without further ado. However, Dr. Stone was not content with official recommendations; he was concerned with the data underlying them. Accordingly, he and his fellow radiologist, Dr. Simeon T. Cantril of the Health Division, launched a comprehensive review of everything previously published on radiation hazards and safeguards.

Their findings were hardly reassuring.

History of the "Tolerance Dose"

Much of the background information that Drs. Stone and Cantril needed had already been assembled by a young research fellow at the National Cancer Institute in Bethesda, Maryland, Dr. Paul S. Henshaw, and had been published in the June 1941 issue of the *Journal of the National Cancer Institute.*

The first effort to determine a "safe" or "harmless" dose of radiation, Dr. Henshaw reported, had been a suggestion offered by the Boston dentist, Dr. William Rollins, back in 1902 (see above, page 182). However, Dr. Rollins's suggestion had been ignored, and Dr. Henshaw found no further effort along this line for the next 22 years.

Then in 1924 an American physicist, Dr. Arthur Mutscheller, had read to the American Roentgen Ray Society a highly influential paper entitled "Physical Standards of Protection Against X-Ray Hazards." [3] Dr. Mutscheller's 1924 study, interestingly enough, had grown out of precisely the same problem with respect to X-ray machines that Dr. Stone and his associates were facing with respect to Fermi's atomic pile 18 years later: how thick a shield was required to safeguard employees? "In order to be able to calculate the thickness of the protective shield," Mutscheller declared in 1924, "there must be known the dose which an operator can, for a prolonged period of time, tolerate without *ultimately* suffering injury."

Mutscheller's solution was in principle quite plausible. He visited "several typical good installations" where radiology was being practiced, and measured the level of radiation actually present in the working areas. From this he estimated the monthly radiation dose received by the radiologists and their staffs. Then, since none of the workers in the installations where he had made his measurements appeared to have suffered any damage, Mutscheller proposed that the doses that they were currently receiving be accepted as an "entirely safe" tolerance dose. To quote from his 1924 paper:

"Thus it seems that under present conditions and standards accepted at present, it is entirely safe if an operator does not receive every 30 days a dose exceeding 0.01 of an erythema dose, and from the present status of our knowledge this seems to be the tolerance dose for all conditions of operating roentgen-ray tubes for roentgenography, roentgenoscopy, and therapy." Translated into 1942 terminology, Mutscheller's proposed tolerance dose was roughly equivalent to 0.2 r per day.

Dr. Mutscheller himself made no extravagant claims for his rough rule-of-thumb estimate. It was derived, he stressed, "from the average of a limited number of typical examples and is perhaps not sufficiently checked biologically; so it may happen that in the future this dose will be changed either to a larger or a smaller practical tolerance dose."

Dr. Mutscheller's new concept had been very much needed in radiology, and it was eagerly seized upon. Several other researchers in the United States and Europe repeated his measurements in their own and in a few neighboring installations and published their own rough calculations. The eminent British physicist Dr. G. W. C. Kaye averaged these various rough estimates and announced his own recommendation based on them in an influential textbook on radiology published both in England and in the United States in 1928.[4] His recommendation was very close to Mutscheller's. Since Dr. Kaye held prominent positions on both the British and the international X-ray protection committees, his opinion carried great weight. In 1934 the International Commission accepted Dr. Kaye's recommendation that 0.2 r per day be adopted as the tolerance dose—based as it was on Mutscheller's measurements in "several typical good installations" plus a limited number of similar measurements by others.

The 1936 recommendation of the U.S. Advisory Committee did not rest on broader data or more cogent reasoning. When Dr. Stone subsequently asked members of the committee why they had cut the recommended tolerance dose from 0.2 to 0.1 r per day, he was told "this was done because it was felt that with the more penetrating radiations from higher voltage machines coming into more general use, a smaller surface dose was necessary...."[5]

In brief, to quote Dr. Stone, the tolerance-dose recommendations generally accepted in 1942 "rested on rather poor experimental evidence" and it was all too clear that "the scientific data...were very limited."[6]

Two further considerations, moreover, made the generally accepted recommendations seem even frailer reeds to support the Metallurgical Laboratory's radiological health program.

First, a number of published reports reviewed by Drs. Henshaw, Stone, and Cantril cast grave doubt on the assumption—uncritically accepted by Mutscheller, Kaye, the International Commission, the U.S. Advisory Committee, and almost everyone else—that the levels of radiation to which radiologists and their assistants were currently being exposed were in fact "entirely safe."

In 1924, for example, 2 years before his own death from cancer, one of America's foremost radiologists, Dr. Russell D. Carman of the Mayo Clinic, had read to the Radiological Society of North America a paper entitled "Occupational Hazards of the Radiologist," [7] which summarized a wide range of evidence indicating that radiologists were in fact being damaged by the radiation they were then receiving. Three years later another prominent American radiologist, Dr. Preston M. Hickey, editor of the *American Journal of Roentgenology,* had made a study of the problem at the request of the Sex Committee of the National Research Council. He sent questionnaires to all American radiologists, and 377 replied. Of these, 138 (36.6 per cent) reported that their marriages were sterile. Among the 262 children born to the responding radiologists before their fathers took up radiology, the abnormality rate was 2.6 per hundred; among the 412 children born afterward, the abnormality rate was 4.0 per hundred.[8] Dr. Hickey's study was based on a small sample, of course, and it was subject to all the shortcomings of the questionnaire method, but it hardly increased Dr. Stone's confidence in the assumption that the doses currently being received by radiologists were *ipso facto* "entirely safe."

An association between radiation and leukemia was also suspected in 1942. Dr. Henshaw of the National Cancer Institute had suggested this possibility in his June 1941 paper, and in a 1942 "general review" of the effects of radiation on normal tissue, prepared under the auspices of Dr. Shields Warren of the Harvard Cancer Commission, Dr. Charles E. Dunlap had reviewed 24 published cases of leukemia following chronic exposure to radiation.[9] Of the 24 victims, 20 were "roentgenologists, radiologists, and their assistants, who presumably had been working with roentgen rays." Dr. Dunlap had cautiously concluded in 1942, "Doubt still exists as to the etiologic role of radiation in the development of leukemia in radiologists, but on the basis of experiments on animals, it appears probable that repeated exposures to small doses of radiation could serve as an exciting or precipitating cause of leukemia."

Another source of doubt concerning the accepted recommendations was a large and growing body of experimental evidence suggesting that the whole concept of a "safe dose" or "tolerance dose" might prove a will-o'-the-wisp. Perhaps there was no absolutely safe dose of ionizing radiation. Perhaps any exposure, however small, might carry some proportionate degree of risk.

The most impressive evidence for this point of view had been published periodically through the years, beginning in 1927, by one of America's foremost geneticists, Dr. Herman J. Müller, working initially at the University of Texas and later at Indiana University. Dr. Müller's work with fruit flies (*Drosophila*) had shown beyond any doubt that radiation of the gonads produces mutations which make their presence known in subsequent generations. His work has been confirmed in mice and other mammals. So far as the evidence available in 1942 revealed, the number of mutations produced was strictly proportional to the dose administered. In a 1933 paper, addressed specifically to radiologists and published by Dr. Otto H. Glasser in his *The Science of Radiology*, Dr. Müller had presented evidence for his conclusion that "even the extremely small amount of gamma and cosmic radiation present in nature must be producing some mutations." Dr. Müller had concluded with an eloquent plea for radiological caution: "We must remember that that thread of germ plasm which now exists must suffice to furnish the seeds of the human race even for the most remote future. We are the present custodians of this all-important material, and it is up to us to guard it carefully and not to contaminate it for the sake of any ephemeral benefits to our own single generation."

Dr. Stone and his associates were well aware in 1942 of Dr. Müller's work. They were concerned, too, that presumably trivial exposures to ionizing radiation might increase, however slightly, the risk of leukemia or other forms of cancer. Dr. Henshaw had searched the literature for reassurance on this point when preparing his June 1941 paper, but had found none.

These possibilities, it was clear, had not been taken into account when the 0.2 and 0.1 r per day tolerance dose recommendations were being arrived at.

Dr. Stone's Three Historic Recommendations

Dr. Stone's position in the fall of 1942 was thus hardly an enviable one. Adequate evidence on which to base prudent decisions was simply not available—yet, with actual construction of the first pile scheduled to begin soon, the decisions could not be postponed. The lives for which the Health Division was responsible, moreover, were not ordinary lives. Already many of the world's leading physicists were assembled at the site of the first pile, and, if it should prove successful, their number would rapidly swell. "Were they to suffer any serious damage from the peculiar hazards," Dr. Stone later commented, "the United States would suffer an irreparable loss. In the scientific world the loss would be analogous to that of killing the generals in the Army." [10]

Dr. Stone accordingly recommended, and the Metallurgical Laboratory adopted, three basic policy decisions.

First, the generally accepted "tolerance dose" of the U.S. Advisory Committee was to become the Metallurgical Laboratory "ceiling" above which no radiation exposures would be authorized.

Second, the doses actually delivered to personnel were to be held as far as possible below this ceiling.

Third, despite other urgent wartime demands, a relatively large-scale research program was to begin without delay, under Metallurgical Laboratory auspices, to secure the missing data needed for prudent future decisions. In Dr. Stone's words, "It was agreed at that time [1942] that we would be given the opportunity to check our calculations by experiments and so establish the tolerable limits of exposure on solid ground."

The long-range consequences of these decisions can hardly be overemphasized. Radiologists during the 1930's had been concerned primarily with preventing the kinds of radiation damage which had made their appearance in the 1910's and 1920's. Now Dr. Stone was proposing to forestall types of damage which, if they were to occur at all, could not be expected to appear until decades or even generations later. Earlier protective efforts had rested on the firm ground of known cases of radiation injury (see pages 161–173); now Dr. Stone was proposing that even vague suspicions be taken into account until they were proved unfounded. "While many individuals were involved in radiation protection," Dr. Gioacchino Failla told the U.S. Joint Congressional Committee on Atomic Energy in 1960, "Dr. Robert Stone deserves the chief credit in that he set the pattern in the early years of the Plutonium Project." [11]

The first practical demonstration of these principles occurred on December 2, 1942. "On that memorable day," Dr. Stone later wrote, "the first pile went into operation in the west stands of Stagg Field at the University of Chicago. The day was one of great excitement. For the first time health physicists were called upon to determine whether conditions were safe or unsafe around an operating pile. . . . It was soon found that in the control room no appreciable readings on any type of ionization-measuring instruments could be obtained." The pile shield had been designed with a sufficient margin of safety to reduce the emitted radiation to a level too low to be measured.

Subsequently the first pile was operated at higher and higher intensities, from ½ watt on December 2 to a maximum of 200 watts on December 12. No experiments above the 200-watt level were undertaken—not because the pile might not be capable of higher intensities, but because of radiological health considerations.

The same concern for holding radiation dose to a minimum continued throughout the life of the Plutonium Project and spread to the other atomic installations built and operated under the general direction of General Leslie R. Groves of the Manhattan Engineer District, U.S. Army Corps of Engineers, commonly known as "the Manhattan Project." When a 1,000,000-watt pile and associated equipment were being designed for the plutonium plant at Hanford, Washington, for example, 10 months of work went into the design of the shielding. The amount of radiation to be emitted there, it was estimated, would be the equivalent of that from hundreds of tons of radium. General Groves described the policy set at Hanford: "The National Advisory Committee on X-Ray and Radium Protection had established a tolerance dose . . . at one-tenth of one roentgen per day. Because this was not definitely known to be safe, the tolerance dose at Hanford was set at one-hundredth of a roentgen per day. . . . It was calculated that one foot of lead, seven feet of concrete, or fifteen feet of water would provide adequate protection. . . ." [12]

Similarly, when Dr. Stone was called upon to recommend the amount of plutonium to which workers at Oak Ridge and Hanford might prudently be subjected, he recommended succinctly: "The only safe procedure is to see that *none* of it is inhaled or ingested."

At the close of the war, the hitherto secret story of the whole atomic effort was made public in the classic "Smyth Report." The achievements of the Health Division were there summed up in these terms: "The major objective of the health group was in a sense a negative one, to insure that no one concerned suffered serious injury from the peculiar hazards of the enterprise. Medical case histories of persons suffering serious injury or death from radiation were emphatically not wanted. The success of the Health Division in meeting these problems was remarkable. Even in the research group where control is more difficult, cases showing even temporary bad effects were extremely rare. Factors of safety used in plant design and operation are so great that the hazards of the home and the family car are far greater for the personnel than any dangers arising from the plant." [2]

Radiation Biology Research

This enviable safety record resulted primarily from the second of Dr. Stone's three recommendations—to keep actual exposures as far below the accepted tolerance dose as possible. However, it was the third of his recommendations—to initiate a major research program—which was to have the most far-reaching consequences. Many of the foundation stones of contemporary radiation biology, health physics, and radiological health research were hewn and laid in position as a result of wartime projects under the auspices of the Health Division.

Before World War II, a limited number of biologists like Dr. Müller, Dr. Egon Lorenz of the National Cancer Institute, and Dr. Raymond E. Zirkle of the University of Chicago and a limited number of physicists like Dr. Failla, Dr. William Duane of Harvard, and Dr. Otto Glasser at the Cleveland Clinic had been concerned with the basic effects of radiation on living tissue. They had worked with only modest resources, however, and for the most part they had pursued such studies as an interesting avocation during whatever hours they could spare from their regular duties. The Metallurgical Laboratory recruited men of this type for war work in Chicago and at Oak Ridge, attracted new men to the field, and assisted others to continue their researches in their own laboratories on a broader scale and at a more rapid tempo.

Among the first of the studies begun under Metallurgical Laboratory auspices were experiments with doses of radiation delivered daily throughout the life span of laboratory animals. The effects of fast neutrons, slow neutrons, and beta and gamma rays as well as X rays were explored in the course of this work. Out of it grew several new concepts basic to modern health physics: the rem, the rad, the relative biological effectiveness or RBE, and linear energy transfer or LET (see above, page 357). The doses studied ranged from massive amounts sufficient to kill one-half of the animals exposed within a few weeks or months (the LD_{50}) down to the 0.1 r per day which earlier researchers had assumed, without tests, would produce no deleterious effects whatever.

The papers issuing from these studies bore such titles as "Biological Effects of Long-Continued Whole-Body Radiation with Gamma Rays on Mice, Guinea Pigs, and Rabbits," "The Clinical Physiology of Dogs Exposed to Single Total-Body Doses of X-Rays," and "The Hematological Effects of Ionizing Radiations in the Tolerance Range." Several of the studies were concerned with the genetic effects of relatively small doses on the descendants of irradiated animals.[13]

Numerous human studies were also undertaken, including one by Dr. Henshaw to determine the relative frequency of leukemia in physicians. Other human studies bore such titles as "Hematological Studies on Patients Treated by Total-Body Exposure to X Rays," "Blood Changes in Human Beings Following Total Body Irradiation," "Changes in Mean Blood Levels of Metallurgical Laboratory Employees During the First

Year of Employment as Related to Working Conditions," and "Tolerance to Whole-Body Irradiation of Patients with Advanced Cancer." On the "extremely rare" occasions when atomic personnel suffered accidental overexposures, intensive studies were immediately begun and followed up for long periods of time.

In addition to such studies of radiation from external sources, there were even broader programs to determine the effects of "internal emitters"—radioisotopes entering the body through the lungs, gastrointestinal tract, or skin. What proportion of these substances was promptly excreted and what proportion remained in the body? In what organs did they lodge, and how were they distributed in each organ? What effects did their radiation produce? By the close of the war Dr. Stone was able to report:

> There is altogether too large and complex a body of knowledge about the metabolism of these products to make it possible even to scratch the surface in [a] short presentation, but the following few facts will be of interest. Strontium, barium, tellurium, cerium, and iodine can all enter the body by absorption from the gastrointestinal tract. These and many others enter quite readily through the lungs, the amount entering depending upon the chemical compound in which they are found. Strontium, barium, zirconium, yttrium, and others locate quite selectively in the bones, and many of them stay for long periods of time. Lanthanum, cerium, and tellurium show no significant degree of selective localization in any tissue and are rather rapidly eliminated. That iodine is selectively absorbed by the thyroid was known before the war. The lungs retain some of the inhaled radioactive elements for considerable periods of time and thus are exposed to the radiations even if they are only weak beta radiations.[6]

The wisdom of Dr. Stone's initial decision to "check . . . calculations with experiments" was repeatedly demonstrated. Preliminary theoretical studies, for example, had led to the conclusion that the *slow* neutrons emanating in large quantity from the pile would be relatively harmless, since they would soon be captured by hydrogen atoms. The only anticipated radiation effect on human tissue from slow neutrons was the emission of a gamma ray at the moment of capture. "Experimental work has shown," Dr. Stone reported in 1945, "that this is not true but that only about one-quarter of the effect in small animals can be attributed to this gamma radiation. . . ." Slow neutrons entering animal tissue, it was discovered, also transmuted nitrogen to carbon, and the "nuclear recoil" associated with this transmutation produced unanticipated physiological effects. Similarly, experiments with plutonium led to surprising and highly significant results. "On the basis of its alpha activity and long half-life it was estimated that it would be about one-fiftieth as dangerous as radium," Dr. Stone reported in 1945. "For acute effects this has been shown to be wrong, and the fact was determined that one microgram of plutonium was about as dangerous as one microgram of radium." [6] The initial error was due to ignorance of the different ways in which radium and plutonium distribute themselves. Both are "bone-seekers"—that is, they deposit themselves preferentially in bone—but the plutonium distribution in the bone, it was learned, is less homogeneous and therefore more likely to produce "hot spots" where the dose to surrounding tissues is far higher than the average.

When the wartime studies were declassified after the war, many of the significant advances in radiation biology were reported to radiologists at the December 1946 meeting of the Radiological Society of North America; the papers presented at this symposium filled the entire September 1947 issue of *Radiology*. The following listing of these papers will indicate some of the major contributors, and some of the centers where Plutomium Project research was pursued:

> "Components of the Acute Lethal Action of Slow Neutrons," by Raymond E. Zirkle, University of Chicago, working at the Clinton Laboratories of the Plutonium Project, Oak Ridge, Tennessee.
>
> "Biological Studies in the Tolerance Range," by Egon Lorenz, W. E. Heston, Allen B. Eschenbrenner, and Margaret K. Deringer, National Cancer Institute, Bethesda, Maryland.
>
> "Hematological Effects of Ionizing Radiations in the Tolerance Range," by Leon O. Jacobson and E. K. Marks, University of Chicago, working in the Metallurgical Laboratory.
>
> "Clinical Sequence of Physiological Effects of Ionizing Radiation in Animals," by C. Ladd Prosser, with contributions by E. E. Painter, Hermann Lisco, Austin M. Brues, Leon O. Jacobson, and M. N. Swift, all working in the Metallurgical Laboratory.
>
> "Effects of Total Surface Beta Irradiation," by John R. Raper, working with K. K. Barnes, R. E. Zirkle, J. E. Wirth, and H. J. Curtis at Clinton Laboratories, Oak Ridge, Tennessee.
>
> "Metabolism of the Fission Products and the Heaviest Elements," by Joseph G. Hamilton, University of California.
>
> "Histological Changes Following Radiation Exposures," by William Bloom, University of Chicago, working at the Metallurgical Laboratory and Clinton Laboratories, Oak Ridge, Tennessee.
>
> "Biological Effects of Pile Radiations," by Paul S. Henshaw, E. F. Riley, and G. E. Stapleton, Clinton Laboratories, Oak Ridge, Tennessee.
>
> "Carcinogenic Properties of Radioactive Fission Products and of Plutonium," by Hermann Lisco, Miriam P. Finkel, and Austin M. Brues, Metallurgical Laboratory and Argonne National Laboratory, Chicago.

Health Physics Progress

In addition to these and many other research projects in radiation biology, major progress was made in health physics under Health Division auspices.

Building radiation safeguards into the initial design of all equipment was one part of the mission of Dr. E. O. Wollan, Dr. Karl Z. Morgan, Herbert M. Parker, and other health physicists on the staff. Training all personnel to follow prescribed precautions was a second, and monitoring all radiation areas to determine radiation levels a third. The monitoring was not as simple as it sounded. The radiation-measuring instruments available in 1942 were of relatively primitive types. Few were capable of measuring with reliability doses as low as those which concerned the Health Division, and there were special problems with the measurement of neutrons and other recently discovered types of radiation. Many new or improved types of measuring instrument were developed by the health physicists. Some were given fanciful names; meters known as Pluto and Zeus, for example, were followed by a combination meter known as Zuto. A light portable meter became known as the cutie-pie, and a device for measuring radioactive dust in the atmosphere was dubbed the "sneezie." Film badges to be worn by individuals to record their personal doses—pioneered a generation earlier (page 169)—were reintroduced and improved; compact, direct-reading ionization chambers shaped like fountain pens, to be carried in pockets, were developed. Thus, the progress of health physics went hand in hand with the progress in radiation biology.

Much of this work was conducted, of course, at the major atomic installations, but projects under the auspices of the Health Division were also launched at many other research centers, including the Radiation Laboratory of the University of California, the National Cancer Institute, the Chicago Tumor Institute, Memorial Hospital in New York City, the University of California Hospital, Michael Reese Hospital in Chicago, and others.

With the end of the war, moreover, these projects did not cease. In 1946, the newly formed U.S. Atomic Energy Commission (AEC) took over the operations of the Army's Manhattan Engineer District, and in a series of notable decisions the AEC not only continued but greatly expanded the radiation biology and health physics research programs of the old Health Division. Vast new resources became available as a result of the high prestige of the nuclear sciences and congressional willingness to appropriate generously for anything associated with "the atom." Scientists leaving the wartime agencies took back to civilian centers the new techniques of radiation research and initiated new projects. The AEC supported many of these extramural projects, as well as many undertaken in the great new national laboratories developed during and after the war, including the Argonne National Laborarory and Argonne Cancer Research Hospital, the Brookhaven National Laboratory, the Los Alamos Scientific Laboratory, the Oak Ridge National Laboratory and Oak Ridge Institute of Nuclear Studies (now Oak Ridge Associated Universities), and the Ernest O. Lawrence Radiation Laboratory of the University of California.

As a direct result, research in radiation biology and health physics ceased to be the part-time hobbies of a few dedicated pioneers and became flourishing scientific specialties. By 1960, the AEC alone was budgeting $49 million for "research programs in biology and medicine," the bulk of it addressed to precisely the problem which had concerned Dr. Stone in 1942, "radiation protection standards."

AEC Research Budget in Biology and Medicine
Fiscal Year 1960

I.	Program Activities Related to Radiation Protection Standards		$37,548,236
	Research related to radiation standards of permissible exposure	$21,694,736	
	Research involving environmental contamination	7,041,700	
	a. Fallout studies	$4,637,000	
	b. Ecology, marine sciences, waste disposal, micrometeorology	2,404,700	
	Research related to treatment of radiation injury and alteration of radiation effects	2,356,200	
	Radiological Physics, Radiation protection, Instrumentation and measurement	6,455,600	
II.	Research Activities Not Directly Related to the Development of Radiation Standards		11,451,764
	Research in chemical toxicity and other biomedical problems	1,266,000	
	Cancer research	4,631,000	
	Research on radioactive tracer techniques and other beneficial applications of atomic energy	5,554,764	
Total			$49,000,000

In addition to work done within AEC establishments, the AEC's Division of Biology and Medicine reported 561 research contracts totalling nearly $15 million with scores of other institutions; merely listing these undertakings filled 25 pages of the AEC's 1959 *Annual Report*.

Research in related areas was also being pursued and supported by the

National Institutes of Health and, on an increasing scale after 1959, by the Division of Radiological Health (later the National Center for Radiological Health, now the Bureau of Radiological Health) of the U.S. Public Health Service.

The basic radiation phenomenon—the effect produced when a quantum of radiant energy interacts with an atom—remained, of course, in the domain of the nuclear physicists, but the health sciences were concerned with every subsequent level of radiation effect. Many of the studies during the 1960's, for example, were focused on what happens when a quantum of radiant energy, such as an X-ray photon, interacts with a chemical molecule, especially a molecule of biological interest such as a protein or enzyme. Of the greatest interest were studies on the interaction of radiation with molecules of DNA (deoxyribonucleic acid), which recent studies had shown to be the "hereditary material" that Dr. Müller had sought to protect in his eloquent 1933 plea. Also of special interest were the "free radicals" abundantly released when ionizing radiation strikes water molecules and molecules of some other kinds. These free radicals, it was learned, are highly active chemically and interact vigorously to produce changes in nearby molecules of physiological interest.

At the next level of complexity, radiation biology studied the impact of ionizing radiation on single cells. Bacteria, yeasts, and other one-celled plants and animals have been irradiated by the billion in these experiments, and much has been learned about the ways in which one quantum of radiation reacting with one atom inside a cell may trigger further interactions which may alter not only the cell but its descendants. Many special kinds of cells—blood cells, marrow cells, nerve cells, ova, and spermatozoa, for example—have been subjected to this kind of study, both in test tubes and in living animals. Of special interest during the 1960's were the studies of what happens when ionizing radiation is absorbed by *human* cells grown in tissue cultures.

The effects of radiation on chromosomes within living cells, first noted in 1905, are now being studied on a broad scale, using various types of radiation delivered at various rates. Also, research is continuing on the effects of ionizing radiation on far more complex organisms—on *Drosophila* and other rapidly breeding insects, on mice and rats, guinea pigs, rabbits, swine, dogs, cats, and monkeys—and on their descendants. Special studies are concerned with the radiation of old animals, young animals, and fetuses still in the uterus. Notable among the many large-scale projects under way are the studies of the genetic effects of quite small doses of radiation by Dr. W. L. Russell and his associates at the Oak Ridge Institute of Nuclear Studies, and the parallel studies of the effects of small doses on animal fetuses by Dr. Liane B. Russell, also at Oak Ridge. Like many other projects of the 1960's, these studies by the Russells stem directly from work initiated between 1942 and 1945 under the auspices of the Health Division of the Metallurgical Laboratory.

All such test-tube and animal experimentation, however, must ultimately be confirmed or modified by findings on human subjects. Hence, human studies have also been intensively pursued.

One classic series of such studies concerned women working in factories where watch dials and instrument dials were painted with compounds containing radium or other radioactive substances, especially mesothorium. Some of the dial painters were accustomed to point the tips of their brushes by drawing them between their lips. The vast bulk of the radioactive material thus ingested—98 per cent or more—was soon excreted again, but the balance lodged in the bones and remained for many years. In the fall of 1923, a New York City dental surgeon, Dr. Theodor Blum, examining a young woman with necrosis of the bone of the jaw, learned that she had been a dial painter, and leaped to the correct conclusion that this must be a case of radiation necrosis; he called it "radium jaw." [14] Other cases soon followed. In 1925 Dr. Harrison S. Martland of Newark, New Jersey, reported the first fatal case of anemia among these dial painters,[15] and in a distinguished series of papers published between 1925 and 1939[16] he followed the tragic course of many of these girls and young women through destruction of soft tissue and bone to anemia, leukopenia, lowering of bodily resistance to infection, generalized bone necrosis, osteogenic sarcoma (bone cancer), and other fatal terminations. Following World War II, interest in these cases revived, and an intensive nationwide search for survivors was launched. More than 200 were identified and remained under observation for late effects during the 1960's.

The dial-painter studies were limited by lack of knowledge of the individual doses received and by the fact that the radium ingested was mixed with other radioactive substances. Hence, studies were also launched of a group of mental hospital patients—many of them diagnosed as schizophrenics—given oral doses of radium in 1931 as a form of therapy. For these patients the doses and dates of administration were precisely known, and many were still available for follow-up studies during the 1950's. Similarly, studies were undertaken of many thousands of patients subjected to X-ray therapy during earlier decades, especially infants and children irradiated for enlarged thymus glands and young men irradiated for anklyosing spondylitis, a crippling form of arthritis.

The AEC established a continuing Atomic Bomb Casualty Commission to study the effects of radiation on the surviving inhabitants of

Hiroshima and Nagasaki, and Japanese physicians also studied these survivors. Studies were made of Japanese fishermen, inhabitants of the island of Rongelap, and United States military personnel accidentally exposed to radiation during the testing of nuclear weapons in the Pacific.[17] Also, there were studies of uranium miners in Colorado and elsewhere, many of whom had been exposed to radioactive gases and dusts at various levels of concentration.

Radiologists themselves became the subject of numerous studies, (see page 435), and the most careful comparisons were made between them and other medical specialists with respect to duration of life and causes of death.

Human studies, moreover, were extended downward to doses long considered trivial. In one notable project, for example, Dr. Brian Mac-Mahon of Harvard reported on a population consisting of the 743,243 children born between 1947 and 1954 in 37 large New England maternity hospitals. The average number of diagnostic X-ray films made of the pelvis and other organs during the pregnancies of the mothers of these children was first determined from the hospital records. Next children dying of leukemia and other forms of childhood cancer among the 734,243 were identified from death certificates. The prenatal X-ray exposure of their mothers was then compared with the exposure of the total group of mothers.[18, 19]

Dr. H. J. Müller's 1933 suggestion that even the slight amount of ionizing radiation present in nature might produce mutations was also followed up. There are measurable differences in this "background radiation" from one part of the world to another, and from one part of the United States to another, and efforts were made in the 1960's to determine whether these differences were reflected in either the number of babies born with identifiable genetic mutations or the number born with developmental defects traceable to fetal radiation.

Out of literally thousands of such studies—some test-tube experiments, some animal experiments, and some observations of humans—a comprehensive view of the scope of radiation hazards and their relationship to dose levels and dose rates was during the 1960's gradually beginning to emerge. The answers are not yet all in, and to summarize here in any detail the current state of scientific opinion would serve no useful purpose. However, the ultimate principles which could be derived from the whole broad flow of research were little changed in the 1960's from the principles recommended by Dr. Stone to guide the Metallurgical Laboratory in 1942:

First, prudent maxima for radiation exposure must be established, based on the best available evidence at any time, and these maxima must be revised, downward or upward, as additional data become available.

Second, the exposures to ionizing radiations actually experienced must be kept as far below these maxima as possible or feasible.

Third, further research must be generously supported and conscientiously pursued.

Fallout from Nuclear Weapons Tests

The hazards of ionizing radiation can in some respects be classed with the hazards of air pollution, water pollution, chemical additives introduced into commonly used foods without adequate prior testing for chronic effects, new drugs introduced without adequate testing for possible side effects, the introduction and widespread use of new insecticides and other pesticides, cigarette smoking, and some aspects of the automobile accident problem. All of these came to be grouped during the 1950's under the general heading of "environmental health hazards." Far greater efforts were devoted, however, to studying and curbing the potentially deleterious effects of ionizing radiation, and widespread public concern with ionizing radiation preceded the rise of public concern with the others. This concentration of effort on one type of environmental health hazard can be attributed almost entirely to a series of events which might be labeled "the great fallout controversy" (1954–1963).[20]

When an atom bomb or other fission device is exploded in the atmosphere or above it, one result is the release of enormous quantities of radioisotopes. Many of these fission products soon fall to earth in the form of dust or somewhat larger or smaller particles. Many have a relatively short radioactive half-life and are soon transmuted into harmless stable elements. Some of the yield, however, after circling the earth for months or even years, may descend in a still radioactive condition. When a fission-fusion bomb is exploded, the fission products are joined by large quantities of radioactive carbon produced when the neutrons generated in the explosion transmute atmospheric nitrogen to carbon-14.

The close-range effects of fallout were initially noted when the first nuclear device was tested at Alamagordo, New Mexico, on July 16, 1945. Radioactive dust fell on the backs of 64 cattle tethered not far from the explosion site; many of these animals suffered burns and loss of hair. Later the burns healed and the hair grew in again, but studies were not abandoned. In a typical example of postwar research diligence, the cattle were retired to an Oak Ridge pasture and periodically examined throughout the following years. (In 1960 one of them developed skin cancer in the area burned 15 years earlier.)[21, 22, 23]

Postwar tests of nuclear weapons, accordingly, were planned with the hazards of short-range fallout in mind. Before the 1954 United States tests at Bikini Atoll, for example, vessels were warned to keep out of thousands of square miles of the Pacific, and natives of islands near the test site were evacuated. One Japanese fishing vessel, however, either failed to receive or failed to heed the warning; radioactive dust falling on the vessel contaminated its fish catch and produced radiation sickness among the 23 fishermen. A shift of wind, moreover, carried the dust in an unexpected direction, so that inhabitants of the island of Rongelap and 28 United States service personnel stationed nearby were subjected to appreciable fallout exposure.[17]

These and several later incidents, occurring in the area surrounding the AEC's Nevada Test Site as well as near the Eniwetok Proving Ground in the Pacific, made front-page headlines in the United States, Japan, and other countries, and aroused worldwide concern and apprehension. Soon this concern with immediately perceptible effects was extended to concern with the genetic effects of even very small doses on future generations. There was also worry about the possibility of delayed effects such as leukemia or bone cancer, which might not make their appearance for a decade or more. One of the products released into the atmosphere during weapons tests was strontium-90, a "bone-seeker." Studies of the United States milk supply during the 1950's and early 1960's showed very small but rising amounts of strontium-90 in milk and some other foodstuffs. Iodine-131, known to concentrate in the thyroid gland, was also found in milk and other foodstuffs.

The result was a demand that the nuclear weapons tests be halted, and fallout became an issue in both the 1956 and 1960 political campaigns. Newspaper headlines, selected almost at random, tell the story of this rising tide of concern:

STRONTIUM-90 LEVEL HIGH IN ALFALFA HAY

BABIES' BONES HAVE UP TO 5% MORE RADIATION

U.S. EXPECTS RISE IN RADIOACTIVITY

POTENTIAL DAMAGE TO MAN FROM NUCLEAR
TESTING IS EXAMINED

FALLOUT POLICIES CALLED CONFUSED

JOINT PANEL TERMS GUIDES FOR PROTECTION
INADEQUATE

MINNESOTA FINDS RADIATION IN ITS MILK NEAR
DANGER LEVEL

RADIATION COUNCIL MOVES TO RESOLVE FALLOUT DISPUTE

LINDSAY CHARGES LAG AND CONFUSION ON FALLOUT

FINDS A FAILURE TO ESTABLISH PROGRAM TO PROTECT PUBLIC

PRESIDENT TO RULE ON FALLOUT DISPUTE

A full-page advertisement in many newspapers, calling attention to the effects of fallout on babies and children, invoked the name of America's best-known pediatrician:

DR. SPOCK IS WORRIED

Reassuring articles in some popular magazines—"Let's Stop Talking Nonsense about Fallout"—were accompanied by alarming articles in others—"What We Are Not Being Told about Fallout Hazards."

One of the arguments frequently used to reassure the public about fallout was to describe fallout doses as small compared with the amounts of radiation used in X-ray therapy and even in X-ray diagnosis. This argument soon backfired, however:

X RAYS WORRY PATIENTS

Medical Doctors Are Concerned That the Patient Requiring X-Ray Treatment or Diagnosis May Refuse it Because of His Fear of Radiation Damage

This worldwide concern with weapons-test fallout faded from the front pages after 1963, when an international treaty banning large-scale nuclear tests in the atmosphere was signed by the three major testing powers—the United States, U.S.S.R, and Britain—and by many smaller countries. (France and Red China continued to test on a small scale.) However, many of the steps taken during the controversy continued to have their effects. Expenditures for radiological health research, substantial even before the first fallout headlines, were greatly increased thereafter. New agencies concerned with ionizing radiation hazards were established, and the functions of existing agencies were expanded. Radiation biologists, radiologists, and health physicists emerged from the controversy with a heightened awareness of the public's concern with radiation hazards and of the insistent public demand for adequate safeguards. Standards-setting and regulatory agencies knew that their pronouncements would be subjected to close scrutiny by independent scientists, who would not hesitate to sound the alarm if they found what they thought might be flaws. The result was a general tightening up of standards and an establishment of radiation safeguards on an unprecedented scale.

NEW STANDARDS AND REGULATIONS

Long before the tests on Bikini Atoll alerted the lay public to the fallout problem, however, the first steps had already been taken to translate the new theoretical findings of radiation biology and the new equipment and procedures developed by the health physicists into practical operating safeguards.

The first important step following World War II was a major reorganization and reconstruction of the prewar standards-setting agencies—the International Commission and the U.S. Advisory Committee. This reorganization was promptly undertaken and successfully completed. In 1946 the U.S. Advisory Committee became the National Committee on Radiation Protection and Measurements (NCRP), with a broadened membership and broadened responsibilities. Dr. Stone himself became a member, along with Dr. Karl Z. Morgan and other health physicists experienced in wartime Health Division activities. For the first time, too, geneticists—including Dr. Müller—were recruited for NCRP responsibilities. Thus, the NCRP became the spokesman for the men at the forefront of research. In 1965 its formal status was enhanced by the grant of a Congressional charter, and it became the National *Council* on Radiation Protection and Measurements. Dr. Lauriston S. Taylor of the National Bureau of Standards, who had headed the old U.S. Advisory Committee, presided over the 1946 reorganization and remained head of the NCRP.

The International Commission was similarly reorganized and modernized, and such outstanding experts as Drs. Stone, Morgan, and Müller joined the United States delegation to it. Dr. Taylor continued to head the United States delegation.

Thus expanded and reinforced, both the NCRP and the ICRP proceeded in a series of steps to tighten up prewar recommendations and to enlarge their scope. The old term "tolerance dose" was abandoned because of its association with the outmoded concept of a "safe" dose. A new term which had been adopted by the Health Division during the war, the "maximum permissible exposure" or "maximum permissible dose," was substituted. The 0.2 and 0.1 r per day pre-war ceilings for occupational exposure established in 1934 and 1936 were cut to 0.3 r per *week* and then to 5 r per *year*—roughly a ten-fold reduction from the 0.2 r per day level. New concepts developed by the Health Division, such as the rem, the rad, and the RBE (see page 357), were accepted.

In place of the single ceiling of 0.1 r per day, moreover, a host of subsidiary ceilings was progressively introduced. Maxima were set for particular organs of the body, such as the gonads, the bone marrow, and the lenses of the eye. The maximum permissible doses (MPD's) were translated into maximum permissible concentrations (MPC'S) of radioactive substances in air, in water, in milk, and in other foodstuffs. The principle was recognized that doses received by persons not employed in places where ionizing radiation is used—neighbors, for example—should be held below one-tenth of the MPD for employees.

In recognition of cumulative genetic effects, some MPD's were not set for the daily, weekly, or even annual exposure, but for an individual's accumulated exposure from conception until the age of 30. For types of exposure likely to be experienced by large proportions of the population—millions of people—the 30-year cumulative dose to the gonads was set at 5 r, a far cry from the 900 r permitted during a 30-year period under the old 0.1 r per day "tolerance dose." Even the most outspoken critics of other aspects of United States radiation protection policies have rarely ventured to criticize the MPD's currently recommended by the NCRP.

Neither the NCRP nor the ICRP has regulatory, inspection, or enforcement powers, but in a variety of ways their recommendations have increasingly become the basis for enforceable regulations. The AEC, for example, is the source of most radioisotopes in the United States and licenses radioisotope users. Licensees must be qualified for the work, and must handle materials in conformity with AEC regulations. Enforceable AEC safety regulations also apply to nuclear reactors. The AEC regulations, of course, are based for the most part on NCRP recommendations.

In 1959 the Federal Radiation Council (FRC) was established to supervise the far-ranging activities of the United States Government with respect to ionizing radiation. The "radiation protection guides" (RPG's) established by the FRC were also derived in considerable part from NCRP recommendations.

The relatively strict AEC regulation of the use of *man-made* radioisotopes and of nuclear reactors led, however, to an anomalous situation: no similar machinery existed for the regulation of radiations from other sources such as X-ray machines, radium, and other radioactive substances found in nature. There was criticism, moreover, of the fact that the AEC combined two contradictory functions. On the one hand, it was charged with promoting the fullest use of nuclear energy for peacetime purposes, and on the other hand it was charged with regulating the functions it was supposed to promote. Also, Federal regulation of ionizing radiation clashed with the traditional policy of state and local regulation of other health hazards. As a result of these and other problems, a new trend began to be evidenced about 1959—a trend to view ionizing radiation hazards as similar to other health hazards and hence the proper responsibility of state and local health departments.

One major step in this direction was a 1959 amendment to the Atomic Energy Act authorizing the AEC to turn over to state agencies many of its regulatory powers, provided that the state agencies met specified standards. By 1966, 14 states, representing nearly half the nation's population, had taken over from the AEC control of radiation hazards within their borders under this provision. Almost all of the states had established at least rudimentary staffs concerned with radiation hazards of all kinds—hazards from X-ray machines and radium as well as from nuclear reactors and reactor-made isotopes.

Most states, of course, lacked initially the expertise to perform these functions effectively, but several national programs under way during the 1960's aided them in facing their new responsibilities. To alleviate the shortage of trained manpower, both the AEC and the Division of Radiological Health of the U.S. Public Health Service launched large-scale training programs at every level from post-graduate research to simple technical skills. Further, through grants-in-aid to the states, the National Center for Radiological Health encouraged the search for practical, effective ways of identifying radiation hazards, measuring them, and minimizing or abating them.

The net effect by the 1960's was that vastly more effort was being expended to curb unnecessary exposures to ionizing radiation than to curb the other environmental health hazards mentioned above, such as air pollution, water pollution, chemical food additives, and pesticides, yet these fields were not neglected. In all probability the great fallout controversy had a sensitizing effect on public opinion in these areas as well.

Radiology Meets the Challenge

Radiologists played many roles in the revolutionary changes of attitude toward radiation safeguards described above. They served in the Metallurgical Laboratory where the revolution began, in other segments of the wartime atomic program, and later in the AEC. They served on the ICRP and the NCRP and were active in the programs of the Public Health Service Division of Radiological Health. Leading radiologists were outspoken on issues raised by the great fallout controversy, and, as state and local health departments expanded their concerns with ionizing radiation, radiologists and their organizations advised and cooperated. The most direct immediate concern of the radiologists, however, was to improve procedures in their own offices and in the hospitals where they practiced and to encourage parallel improvements among other physicians using ionizing radiation.

Prior to World War II, for example, there had been very little concern with the dose of ionizing radiation delivered to a patient during the making of a diagnostic X-ray film. The dose required for making an X-ray film was assumed to be trivial. A fluoroscopic examination delivered hundreds of times as much radiation with no apparent harm, and doses thousands of times as large were routinely administered in radiation therapy. The risk that any given patient, or his remote decendants, might be damaged during X-ray radiography was too implausible to be considered—except, of course, by a few geneticists like Dr. Müller. However, the new understanding of and attitude toward ionizing radiation after World War II added a further dimension to the problem. Tens of millions of diagnostic X-ray negatives were being made each year. Thus, even though the risk to a single patient, or to all the patients treated in a year by a single physician, was hardly worth bothering about, the cumulative exposure of the population as a whole could be substantially lowered by lowering the exposure during each of tens of millions of radiographic exposures each year.

Radiologists, accordingly, sought—and found in abundance—techniques for reducing the dose of radiation administered and the volume of tissue irradiated when an X-ray negative is made. Here are some examples[24]:

Higher Voltage

A voltage of 60,000 or 70,000 (60 or 70 kilovolts) was customarily used for many diagnostic exposures prior to World War II. Much of the radiation emitted by a tube at this voltage is too soft to reach the X-ray film; it thus contributes to the patient's exposure without supplying diagnostic information. Merely by increasing the voltage on the tube to 85 kilovolts or higher, the dose administered to the patient's internal organs—the ovaries, for example—could be reduced by as much as 40 per cent.

Filtration of the Beam

Back in the 1900's, Dr. William Rollins of Boston had urged that a filter be introduced into the X-ray beam "to strain out undesirable radiations"—that is, radiation too soft to penetrate the body. Filters thereafter came into common use for therapeutic radiation. After World War II adequate filtration during diagnostic radiology was increasingly stressed; merely placing a thin aluminum filter in the beam, it was learned, could reduce the skin dose by 40 per cent or more, while simultaneously improving the diagnostic quality of the film.

Faster Film

Just as fast photographic film makes possible an acceptable photograph taken in dimmer light, so an X-ray film with a faster emulsion makes possible an acceptable X-ray negative with a smaller dose to the patient. Dosage could be reduced by 40 to 50 per cent or more with the new fast films introduced after World War II.

Full Development

There is in general an inverse relationship between the time that an X-ray film spends in the developing tank and the radiation dose which must be administered to the patient. By improving development procedures, patient exposure could be reduced by 40 per cent or more. Control of development temperature, improved development chemicals, and automatic processing of film also contributed to potential dosage reduction and improved the quality of the film image.

Intensifying Screens

The technique pioneered by Dr. Rollins of sandwiching an X-ray plate in between two intensifying screens was in common use prior to World War II, and the X-ray films used after 1920 were generally coated with emulsion on both sides to take full advantage of the two screens. After the war, improved intensifying screens made possible a still further reduction of dose by 40 to 50 per cent.

Combined Effects

Startling results could be achieved when the various methods of lowering the radiation dose were combined. Here is an example, as calculated by Dr. Walter R. Stahl of the University of Oregon radiology department and reported by the American College of Radiology:

> An ordinary X-ray machine without a filter, operated at 60 kv., with standard-speed film developed for three minutes, used to take a picture of a woman's pelvis, will deliver a dose to the ovaries which, for comparison purposes, can arbitrarily be set at 100 units. By developing the film for five minutes instead of three, or by adding an adequate filter, or by increasing the kilovoltage from 60 to 85, the physician can reduce the dosage to the ovaries from 100 units to about 60. If all three measures are taken, the dosage will fall to less than 30 units. In addition, the use of fast film and a fast [intensifying] screen will further reduce the dosage to 14 units, one-seventh the original level.

Volume of Tissue Irradiated

Dr. Rollins in the 1900's had offered what he called the "first axiom" of radiological protection (see above, page 184): "No X-light should strike a patient except the smallest beam which will cover the area to be examined, photographed, or treated." This axiom was taken seriously in radiation therapy, but prior to 1942 it was generally neglected in the making of X-ray negatives, since the dose delivered was considered too small to worry about. Thus, large volumes of the body might be irradiated even though only a small volume was of diagnostic interest. Following a study of New York City installations, Professor Hanson Blatz reported that in 50 per cent of all chest X-rays, the gonads were included in the direct beam.

Simple ways of reducing the volume of tissue irradiated, such as cones of the proper size attached to the X-ray head, came increasingly into use during the 1950's. This often dramatically reduced the dose to the gonads—to $\frac{1}{300}$th or $\frac{1}{400}$th the unconed dose, for example, in the procedures which Dr. Blatz studied.

As Dr. Rollins had pointed out during the 1900's, however, a cone is less effective than a rectangular device for limiting the beam. Accordingly, another of Dr. Rollins's inventions of 50 years earlier was refined and introduced: an adjustable multi-leaf diaphragm or collimator with a rectangular aperture (see page 184). With some of the new rectangular collimators, a system of lights and mirrors projects a visible image of the beam cross-section on the patient before the tube is turned on, and the technician can then independently adjust the height and the width of the rectangular beam in order to fit it precisely to the region of diagnostic interest.

Finally, to limit radiation to the gonads, leaded aprons and other types of shield came into increasingly common use during the 1950's and 1960's.

Unnecessary Exposures

Yet another approach to dose reduction was the elimination of *unnecessary* exposures. "Be sure that you have a good and adequate reason for *each study*," the American College of Radiology recommended in a 1958 publication addressed to all physicians and dentists, "—a purpose based on sound medical or dental judgment.... Always ask yourself, 'Is this examination important to the health and well being of the person exposed?' "

Stress was also placed on achieving a satisfactory negative the first time, so that "retakes" would rarely be necessary. Several new devices proved helpful in this respect, including the "phototimer" introduced in 1942 by Drs. Russell Morgan and Paul C. Hodges (see page 267). A phototimer automatically shuts off the beam as soon as enough radiation has reached the X-ray film to produce a negative of the desired density. Thus, both underexposures and overexposures requiring retakes are prevented.

The most impressive feature of these and other improvements in equipment and procedures was the fact that they curtailed patient exposure *without reducing the usefulness of diagnostic radiography*. In many cases, indeed, the diagnostic quality of the negative was actually improved. Thus, limiting the beam to the area of diagnostic interest not only reduced the volume of tissue irradiated but also curtailed the fogging of the film by stray radiation.

Lowering the Fluoroscopic Dose

The fluoroscoping of a patient generally requires a dose far larger than that required for an X-ray film; hence, opportunities to reduce the dose during fluoroscopy were also extensively explored.

Some of the techniques for limiting exposure during the making of and X-ray film, such as limiting the beam to the area of clinical interest, filtering the beam, and avoiding unnecessary examinations, were also applicable to fluoroscopy. In addition, safeguards unique to fluoroscopy were introduced.

The NCRP, for example, recommended that the exposure *rate* during routine medical fluoroscopy "should be as low as possible—and shall not exceed 10 r per minute." Many radiologists, by adapting their eyes to the dark for 20 minutes or more before examining a patient, were able to complete most examinations with exposures of only 5 or 6 r per minute. Surveys made in several states during the 1950's revealed, in contrast, that a minority of fluoroscopic machines then in use were delivering 20, 40, or in a few cases even 60 r per minute.

Even at its best, however, fluoroscopy with conventional equipment delivers a far larger dose to the patient than the making of a negative or a series of negatives. Hence, physicians were increasingly advised, and were taught in medical schools, to limit fluoroscopy to "occasions where it is essential rather than merely desirable." Dr. Hodges at the University at Chicago, for example, stressed this cautious approach in the *Journal of the American Medical Association* for February, 1958.

"Like most older radiologists," he wrote, "I formerly used fluoroscopy freely for the diagnosis of fracture and gunshot wounds of the skeleton and the positioning of such parts for filming; for the measurement of the heart and great vessels and the observation of their action; and for the study of the effect of respiratory phase on lungs, mediastinum, and diaphragm. As a matter of fact, until about 25 years ago I believed and taught that it was advantageous to combine fluoroscopy with filming in examinations of practically every part of the body. About a quarter of a century ago, however, I began to be cognizant of the importance of reducing the dose of radiation received by the patient and particularly by the operator, who, unlike the patient, is exposed many times a day, day after day, for months and years. For some decades it has been the policy of our department to restrict fluoroscopy to those situations where it is essential rather than merely desirable.... In the interest of the well-being of patients and staff, fluoroscopy of all sorts should be held to a minimum and that which is done should be done by radiologists."

Image Intensification

During the late 1950's and 1960's however, new devices altered the outlook for fluoroscopy. The basic advance (as noted above, page 266) was the "image intensifier"—a device resembling in some respects the picture tube in a TV receiver. The X rays, after passing through the patient, impinge on the face of a screen and trigger the ejection of electrons, which are then speeded up and focused within the tube by means of magnetic fields. The effect is one of amplification. When these speeded-up electrons strike the phosphor at the output end of the tube, they trigger the emission of light photons which recreate the desired image—but several hundreds or thousands of times as bright as in the case of the conventional fluoroscopic screen. The output of the image intensifier, moreover, can then be picked up by a television camera, further amplified, and viewed by the examining physician without dark adaptation.

Moving pictures can be taken of the output phosphor of the intensifying tube or of the television receiver image, or the moving images may be stored on magnetic tape. This permanently records the changing image and makes possible a further reduction of total dose to the patient, for, instead of prolonging the exposure while he searches various parts of the image or checks for various factors, the radiologist can record a relatively short exposure and then rerun the moving picture film or tape as often as necessary to transfer to his eyes and mind the varied information that it contains. As a further refinement, some cinefluoroscopic installations of this general type synchronize the output of the X-ray tube with the moving picture camera. Rays from the tube pass through the patient in pulses instead of continuously, so that no exposure occurs during the portion of the photographic cycle when the film is not stationary and ready to record the scene. This pulsing procedure, it will be recalled, was another of the dose-reducing measures pioneered by Dr. Rollins of Boston in the early 1900's (see page 187).

Dr. Richard H. Chamberlain, chairman of the University of Pennsylvania radiology department, summed up the advantages of image intensification devices in his testimony on June 6, 1962, before the Joint Congressional Committee on Atomic Energy. "In the better forms," he reported, "radiation dosage can be reduced to one-tenth or even to one-hundredth of former values while obtaining the same or greater diagnostic information than before." The dose to the radiologist himself is reduced to zero or almost zero. The combination of brighter image and lower dose to the patient, moreover, has made it possible for radiologists to develop a number of important new diagnostic procedures which could not have been accomplished at all without image intensification.

Safeguards in Radiation Therapy

Efforts to increase the dose to cancer tissue while sparing normal tissue have already been described (pages 283 and 293–295). These efforts, as has been noted, were moderately successful. But with life itself at stake in the use of radiation for cancer therapy, the hazards of undertreatment or of failure to treat loomed very large. Radiologists accordingly continued to search for the *right* dose rather than the *smallest* dose.

Radiation therapy for benign conditions, however, raised quite different problems—and a substantial proportion of all radiation therapy prior to World War II was for benign conditions. Indeed, as noted above (page 299), radiation was deemed the treatment of choice for more than a hundred benign conditions. *The Science of Radiology* (1933) listed 96 skin diseases alone, from acne to warts, which dermatologists were accustomed to treat with radiation. The *Year Book of Radiology* for 1941 and 1942—a respected compendium of abstracts of outstanding contributions to the world's radiological literature—summarized articles on the use of radiation to treat bursitis, staphylococcic and other infections, pulmonary and other forms of tuberculosis, hyperthyroidism and hyperparathyroidism, angina pectoris, late sequelae of syphilis such as dementia paralytica and tabes, erysipelas, sinusitis, parotitis, mastoiditis, otitis media, lobar and other forms of pneumonia, acute nephritis, Raynaud's disease, many forms of arthritis and rheumatism, high blood pressure, glaucoma, conjunctivitis and other diseases of the eye and its surrounding tissues, persistent nosebleed, psoriasis, salivary fistulas, herpes simplex, ileitis, asthma, hay fever, peritonitis, and tendovaginitis. Several papers reported on the radiation of the ovaries for premenstrual headache, scant menstruation, excessive menstruation, painful menstruation, failure to menstruate, infertility, and other "functional disorders of the female." Several papers reported that diphtheria carriers could be cured by radiation, and several recommended that if a child had one leg longer than the other, the longer leg should be irradiated in order to curb its further growth and achieve symmetry.

The doses administered for these purposes, of course, were substantial—sometimes hundreds of roentgens.

By the early 1960's profound changes had occurred. Neither the *American Journal of Roentgenology, Radiation Therapy, and Nuclear Medicine* nor *Radiology,* for example, carried a single article reccommending or even describing the use of radiation in the therapy of any benign condition during the entire year 1963.

The striking curtailment in the radiation treatment of conditions other than cancer was facilitated by advances in other forms of therapy. The sulfa drugs, penicillin, and other antibiotics and chemical agents made radiation unnecessary for a wide range of infections. The introduction of cortisone and the other steroid drugs provided an alternative to radiation for a wide range of inflammatory conditions. However, much of the credit for this curtailment must go to radiation therapists and dermatologists who voluntarily relinquished a substantial portion of their traditional practice as part of the price paid for the new philosophy of protection against radiation hazards.

Radiation therapy for benign conditions, it is true, was not completely abandoned, but it ceased to be the *first* resort. For the most part it was limited to cases which failed to yield to alternate modes of therapy, and to cases where the medical benefits clearly outweighed the hazards. Far greater attention was paid to the selection of proper radiation—very soft rays for skin conditions, for example, in order to minimize the dosage to internal organs—and to limiting the volume of tissue irradiated.

Radioactive Isotopes

The introduction of man-made radioisotopes for medical diagnosis (see pages 394–399 above) was itself in some cases a dose-sparing measure. Radioisotope procedures for diagnosing such conditions as placenta previa, for example, delivered significantly smaller doses to the mother and fetus than X-ray films made for the same purpose. During the 1960's, moreover, procedures were searched for and found which reduced radioisotope doses even further.

More sensitive radiation detectors, for example, made it possible to localize smaller amounts of a radioisotope, and research was undertaken to adapt image intensification procedures to isotope scanning.

Another significant approach was the introduction during the 1960's of new radioisotopes which delivered much smaller doses than those commonly used in the 1950's, while achieving the same or superior diagnostic results. Radioisotopes with a very short half-life were useful in this respect. An isotope which loses half its radioactivity in 5 or 10 minutes, for example, will in many cases deliver a far smaller total dose than one which delivers the same quality and intensity of radiation but has a half-life of many days or weeks. The problem of handling these short-half-life radioisotopes seemed at first insoluble, for, by the time they were taken from the nuclear reactors where they were produced and shipped to the physician who needed them, they would have lost almost all their usefulness. A solution, however, was found. Many radioisotopes of relatively long life produce short-lived radioactive "daughters" which are potentially useful in diagnosis. These radioisotopes are today produced in nuclear reactors, sealed in special containers, and shipped to medical centers all over the country. En route and after delivery, short-lived radioactive daughters accumulate in the containers. Immediately before a procedure is to be performed, the short-lived radioisotope is extracted from the containers—a process known as "milking the cow"—and administered to the patient. (The milking of radom from radium—see above, page 280—was the first practical example of this procedure.) In addition to making possible very striking reductions of dosage, these short-lived radioisotopes have other advantages. Often it is desirable, for example, to make an isotope test, perform some therapeutic procedure, and then repeat the test to determine the effect of the treatment. This is impossible with many radioisotopes, for the isotope from the first test persists to becloud the second test. With the very short-lived radioisotopes, a retest the next day or even later the same day may be possible.

An example of the "radioactive cow" is tellurium-132, with a long enough half-life to be shipped anywhere. It decays to iodine-132, with a half-life of 153 minutes. When this iodine-132 is used instead of iodine-131 (by far the most commonly used radioisotope for diagnostic purposes) radiation to the patient may be reduced by more than 90 per cent.[25]

Another approach to isotope dose reduction has been through the use of radioisotopes which emit only low-energy gamma rays (as distinct from those which emit high-energy gamma rays plus in some cases beta particles or alpha particles). One example is iodine-125, which has a longer half-life than iodine-132 but achieves a marked reduction of dose as compared with iodine-131 by virtue of its pure low-energy gamma emission. A second example is technetium-99, introduced for a variety of diagnostic purposes during the 1960's. Further opportunities for isotope dose reduction, it seems likely, will appear from time to time, for the number of radiosiotopes available for clinical use by the mid-1960's far exceeded the facilities available for subjecting them to clinical trials.

Spreading the Word

In addition to adopting these and many other dose-reducing procedures in their own offices and in the hospitals where they practiced, radiologists were concerned during the 1950's and 1960's with spreading the message of radiation safeguards throughout the medical profession.

One keynote of this campaign was sounded by Dr. Wendell G. Scott, professor of clinical radiology at Washington University in St. Louis, during his 1958 Chairman's Address to the Section on Radiology of the American Medical Association.[26]

"The problem today," Dr. Scott told an audience composed not only of radiologists but of other physicians who used radiation in their practices, "is one of control of radiations so that man can live safely in the artificial environment which the atomic industrial revolution is creating. In essence, we must prepare now to safeguard a brilliant future by keeping all forms of ionizing radiation at the lowest possible level."

Dr. Scott then reviewed very frankly the new data from radiation biology on both genetic and somatic hazards from radiation, and drew a moral: "These conclusions are not a pronouncement of doom for radiology. They are a challenge and a stimulus to do a better and a more careful job. Just as there are advances in other fields of medicine from the development of new knowledge and ideas, so there are in . . . radiology. New roentgenographic techniques and procedures have to be developed, old ones modified, and others discarded."

The possibility of genetic damage to future generations from gonadal radiation was very much in the news in 1958, when Dr. Scott read his paper. He met this anxiety head-on: "No matter what the present average gonadal dose is, it is too high if it can be lowered."

Then he reviewed the many techniques, described above, for lowering the dose to patients without impairing the diagnostic usefulness of radiation, and sounded a call to action: "With use of present-day developments, radiation dosage from the medical use of X rays can be reduced by 75 to 85 percent."

Dr. Scott did not speak alone. During the next few years much the same message, with individual variations, was repeated literally tens of thousands of times. Dr. Richard H. Chamberlain, chairman of the radiology department of the University of Pennsylvania, when testifying on June 6, 1962, as spokesman for the American College of Radiology before the Joint Congressional Committee on Atomic Energy, was proudly able to report that "since 1957, some 14,898 talks, speeches, programs, papers, editorials, and exhibits" on radiation safeguards had been presented to physicians and the public by 2,500 radiologists. The nation's medical schools had expanded their hours of instruction devoted to radiation protection. A moving picture illustrating radiological precautions and dose-lowering procedures, prepared by the American College of Radiology, had been exhibited hundreds of times to an estimated total audience of 68,000 physicians and others professionally concerned. The leading radiological journals, the journals of other specialties, and the *Journal of the American Medical Association* had published hundreds of articles on why and how to curtail patient exposures to radiation. A basic handbook[27] on how to reduce exposure was prepared by the ACR in 1958 "for users of X rays in the healing arts"; by 1966, some 350,000 copies of this "Practical Manual," in Spanish and Portuguese as well as English, had been distributed. Other medical organizations and specialist societies joined in this campaign. The message of dose reduction and other radiological safeguards was brought home not once but repeatedly to every physician, dentist, and technician using ionizing radiation.

Paralleling this nationwide campaign was a program of local "surveys" pioneered by a number of state and local health departments, with support from the Division of Radiological Health of the U.S. Public Health Service. An example was the survey in Polk County, Florida, conducted by the Florida Board of Health from September 1961 to August 1963 with PHS funds and consultants. The names and addresses of hospitals, physicians, dentists, osteopaths, and chiropractors using X rays were first secured, and permission to visit their installations was requested. (Only six out of 241 requests were refused.) Radiological health personnel then made the rounds of the installations and checked such critical matters as the size of beam and the presence of adequate filtration. (Some of the surveys went much further, checking tube voltage, film type used, speed of intensifying screens, development time, fluoroscopic output per minute, etc.) The findings were discussed with the physician or other person in charge, and a written recommendation for improvements was left with him. After 3 months, another visit was paid and a recheck made; if improvements had not yet been completed, a second recheck followed 3 months later.

Subsequent analysis of the results provided a rough gauge of the effectiveness of the survey approach. During a 4-week period prior to the survey, the data indicated, an estimated 3,257 Polk County patients had received an unnecessarily large exposure due to readily correctable factors. (In three-quarters of the cases, too large a beam was the problem.) After the second round of follow-up visits, only 232 patients were receiving an unnecessarily large exposure. Thus, the improvements achieved between survey visits had lowered the radiation exposure for 92.8 per cent of all patients.[28]

Progress Made and Outlook for Future Progress

One interesting measure of the progress made in curbing unnecessary radiation exposure concerns the life span of radiologists themselves. Dr. Shields Warren of the New England Deaconess Hospital and the Harvard Cancer Commission, and his associate Olive M. Lombard, reported on this in the *Archives of Environmental Health* for October 1966.

Among certified radiologists dying between 1934 and 1939, they noted, the average age at death was 56 years—much lower than for white males over 25 in the general population. Thereafter the average age at death rose to 59 (1940–1949), to 64 (1950–1959), and to 70 after 1960. By then, radiologists were actually living somewhat longer than white males over 25 in the general population. The improved longevity of radiologists almost certainly reflected in large part a lowering of radiation exposure.

During the 1940's, the report noted, 11 certified radiologists died of leukemia. This was a small number, but it was 8 times the number to be expected on the basis of nationwide leukemia rates. During the 1950's, the leukemia death rate among certified radiologists fell to only about 4 times the rate for the general population—another example of lessened risk following reduction of exposure.

To secure data concerning patient exposure levels, a nationwide "X-Ray Exposure Study"[29] was launched in 1964 by the U.S. Public Health Service in cooperation with the American College of Radiology and others. This PHS study began with visits to a cross-section of American homes during the period April to June 1964. Data on X-ray exposure were collected from 10,000 households comprising approximately 32,000 men, women, and children. Like the similar 1961 PHS population study (see above, pages 214–215), this 1964 study turned up some startling figures.

It was estimated, for example, that 506 million X-ray films were exposed during the year, of which 232 million were radiographic, 227 million were dental, and 48 million were "spot films" taken during fluoroscopic examinations. There were an estimated 10.5 million fluoroscopic examinations and 3.5 million X-ray therapeutic procedures. The estimated annual number of medical X-ray visits per year had increased from 47.9 per 100 people in 1961 to 49.8 per 100 in 1964; more numerous abdominal procedures accounted for much of the increase. Dental X-ray visits declined a bit, from 27.4 per 100 in 1961 to 26.8 per 100 in 1964. Data on parts of the body exposed and on the hospital, office, or other place where the exposure occurred were collected.

During the second phase of the study, data were collected from the radiologists and other physicians, the dentists, and the chiropractors, chiropodists, and podiatrists who had performed the procedures reported in the population study. These data were of two kinds. First, the professional men were asked to report the details of each exposure—film size, collimation, voltage, amperage, etc. Second, they were asked to expose a specially designed film pack under conditions similar to the exposure given the patient during the reported procedure.

Several major studies were necessary to assure proper evaluation of these film packs when they were returned to the Public Health Service. At the Johns Hopkins, for example, a conventional X-ray table top was divided into 3,000 distinct "locations." Thirty patients of varying height and weight were then X-rayed, using beams of four different degrees of quality or "hardness" and five different angles of projection. More than 20 million dosimetric measurements of exposure at the 3,000 locations were then made on the resulting film packs, at the rate of 1,000 measurements per second, by means of advanced computer techniques. Computer analysis of the results made it possible to estimate, from each film pack, the dose delivered to the male or female gonads in the course of the examination. A similar technique for fluoroscopic examinations was developed at Emory University.

Some results of the study were announced in a 218-page Public Health Service report entitled *Population Exposure to X Rays, U.S. 1964,* by Joseph N. Gitlin and Philip S. Lawrence. This report noted, for example, that too large a beam continued to be a major factor in unnecessary X-ray exposure. "More than one-half of all the radiographic films recorded in the study had a beam area in excess of the reported film area plus a 25-percent allowance. More than 25 percent of these exposures were associated with beam areas that were two or more times larger than the film area plus the allowance." Since the portion of the beam which does not strike the film is inherently useless, the need was demonstrated for further emphasis on the "first axiom" of radiological protection announced by Dr. William Rollins back in 1901 (page 184): "No X-light should strike a patient except the smallest beam that will cover the area to be examined, photographed, or treated."

Dentists came out rather well in the study. Approximately 80 per cent of the dental exposures recorded were within the 3-inch maximum beam diameter recommended by the National Committee on Radiation Protection and Measurements, and the report noted other indications of "a continuing upward trend in the proportion of dental X-ray examinations within recommended beam diameters."

Hospitals and radiologists also came out rather well. Mr. Gitlin and Dr. Lawrence reported that "abdominal examinations performed in hospitals, private group practices, and by radiologists in private offices involved approximately one-half the mean exposure per film compared to those performed in the private offices of other practitioners."

Ever since the great fallout controversy (page 419), both scientific and popular attention had been riveted on the potential genetic significance to future generations of X rays delivered to the male testes and female ovaries. The 1964 PHS population exposure study made it possible for the first time to estimate the "genetically significant dose" or GSD being received by the American public at large.

To calculate the GSD, PHS specialists began with the average gonadal dose delivered during a specified type of examination to a patient of each sex and age group. These doses were then "weighted" by the number of people receiving each type of examination and the number of future children they could be expected to produce. Thus, a relatively small gonadal dose to millions of young men and women contributed more to the GSD calculation than a heavy gonadal dose to a few thousand men and women, and a modest dose to a boy or girl of 15 outweighed an enormous dose to a woman past the child-bearing age.

The results, as reported in the February 1968 issue of *Radiology* by Dr. Richard L. Penfil and Morton L. Brown of the PHS National Center for Radiological Health, were startling in a number of respects. For example:

1. The genetically significant dose for the United States from diagnostic medical procedures was estimated on the basis of 1964 data as 55 millirads—about $\frac{1}{20}$ rad—per person per year. This estimate was reassuring in several respects. It was less than had generally been expected. It was within the range of levels reported from Sweden, Japan, and other industrially advanced countries, although differences in methodology made precise comparisons difficult. Also, it was less than half the estimated GSD produced by natural background radiation—120 milli-

rads per person per year. Thus, reducing the *medical* GSD to zero would reduce the *total* GSD by less than one-third.

2. The overwhelming bulk of the genetically significant dose—about 96 per cent—came from diagnostic films. Only 4 per cent came from fluoroscopy (including spot films taken during fluoroscopy). Photofluorography contributed less than 1 per cent. Dental exposures were not included in this portion of the study, but the report described the contribution of dental examinations to the GSD as "minimal."

3. By far the largest part of the genetically significant dose was being received by males—82 per cent of the total. Females received only 16 per cent of the GSD, and fetuses about 2 per cent. This was particularly astonishing because the male testes can be shielded from the direct beam during several kinds of abdominal examination which *necessitate* direct radiation of the ovaries. The authors attributed the relatively low female exposure to the fact that the ovaries are buried within the body and are therefore partially shielded by overlying tissues.

4. The age distribution of the GSD also proved a surprise. From birth to age 15 the dose was quite small (7 per cent of the total) because exposures were relatively rare. Patients aged 15 to 29 accounted for 71 per cent of the GSD at all ages—largely, of course, because their childbearing years were still in considerable part ahead of them, so that even a modest exposure contributed significantly to the GSD. Indeed, 60 per cent of the total GSD at all ages for both sexes was received by boys and men aged 15 through 29. Men and women past 29 received only about 20 per cent of the total GSD.

These and other findings, of course, gave radiologists and radiological health authorities many helpful pointers in their efforts to reduce the GSD still further. However, one finding overshadowed all the others in practical significance. *Merely by limiting the beam size to the size of the film, the report stressed, the national GSD could be cut from 55 to 19 millirads per person per year—a dose reduction of almost 70 per cent.* Virtually all of this dose reduction, the report added, would be traceable to "exclusion of the testes from the primary beam in examinations of the abdomen and pelvis."

The 1964 PHS population exposure study thus marked a turning point in the history of radiation safeguards. It indicated that the hazard to future generations against which Dr. Müller warned radiologists back in the 1930's (page 408) is today being held within bounds—and it pointed the way to still more strenuous efforts to reduce the genetically significant dose, largely by a more rigorous adherence to Dr. Rollins's first axiom.

REFERENCES

1. HEWLETT, R. G., AND ANDERSON, O. E., JR., *The New World.* The Pennsylvania State University Press, University Park, 1962.
2. SMYTH, H. D., *A General Account of the Development of Methods of Using Atomic Energy for Military Purposes* (the "Smyth Report"). U.S. Government Printing Office, Washington, 1945.
3. *Amer. J. Roentgen., 13:* 65–70, 1925.
4. KAYE, G. W. C., *Roentgenology: Its Early History, Some Basic Principles, and Protective Measures.* Paul C. Hoeber, Inc., New York, 1928.
5. *Radiology, 58:* 639–660, 1952.
6. *Proc. Amer. Phil. Soc., 90:* 11–19, 1946.
7. *Radiology, 3:* 408–417, 1924.
8. *Amer. J. Roentgen., 18:* 458–462, 1927.
9. *Arch. Path. (Chicago), 3:* 562–608, 1942.
10. STONE, R. S., *Industrial Medicine on the Plutonium Project,* pp. 9–10. McGraw-Hill Book Company, New York, 1951.
11. Joint Committee on Atomic Energy, 86th Congress, 2nd Session, *Selected Materials on Radiation Protection.* U.S. Government Printing Office, Washington, May 1960.
12. GROVES, L. R., *Now It Can Be Told: The Story of the Manhattan Project.* Harper & Row, Publishers, New York, 1962.
13. STONE, *op. cit.,* pp. xxi–xxiv.
14. *J. Amer. Dent. Ass., 11:* 802–805, 1924.
15. *JAMA, 85:* 1769–1776.
16. MARTLAND, H. S., *Collection of Reprints on Radium Poisoning.* U.S. Atomic Energy Commission, Oak Ridge, Tennessee, 1951.
17. LAPP, R. *Voyage of the Lucky Dragon.* Harper, New York, 1957.
17. LAPP, R., *Voyage of the Lucky Dragon.* New York, 1957.
18. *J. Nat. Cancer Inst., 28:* 1173–1191, 1962.
19. *Science, 140:* 1102–1104, 1963.
20. FOWLER, J. M. (ED.), *Fallout, A Study of Superbombs, Strontium 90 and Survival.* Basic Books, Inc., Publishers, New York, 1960.
21. *JAMA, 179:* 210–214, 1962.
22. *J. Amer. Vet. Med. Ass., 140:* 1051–1055, 1962.
23. *Arch. Path. (Chicago), 72:* 175–190, 1961.
24. *Public Health Rep., 75:* 652–658, 1960.
25. *J. Nucl. Med., 3:* 352–359, 1962.
26. *JAMA, 170:* 421–428, 1959.
27. American College of Radiology, *A Practical Manual on the Medical and Dental Use of X Rays with Control of Radiation Hazards.* American College of Radiology, Chicago, 1958.
28. U.S. Public Health Service Publication No. 999-RH-8, U.S. Government Printing Office, Washington, 1964.
29. U.S. Public Health Service Publication No. 1519, U.S. Government Printing Office, Washington, 1964.

Epilogue—The Future of Radiology

by Kenneth L. Krabbenhoft, M.D.

> "History has its foreground and its background, and it is principally in the management of its perspective that one artist differs from another. Some events must be represented on a large scale, others diminished; the great majority will be lost in the dimness of the horizon, and a general idea of their joint effect will be given by a few slight touches."—*Macaulay*

Radiology has advanced relatively more rapidly than other branches of medicine in its short period of existence. Modern medical practice would be impossible without its methods of study. As an example, increased precision of diagnosis has resulted in fewer exploratory surgical procedures. In some surgical practice, particularly cardiovascular, precise anatomic and functional information is necessary before a procedure can be attempted.

The science and art of radiology is slightly less than 75 years of age, and thus some radiologists still active were born before Roentgen's epic discovery in 1895. The first equipment was primitive compared to presently available equipment, which permits such technical achievements as high-speed serial roentgenography and cineroentgenography with bi-plane and even stereoscopic recording. The history of powered flight encompasses a slightly shorter period of time than that of the application of ionizing radiations in medicine but represents a parallel in rate of technological achievement, leaping from primitive early beginnings to present lunar flight and possibly to interplanetary travel.

However, for those who would be unduly impressed with present-day accomplishments, history in review is humbling, giving a realistic perspective of our profession and our position within it. As an example, the concept of teletherapy may be thought new and related to the nuclear era, but it originated in 1906. The principle of rotational therapy was originally described in the early 1900's. A method for localizing foreign objects within the eye was first devised in 1902 or 1903 and is used with little alteration to this day. Many similar examples of early insight could be cited.

Until two decades ago, radiology was largely practiced by general radiologists, with a few concentrating on either its diagnostic or therapeutic aspects. Early radiologists gravitated from other and usually broader disciplines to this new field. Some radiologists today have developed into sub-specialists, as demanded by the over-all increasing scope of this specialty. Nuclear radiology has developed since World War II, and more recently the subjects of pediatric radiology, neuroradiology, cardiovascular radiology, and angiography have become more clearly defined. Profound effects on training programs as well as on patterns of professional certification may ensue.

Radiology is one of the medical specialties combining the physical, scientific, and clinical aspects of medicine. An early heavy dependence on physics and mathematics led to close cooperation among the physicist, engineer, and physician-radiologist. The position of the radiological physicist has remained critically important, standing shoulder to shoulder with the clinical radiologist.

The gap between discovery and clinical application is closing. Financial support from many sources for medical research has encouraged the design, development, and production of expensive, highly complicated medical instrumentation. Industrial concerns have invested in research and development, and some have organized medical divisions, based upon the projection that health is becoming one of the major industries in our country. The use of electronic and other complicated kinds of instruments will extend the physician's usefulness by increasing his efficiency and allowing him to treat more patients better. Radiology is the most deeply committed of the medical specialties to the physical sciences, a natural commitment in view of its historic origins. The radiologist must be the most extensively prepared physician in mathematics and physics. At the same time, radiology in practice demands a broad knowledge of the entire field of medicine for effective consultation with other specialists and generalists. The need for relating to patients personally to allay fear, build confidence, and assure comfort is as important as in the practice of other specialties of medicine.

In this age of increasing technological achievement, unlimited career opportunities for professional and nonprofessional health personnel exist. It is estimated that an annual increase of 7 or 8 per cent in the demand for radiological service occurs, and that the present number of 7,000 radiologists should be increased to 25,000 by 1970 and 28,000 by 1975. The provision of medical service is a proliferative phenomenon, forcing an assessment of priorities, since a finite amount of money and other resources is an inescapable reality. In certain age groups, radiological procedures are more frequently needed. The percentage of the United States population over the age of 65 increased from about 3 per cent to 9 per cent in the past decade, with a concomitant increase in the incidence of geriatric disorders. The possibility of using existing facilities on a 7-day-per-week basis and the extension of group practice could result in more efficient utilization. We may expect a relative increase in financial support for teaching in the future in addition to that directed to research.

The development of Regional Medical Programs for centralization and concentration of highly technical patient-care facilities will lead to higher degrees of specialization. Highly specialized procedures in diagnostic radiology, the development of complicating scanning and imaging devices in nuclear radiology, and the installation of costly megavoltage equipment for radiation therapy necessitate some centralization of services, making better equipment and facilities available.

Having viewed briefly some aspects of radiology, a look at each of the major specialties within radiology—*i.e.*, roentgen diagnosis, radiation therapy, and nuclear radiology, and their allied disciplines of radiological physics, radiation biology, radiation chemistry, and radiation pharmacology—will be of interest in prospect of the future. Radiological equipment and electronics, computer technology, and new techniques may apply to more than one of the specialty fields and therefore are considered separately. Administration and practice, as well as the organizations within radiology, will undergo change in response to socioeconomic and technological influences. The interests of medical education will be served in part by new publications. The problems of manpower as related to professional and allied health personnel and their education will constitute one of the major concerns for the future. Finally, our challenges for the future are shared with the entire medical profession and the health care system in meeting basic responsibilities for the provision of care, teaching, and research.

Roentgen Diagnosis

Roentgen diagnosis, or diagnostic radiology, the largest of the specialties within radiology, applies the analytical approach of the diagnostician to disease recognition in recorded roentgenographic images. In earlier years, this method of study was primarily morphologically oriented to the clinical recognition of disease entities. More recently, functional and physiological methods of study have received emphasis. Critical analysis has been applied to every step in the practice of radiology, from producing the X ray to delivering an interpretation to the referring physician. This has entailed study of the neurophysiology of vision and psychological influences on the radiologist in addition to technical aspects of the method. Many applications of computer technology are being used and will become increasingly important in the future. A detailed accounting of the vast field of roentgenological diagnosis would be impossible, but we can cite certain developments which have occurred rapidly and will undergo further improvement.

Recognition of new disease entitites continues. Rubella embryopathy and the Wilson-Mikity syndrome are examples of newly recognized diseases. The correlation of radiological diagnosis with chromosomal aberrations has permitted more accurate classification of some hereditary and congenital conditions.

Iatrogenic conditions, such as lung fibrosis resulting from radiation over the chest, have been known for several decades. Recently, the development of lung fibrosis as the result of certain chemotherapeutic agents and of fibrous alveolitis due to a variety of etiologic agents is being recognized. Esophagitis on the basis of monilial infection due to antibiotic therapy, and aseptic necrosis of the femoral head resulting from corticosteroid therapy, are other examples. Similarly, the interstitial calcinosis of excessive vitamin D therapy, small bowel ulceration due to the oral administration of certain medications, and retroperitoneal fibrosis, previously considered idiopathic but now possibly attributed to medication, are further examples.

Fluoroscopy, now principally performed with image intensification, is employed to a lesser degree than before. It is used only where functional evaluation is a necessary part of an examination, but may be omitted where the detailed roentgen image serves better. A decrease in radiation exposure has resulted.

Application of cineradiographic methods to gastrointestinal examination permits better functional appreciation of this system and some of its disorders.

Opacification studies, which in the first decade following discovery of the roentgen ray were confined to natural contrasts of body tissues, have been highly developed. Earliest attempts involved the oral ingestion of opaque meals to visualize the gastrointestinal tract (see page 117). Today, with a variety of iodinated contrast media and other substances, virtually every accessible portion of the body may be visualized, and the search for ideal contrast media is constant. Bronchography is an excellent example of the attempt to find a contrast medium which has optimal physical characteristics but which evokes a minimal pulmonary reaction. To date, the ideal agent has not been found.

Of particular note in this regard are the techniques of angiography, which have vastly extended our diagnostic capabilities. Improvement of contrast media with lesser toxicity, permitting selective opacification of vascular structures with larger injected volumes and consequently better anatomic visualization, has provided both morphological and physiological information previously unavailable. By intravascular catheter placement under image-intensification fluoroscopy, detailed demonstration of the arterial and venous systems of parenchymatous organs, including the brain, lungs, liver, spleen, and other visceral structures, has been achieved. The accuracy of diagnosis permitted by these and other studies has had a profound effect on medical and surgical practice and is one of the bases for the indispensability of radiological methods in practice today. The contribution of angiography in the evaluation of hypertension and atherosclerosis is of particular importance. It is in such conditions that the multi-disciplinary or team approach is most effectively employed. This is exemplified in the study of renal vascular hypertension, where a multiplicity of radiographic and nuclear radiological procedures, *i.e.,* intravenous urography, drip-infusion pyelography, intravenous nephrotomography, isotope renography, aortography, and selective arteriography of renal vessels, are carried out in conjunction with the internist, urologist, and other interested specialists. More recently, the investigation of hypertension has been aided by retrograde inferior vena caval catheterization with collection of samples from the adrenal vein for analysis of renin content. These methods of study may lead to identification of the patient with surgically correctible hypertension.

The team approach is employed in neuroradiological investigations in conjunction with the neurologist, neurosurgeon and other interested specialists. Simultaneous or consecutive biplane techniques in visualizing cerebral vessels make possible a higher degree of diagnostic accuracy.

Recently, arteriographic evaluation of spinal cord angiomas and venous catheterization of basilar venous sinuses of the skull have been performed.

Many opacification studies are combined with rapid filming or cine-radiographic techniques, the latter capable of stereoscopic recording. Fine details of arterial anatomy are particularly important in such organs as the heart, where the coronary arteries can be selectively catheterized and visualized in this manner. Precise angiocardiographic information is essential to the surgeon in the treatment of congenital and acquired heart disease, and without this information many such surgical procedures would be extremely hazardous if not impossible.

The stomach has been studied with a combination of contrast methods by coating its mucosal surface with barium, filling the gastric lumen with air, and at the same time performing arteriography of the celiac artery. Similar triple-contrast techniques have been applied to the urinary bladder. A great achievement would be the application of this kind of study to the heart, but at present this appears technically impossible.

The team approach is of importance in the early detection and evaluation of breast cancer, and renewed interest in the roentgenographic examination of the breast—mammography—has contributed to earlier diagnosis and more effective treatment. The surgeon, radiologist, and pathologist, in concert with the epidemiologist, biostatistician, chemotherapist, and endocrinologist, are attempting to improve survival statistics in this manner.

Even the delicate, fragile lymphatic system has been brought into radiological view with the technique of lymphography. The exact value of this method and its limitations in scope of demonstration, accuracy of diagnosis, and contribution to therapeutic procedures continue to be investigated.

Exhaustive studies are directed to the complications of these involved methods of study and, in the case of contrast media, have involved the pharmacologist and biochemist in assessing the effect of these substances on the blood, brain, and other portions of the central nervous system, as well as the kidney. Embolic phenomena related to lymphangiography and thrombus formation as the result of intravascular procedures are other examples of hazards under scrutiny.

Body-section roentgenography has been significantly improved with the development of an instrument capable of linear, elliptical, circular, hypocycloidal, and circular zonography, producing greater radiographic detail in the demonstration of such fine structures as the auditory ossicles.

Intrauterine fetal transfusion and gastric camera guidance with television fluoroscopy will probably be employed with increasing frequency.

Subtraction techniques by photographic or television systems, and in some instances by second-order methods, can be employed for extended diagnostic accuracy in certain opacification studies.

Fractional focal spot X-ray tubes producing finer image detail have made possible magnification radiography in the living patient. Similar techniques of microradiography result in detailed analysis of pathological specimens.

Greater utilization of computer techniques will bring a systems-analysis approach to diagnostic processes, with resultant conservation of professional time and clarification of diagnostic logic. Duplication of single observations and simple probability diagnosis are possible and will provide diagnostic clues, handle data consistently, and perform repetitive tasks better. Although the computer is not capable of creative activity, the radiologist will thus be freed for such endeavors. These techniques relate to the storage, retrieval and probability aspects of computer technology.

Interesting future developments may include the application of radio frequencies, sterotaxic procedures, laser beams, and possibly the neutron gun in diagnostic and surgical techniques.

Radiation Therapy

Radiation therapy, that portion of radiology oriented to the treatment of predominantly malignant disease with ionizing radiations, is most commonly applied in the form of an X ray or teletherapy radionuclide beam. Intracavitary insertion of treatment cones or of naturally and artificially radioactive substances is another method of application. Interstitial implantation of radioactive sources is also used. The radiation therapist's approach is primarily one of synthesis, whereby a given lesion is treated by radiation alone or in combination with surgical, chemotherapeutic, hormonal, and immunological methods. In the 1930's, machines capable of delivering beams in excess of 1,000,000 electron volts of energy became available, as has been recounted above (Chap. 23). Before that time, equipment was undependable and capricious. At about this time more precise radiation dosimetry was developed. During the 1930's, most studies were oriented to accuracy of dose assessment and clinical investigation of optimal methods of combined treatments. In the 1940's higher-energy units became available, including the betatron, generating beams up to 24 and 31 million electron volts. The bone-sparing, skin-sparing, and increased depth-dose characteristics of these energies made treatment-planning simpler and resulted in more effective curative and palliative treatment. Since World War II, teletherapy units of cobalt-60, cesium-137, and some other elements have been made available, and, in many present installations, a variety of treatment facilities exists for the optimal application of irradiation to various anatomic areas and different kinds of neoplastic disease.

Presently, high-voltage accelerators with energies of 4 to 8 million electron volts are gaining in use, and treatment with the electron and heavy-ion beam may be employed where such equipment is available. In the future, regional treatment centers will make such treatment facilities available to growing numbers of patients. An increase in combined methods of treatment, employing chemotherapeutic agents, hormonal substances, and in some instances immunological methods, requires the radiation therapist to work closely with specialists in other disciplines. Greater precision in dosimetric determination is made possible by computer applications; enhancement of the radiobiological effect by the administration of oxygen and other substances under atmospheric or hyperbaric conditions is undergoing evaluation and will continue to be an important field of study. There is, as yet, no definite consensus on the ideal relationship of time and dose in regard to the fractionation and protraction of irradiation.

Total-body radiation in the treatment of generalized neoplastic disease has been used for some time but is undergoing a revival of interest and has been particularly effective in certain types of lymphoma.

In applying the principles of radiation biology, the application of treatment under hyperbaric oxygen conditions—or by the intravenous administration of hydrogen peroxide in other instances—and attempts at enhancing the radiotherapeutic response with chemotherapeutic agents are undergoing study. Neutrons and pi mesons have been found capable of overcoming the resistance of hypoxic cells because of a higher linear energy transfer. The provision of these sources of energy, however, is complicated by the bulk of the machines needed for their production, with a resultant decrease in flexibility for biological and clinical application. Through the cooperation of the radiation therapist, the physicist, the radiobiologist, and the engineer, however, some of these problems are certain to be overcome.

In determining dose-survival curves, loss of cell viability can be determined by cell-culture techniques, by the study of stem cells in the bone marrow and blood, and by the study of cancer cells. These studies will become more important in determining optimal methods of cancer treatment and in determining acceptable levels of radiation exposure. Relative sensitivity of mammalian cells and bacteria can be observed; the differential radiosensitivity of normal and malignant mammalian cells to X radiation and gamma radiation has been found to be somewhat lower than previously thought. This may modify overaggressive treatment plans in the future. The development of microcinematography, techniques of radioactive tracer study, and cytogenic analysis in assessing response to ionizing radiation will contribute to future concepts of radiation therapy and problems of radiation protection.

It was early appreciated that higher energies were not the final answer in the search for more effective treatment. Accurate evaluation of the clinical stage of disease and an understanding of the tumor-host relationships are important factors in selecting methods of treatment. In spite of sophisticated equipment indispensable to adequate treatment, the well-trained and experienced radiation therapist remains the most important element.

Nuclear Radiology

Nuclear radiology is the most recent of the three specialties within radiology. It is that segment of medical practice employing radionuclides (radioisotopes) in diagnosis and treatment. With the discovery of artificial radioactivity in 1934 (see Chap. 25), the door was opened to the production of a huge variety of these radioactive substances, which now number in the thousands. Many of these are of no practical use in medicine due to unacceptable half-lives, radiation characteristics, or biochemical characteristics. In the 1930's and early 1940's these materials were in short supply, produced in a costly manner with particle accelerators and therefore limited to research applications. Since World War II, economical manufacture of radionuclides with nuclear reactors has made radioactive substances of variable characteristics available in necessary quantities to permit wide clinical application. Some radionuclides of desirable biochemical and physical characteristics, such as carbon-11 and oxygen-15, must be produced by particle bombardment in accelerators. Applications of these elements are at present limited to a few centers located near these costly installations. The human body is mostly made up of approximately 15 elements, and, of these, oxygen and nitrogen have the least usable isotopic forms for clinical and research application. In the future, major medical centers may have cyclotrons for the purpose of producing short-lived isotopes. Three such units are already installed or are being installed in medical centers. In addition to making short-lived materials available, wider use of neutron-activation analysis would be possible in this setting. In this approach, elements within biological specimens are made radioactive, enabling them to be detected even though they are present in quantities too small to be measurable by chemical means. Multi-phasic screening methods with isotope techniques will have wider application in the future.

It has been estimated that 1500 to 1600 radionuclides were known in 1961, and of these approximately 300 may have medical usefulness. Of these, about one-sixth have popular applications.

A significant technological step forward has occurred with the availability of radionuclide generators ("cows") containing a radionuclide of moderately long half-life which, in the course of its decay, produces daughters of short half-life which can be extracted daily ("milked"). The technical advantage of short-lived radionuclides lies in a reduction of radiation to the patient, permitting larger doses and therefore more reliable counting statistics. At present, it is estimated that as many as 118 radioisotope cows are possible. Of these, four to seven may have immediate application, and at least one of these—molybdenum-99 decaying to technetium-99m—has been employed extensively. Coupled with newer detection devices, imaging apparatus, and the use of computer technology, these substances have introduced valuable techniques for the dynamic evaluation of organ function.

Isotope methods, despite their radioactive character, deliver an amount of radiation determined to be within safe limits. In most instances this is less than environmental background. These procedures may be less expensive in time or money, more precise and more informative, easier to perform and esthetically more acceptable, or safer than biochemical or other methods of study employing contrast media. Even if they do not replace other methods of study, isotope techniques may still provide valuable auxiliary or screening information in relation to them.

In diagnostic applications, metabolic physiological localization, distribution of labeled organic metabolites, dilution techniques, and flow measurements long encompassed the types of study employed. To these may now be added physical placement by intravascular injection of aggregated labeled materials of appropriate size for temporary capillary entrapment. This technique has been used in the study of lung perfusion and, more recently, of the brain. The dynamics of cerebral circulation will be evaluated in this and other ways in the future.

Double- and triple-isotope techniques have also been conceived and may be expected to increase in number. By selecting labeled organic materials and those which localize by physiological activity, three parameters of renal function have been evaluated in immediate sequence. One substance, not selectively excreted, measures vascular flow rate; another, selectively secreted by renal tubules and filtered by glomeruli, measures excretory capability; and a third concentrates in renal tubules to evaluate renal morphology.

A similar technique in the evaluation of upper abdominal masses employs a labeled substance concentrated in the liver, another concentrated in the pancreas, and still another deposited in the kidney. Application of video tape-recorded data subtraction can alternately display and separate the above images. A dual-isotope system permits electronic subtraction of one energy from another to evaluate lesions within the liver parenchyma.

Lung perfusion with trapped aggregates coupled with ventilatory evaluation by inhalants is a further example of physiological evaluation made possible by radionuclide methods.

Scanning or imaging techniques (which have been referred to as emission radiography, as opposed to the transmission radiography of the radiological method) for the study of many major parenchymatous organs in morphological and functional evaluation have been made possible by rectilinear scanners and stationary camera imaging devices. The development of the scintillation crystal is as basic to these techniques as the development of the X-ray tube has been to radiology. Rectilinear scanning techniques have been relatively slow in recording time, but, with the production of several designs of cameras and their coupling to magnetic tape and electronic recording systems, this type of organ recording has reached the speed of fraction-of-a-minute and even second exposures, thus extending functional evaluation. Rapid recording of dynamic phenomena by this method has been referred to as the emission counterpart of transmission cineradiography and has been applied to the study of cerebral, renal, and cardiac circulation. A digital computer attachment can store data, permitting recall for observation and manipulation with quantitation of static and dynamic studies. These designs link individual crystal elements to a computer memory, and, whereas these studies were formerly of a qualitative nature, they are now capable of quantitation, since numerical values can be applied to raw data which can be displayed in different forms and degrees. When recalled from video tape storage and replayed on a television monitor system, images can be recorded with filming techniques. In the evaluation of renal function, digital computer vascular background subtraction can be applied to increase accuracy and permit quantitation. All these types of dynamic study must be regarded as in the infancy of their development and will multiply in both sophistication and number.

Therapeutic application of radionuclides has depended on biochemical concentration, as with radioiodine in the treatment of thyroid disorders, and on physical placement, as in the intracavitary injection of colloidal radioactive suspensions or the interstitial or intracavitary insertion of seeds, grains, pellets, cylinders, etc. Teletherapeutic application of radioactive substances falls under the subject of radiation therapy and has been considered in that discussion. Early predictions of the effectiveness of treatment of certain neoplasms has been disappointing. Only 10 to 15 per cent of thyroid cancers function sufficiently well to concentrate radioactive iodine for treatment. Recently the intravascular injection of radionuclide-labeled materials and the labeling of antibodies has carried irradiation more selectively to the tissue of interest. We may expect further development of these antibody techniques. Intravascular microspheres, possibly combined with magnetic localization and isotopic labeling, may find diagnostic and therapeutic use.

Whole-body radiation counters, originally very costly, are being designed more simply and less expensively and will become more widely available. Whole-body counting techniques have broadened our understanding of intestinal absorption, metabolic phenomena, body content of certain elements in the evaluation of obesity, and genetic abnormalities (potassium-40 content in muscular dystrophy and iron-59 absorption in hemochromatosis). Valuable information relative to body burdens of radioactive substances has been gained by these techniques as well.

In the nuclear radiological department of the future, we may expect to find not one but several types of scanning and imaging devices. Design of these units must be oriented to certain specific applications. A scanner ideal for liver recording may not be ideal for brain recording, and vice versa.

As nuclear radiology becomes more involved with dynamic studies, imaging instrumentation, video tape recording, variable playback, and photographic recording will be further developed. Observations at as short as 0.1-second intervals have been made, bringing rapid-motion study with emission radiography into reality. Research efforts, as reflected in improvement of equipment, will be oriented to improved recording media of various kinds. The substitution of chromium dioxide for iron oxide in the manufacture of magnetic recording tape is an example.

RADIOLOGICAL PHYSICS

The application of ionizing radiation in treatment requires precise dosimetric calculations and accurate treatment planning. Clinical evaluation is made by the therapist who, in consultation with the radiation physicist, carries out the treatment plan. A great debt is owed the radiation physicist. Roentgen himself was a physicist. The development of better methods of dosimetry is largely attributable to the physicist, as are many inventions of equipment and technique. He is essential to the guarantee of radiation safety in diagnostic roentgenology and to dosage calculation as well as other aspects of nuclear radiology.

Adaptation of physical science techniques to the life sciences will continue in the future, as has occurred in the past. The close cooperation of the radiation therapist and the physicist will continue and increase in the future. The clinician relies upon the physicist for accurate scientific orientation, and the physicist in turn relies upon the therapist for clinical direction.

RADIATION BIOLOGY

The radiation biologist is interested in the effects of ionizing radiation on living organisms at both the cellular and organic level. Much of his information has been derived from animal experimentation, accidental human exposure, and clinical observation. Extrapolation of these data has led to determination of safe exposure levels. Emphasis on the cellular level of effect has increasingly been oriented to molecular biology. The application of zonal ultracentrifugation, originally employed for isotope-separation techniques, holds promise for better understanding of human disease at the molecular level.

RADIATION CHEMISTRY AND RADIATION PHARMACOLOGY

The work of the radiation chemist has divulged in part the character of chemical change occurring in body fluids as a result of exposure to ionizing radiations. These effects are then related to histological and physical phenomena. Interdisciplinary studies will continue and probably increase as the search for better understanding of basic radiochemical and radiobiological phenomena proceeds. The radiation pharmacist or pharmacologist, in collaboration with physicians searching for improved radiopharmaceuticals, has manufactured several radionuclides and labeled substances, extending the application of nuclear radiological techniques.

RADIOLOGICAL EQUIPMENT

Although equipment is usually designed for use in one of the major sub-divisions of radiology, such as Roentgen diagnosis, radiation therapy, or nuclear radiology, certain general considerations can be directed to the problem of equipment as it applies to all of radiology. That there has been a technological explosion in the past several decades is obvious. Most major research efforts today require an interdisciplinary team approach due to the complexity of inventions, the costliness of development, and the accumulation of vast amounts of knowledge. This forces a degree of specialization which destroys broad and interdisciplinary orientation. For example, crystals can be made by chemists, but of necessity are measured by physicists who in turn do not know how to make them. Furthermore, the gap between conception of a basic discovery and the manufacture of a finished product requires a theoretically oriented scientist for the former and applied scientists for the latter. All of this means that equipment design for the future will become more costly and will depend primarily upon corporate and Federal financing.

Electronic developments have been of particular importance to radiology with the use of television for administrative, educative, and technical applications. Some applications of television are listed below which are presently employed in institutions and will become commonplace in the future.

1. The remote fluoroscopic examination of patients will serve to further reduce radiation exposure of personnel.

2. Components applied to data retrieval and manipulation from video tape storage with contrast enhancement, subtraction, reversal, and alteration of images are other uses. Video tape recordings and television replay may decrease conventional fluoroscopy and ordinary spot filming in some installations.

3. Coupled with computer elements for retrieval of stored information, diagnostic differential capabilities broaden, and data can be transmitted immediately.

4. In administration, patient traffic control, scheduling of examinations, departmental surveillance, and speed of communication and consultation can all be improved by closed-circuit television systems. These can be coupled with computer elements as well.

5. Instant communication among areas of the hospital such as the operating room, emergency room, admission areas, and patient care areas will result in reduction of hospital costs.

6. Closed circuit communication among hospitals, auditoria, and medical schools will provide teaching aids.

Increasing cooperation between equipment manufacturers and representatives of the profession will occur in translating clinical needs into finished hardware. Some radiological societies have formed committees to serve this purpose. Technical improvements in diagnostic equipment will respond to demands of angiographic and other techniques. Image intensifiers, television applications to fluoroscopy, cineradiography, and video tape recordings are relatively new developments which may be expected to undergo significant improvement.

Radiographic tube design, with fractional focal spot apparatus and improved generator circuitry capable of increased loads, has extended fine-detail radiography. Other radiographic tubes and generators of high load capability have extended the technical effectiveness of rapid serialography and cineradiography. More radiological departments of the future will be equipped with electrical power capable of serving three-phase equipment.

Mobile X-ray units have been designed beyond many hospitals' present electrical capability to supply them. Condenser-discharge generators and field-emission units have been developed which are independent of immediate electrical power. It is predicted that the focal spot may be reduced to a diameter of 20 microns, which would provide sufficient radiographic detail for magnification of structures such as bone and soft tissues. In this design, described by Dr. Michel Ter-Pogossian, electrons are produced at the cathode by volatizing its surface by means of a laser pulse. High X-ray output results by producing the X radiation before the target is destroyed. With relatively low kilovoltage and exposures as short as a few microseconds, this apparatus permits radiography of the thickest body parts using a disposable tube comparable to a photographic flash bulb. Simplicity of design and restriction of use to highly specified purposes may make such a tube practical.

A self-contained radiographic unit which has been used in industry has recently been designed for medical use in the examination of post-operative specimens and for teaching radiographic technique. The unit, operating on ordinary 110- to 220-volt alternating current has a fine focal spot of 0.5 millimeter and a beryllium window, making possible radiography of high definition.

COMPUTERS

Computer technology, already important in science and industry, is being rapidly integrated into medical care. Cost of these systems is high, but will become relatively less in the future through increased efficiency. Even if actual reduction in cost is not achieved, it will help to hold the line and contribute to more comprehensive care. It has been said that 50 million electrocardiograms are recorded each year in the United States, and that these ultimately will be programmed to computer analysis.

Increasing reliability of computers and vast extension of their capabilities will occur. First-generation computers built in the early 1950's with vacuum tubes were volatile and subject to change, drifted, and were unstable. Like the first Van de Graaff electrostatic accelerator, they required a very large housing (the Van de Graaff accelerator was first built in an airplane hangar—see above, page 340—but today is contained in a steel pressurized tank of approximately 3 by 8 feet). Second-generation computers were developed in the mid-1950's with a change to solid-state circuitry, and these computers had a core memory. They were very reliable, but their design changed rapidly. The present third-generation computers are highly reliable. Solid-state and integrated circuitry is employed, greatly increasing potential applications. Present computers operate with a response time of 4 to 5 nanoseconds, and it is predicted that by the 1970's computers of greater capability will respond with times of 1 nanosecond.

It has been estimated that the human mind has a capacity of about one septillion (1,000,000,000,000,000,000,000,000) computing elements, compared to present electronic computers with estimated capacities of ten thousand to ten million (10,000,000) units. Digital magnetic tape and other media for recording are constantly being improved for the storage of unbelievable quantities of information on small areas. The computer is faster, less forgetful, and less subject to error in its computations than is the human mind. However, it is less flexible and has little or no creative ability. It is clear, then, that with effective programming the computer can be used to perform repetitive tasks. Evaluation and interpretation of medical data will remain the province of the competent physician with the necessary knowledge and experience to practice his art.

Computer techniques as applied to coding, transmitting, storage, and retrieval of radiological data have been brought to a point of practical utilization in some research settings and may be expected to have wider application in the future.

At present, four major health-activities areas are medical facilities, clinical work, research, and health education. Communication to and from laboratories and provision of management needs are computer capabilities relative to medical facilities. Clinical work can be computer-assisted in rendering reports and in some laboratory automation. Statistical problems of research and machine-assisted instruction in health education are other areas of computer technology that can be effectively applied to the practice of radiology.

On-line computer availability for transmitting X-ray reports will result in incalculable savings of personnel and time. The physician, in order to make use of these advancements, must learn the language of the biomathematician, who in turn must learn the physician's language. Appropriate programming language is basic to efficient use and to satisfactory application of these techniques. Computer-aided diagnosis, radiation dosimetric calculation, synthesis, storage, and retrieval of information in applications to nuclear radiology are but some of the present and projected uses. Digital computation is of undeniable value in nuclear radiology and will become increasingly important. In addition to educational use and storage and retrieval of information, accurate determination of radionuclide inventories will be simplified. These techniques will find increasing application to physiological function studies, to radioisotope scans, and to systems analysis in over-all laboratory operation. The latter role of the digital computer can be expanded to encompass the entire radiology department, the general hospital, the medical center, and the modern medical school.

Computers can speed the learning process through interaction of the student and the computer, and they make possible quick transferance and retrieval of information in library systems. They can relieve administrative burdens, and as an instructional tool they tailor courses to individual student speeds of response and learning.

It has been advised that computer orientation of health workers be started with relatively simple modular programs, building these into series preparing for total integration of hospital systems. Such a complicated system can only be created by combining operable sub-systems.

Computer costs may be prohibitive for some installations from the standpoint of hardware. Smaller computers, however, may be linked to larger ones with large memory banks. This service may be obtained in the future as we now purchase electric power, heat, and other central services.

As applied to screening methods, multiphasic computer evaluation, including radiological screening, may be directed to large-scale prevention and detection of disease.

NEWER TECHNIQUES

Newer techniques of study employing ionizing radiations and other forms of electromagnetic energy are undergoing development and critical analysis.

Xerography employs X radiation directed to a charged selenium plate which is subsequently dusted with powder to create an image. Radiographic film is unnecessary. Mammographic screening may be easier and more accurate if this equipment can be improved and marketed.

A miniature-anode radiographic tube has been developed for intracavitary insertion and "inside-out" panographic wide-angle roentgenography of the teeth and mandible.

Thermography, a method of recording infrared radiations, has been used in the study of malignant and other lesions associated with increased vascularity and therefore increased heat emission. The advantage of such a technique lies in its nondestructive character, obviating radiation exposure. Generally, it may be said that present hardware is inadequate to the task but that improvements may result in a wider application of this technique, possibly for screening methods.

Doppler ultrasonography has been employed as a transmission or a tomographic technique with compound scanning. Echoencephalography has been applied to the evaluation of intracranial lesions which cause displacement of midline structures.

Three-dimensional electron micrographs have recently been made of cancer cells. Holographic image restoration and three-dimensional holographic movies pose possible interesting techniques for the future. Holography makes use of the coherence and monochromatic characteristics of a laser beam for recording permanently on film a "photographed" object. This presently experimental technique may one day be adapted to radiological methods for three-dimensional visualization and reproduction.

Proton radiography employing energetic particles from an accelerator has been used to produce radiographs with unusually high contrast but with poor spatial resolution. This is at present a research technique with possible industrial applications and future medical implications.

Neutron radiography may have some medical application because materials which are relatively opaque to X rays or gamma rays are usually transparent to the passage of neutrons. Neutron therapy may be improved and made useful despite early poor experience described in Chapter 24.

In nuclear radiology, isotope placentography can be performed with minimal radiation exposure to the patient and fetus, and in some instances this technique more accurately localizes the position of the placenta. Isotope encephalography can provide valuable information as to the status of cerebrospinal fluid flow which cannot be obtained in any other way.

Thermoluminescent dosimetry has resulted in practical intracavitary dose measurements under actual treatment conditions, leading to better estimation of optimum dose.

RADIATION PROTECTION

It is important to realize that concerns for human radiation exposure must be divided into those of somatic and genetic implications.

Radiologists have long been cognizant of the potential harmful effects of ionizing radiations and have employed protective measures. Increasing public awareness and broader medical and dental use, along with the "great fallout controversy" described in Chapter 26, have more recently focused attention on this problem. Unfortunately, needless alarm has arisen from inaccurate implications embodied in testimony before legislative committees as to the magnitude of this hazard and the degree of damage to be expected.

Stringent care should always be exercised, particularly where genetic exposure is of concern. Theoretical hazards, however, should never preclude studies indicated on the basis of sound clinical judgment. Although there is an acknowledged link between exposure to ionizing radiations and potential damage to body and reproductive cells, these are theoretical and "possible," not actual and "probable," in diagnostic applications. Properly executed radiological examinations should not be postponed or omitted where they are indicated. In the future, close surveillance of radiological facilities will continue to minimize exposure of patients. It is equally important to study other sources of environmental hazards capable of producing genetic damage. Potentially genetically injurious chemicals and other substances in our environment could be more important than radiation exposure in some instances.

ADMINISTRATION

Demands for radiological services are proliferating at an estimated annual rate of 7 to 8 per cent, with consequent stress on institutional, private office, and manpower resources. In an attempt to use available facilities more efficiently, proposals have been made for the provision of 24-hour service on a 7-day-per-week basis. In certain central locations, such organizational solutions may be necessary. This concept has already been applied to emergency services and in one instance, at least, to a special procedures facility. Accident victims arriving by air within minutes of injury are definitively studied for recognition of aortic rupture or other internal injury and undergo corrective surgery within 1 or 2 hours. Increasing urbanization, large numbers of physicians in group practice, and heavier emphasis on institutional practice are factors which will effect administrative changes. The radiologist will be relieved of repetitive and administrative tasks as appropriate personnel can be trained. He will then be free to concentrate his efforts on creative tasks and to exercise judgment in those problems which he is uniquely qualified to handle.

Administration has been improved by the advent of automatic film processing, mechanized film handling, and application of computer technology to appointment systems and to storage, retrieval, and transmittal of information. In radiology, an area of medicine particularly well suited to technological adaptation, these techniques will be quickly implemented on a broad scale, having been studied extensively in some areas and found to have proved worth.

Mass public-health screening oriented to certain diseases commoner in older people, *e.g.,* arteriosclerosis, hypertension, and some neoplasms, will place a heavier load on the radiologist for definitive studies.

Organizations

In the past two or three decades changes within existing societies have occurred, as compared to an earlier period in which new organizations appeared. The American College of Radiology has undergone many changes, recently reorganizing existing state and local societies into component chapters of the national organization. Presently, organizational changes in the American Medical Association are under study which may have an effect on the American College of Radiology and other radiological organizations.

As we have seen in the past (Chap. 21), amalgamations, mergers, and discontinuance of old and creation of new societies have occurred and will undoubtedly continue in the future. New societies may be expected to develop out of the emergence of specialty groups within radiology.

Continuing education, new techniques, and exchange of ideas will continue to spark interest in national and international scientific meetings.

The American College of Radiology cooperates with the American Society of Radiologic Technologists in support of the American Registry of Radiologic Technologists, the voluntary certifying body for technicians. New and better job descriptions and more realistic economic standards have emerged from these cooperative efforts. In some states licensing of technicians has been inaugurated.

Legislative control of radiation exposure to the population has been guided in part by testimony from radiologists representing professional organizations. Proposed legislation relating to the shipment of radioactive substances and to radiation exposure from electronic devices has been clarified for the information of legislators and the benefit of the public.

Organizational representation is important where questions arise relative to professional status of radiologists and the relationship of radiology to medicine in general. Within the past two decades, it has been necessary to reaffirm that the practice of radiology is, in fact, the practice of medicine. This may appear odd, in view of the educational training of radiologists. Following graduation from an approved medical school (the same as other physicians) and an internship, three or more years are spent in residency training, yet the need for clear definition of the professional character of our practice has occurred, and similar questions may be expected to arise in the future.

PUBLICATIONS

As I have reported elsewhere,[1] more than 50 journals of radiology or allied sciences were published over the world in 1962, exclusive of a large number of pre-existing publications which had been absorbed by some of those listed. In addition, over 60 titles in the world literature had been abandoned without incorporation into other publications. In the United States alone, the explosion of knowledge and of the volume of published material in the past 8 years is manifested by the appearance of texts, monographs, and published symposia in large numbers and by the emergence of three important new journals. *Radiologic Clinics of North America* first appeared in 1963, *Investigative Radiology* first appeared in 1966, and *Seminars in Roentgenology* was also first published in 1966. As the extent of our knowledge and the volume of research increases, we may expect further expansion of radiological publications.

Manpower: Professional and Allied Health Personnel; Education

In meeting professional and allied health personnel needs for the future, problems of recruitment, facilities, and education loom large on the horizon. Dr. C. Allen Good, addressing the American Roentgen Ray Society as its president in 1967, called attention to the ferment in medicine today. Changing curricula in medical schools, the effect of the Millis Commission report to the American Medical Association (Citizens Commission on Graduate Medical Education) recommending abolition of the internship and other changes, the development of Regional Medical Programs under Federal government auspices, and specialty boards making plans for recertification are but some of the signs of disquietude. The third NACOR report in 1966 (National Advisory Committee on Radiation) noted the scarcity of radiologists, the need for the development of specialists within diagnostic and therapeutic radiology, and the possible advantage of separating diagnosis and therapy. Nuclear radiology requires more trainees as well.

In meeting some of these problems, Dr. Good advises that the intern year may be replaced by an "internship in radiology." The residency program could then be 2 or 2½ years in duration, followed by certification. A sub-specialty interest could then be pursued. Other programs of training could equip radiologists for general community radiological practice. Continuing medical education in radiology poses the same challenge as that faced throughout medicine.

Now is the time to prepare health personnel with combined medical and computer orientation. The need already exists and will increase sharply in the future. Better physics, mathematics, and electronics education will be needed by doctors of medicine and particularly radiologists in an age of instrumentation.

Institutes for the training of allied health personnel, with rotation of trainees through affiliated hospitals, are being organized and will increase in number. Some of the routine examinations presently performed by radiologists may of necessity be performed by nonradiologists, freeing the radiologist for special procedures. This will apply to administrative as well as technical tasks. It is predicted that undergraduate and graduate medical education will require a broader orientation to radiology. It is important that the young physician receive hospital exposure to this indispensable specialty of medicine. Being introduced in this manner will familiarize him with radiology and may generate an interest in making it his career.

Compounding the problems of greater service loads, teaching requirements, and research commitments (factors common to all of medicine) is the increasing length of residency training made necessary by the greater span of knowledge and experience. New approaches to residency training in radiology will be forced by the specialty's rapid growth and changing practice patterns.

Training of personnel in allied health fields will be accelerated in coming years. A shortage of technicians has been attributed in part to a failure on the part of the medical profession to make these jobs attractive. A National Conference on X-Ray Technician Training in 1966 explored our present situation and made recommendations. An American Medical Association Commission to Coordinate the Relationships of Medicine with Allied Health Professions and Services has appointed a Study Committee on Radiology and other committees on anesthesiology, ophthalmology, orthopedic surgery, pathology, and physical medicine to explore more effective relationships between these groups.

Regional planning of institutional needs will take into account the high cost of new equipment. At a time when greater reliance must be placed on technology and automation in medical diagnosis, in storage and retrieval of information, and in research, re-emphasis of clinical teaching and research is imperative.

CHALLENGES FOR THE FUTURE

The challenges facing radiology in the future are those facing all of medicine and additionally involve development of safer and more effective methods of diagnostic examination and the conception of better methods of treatment. Complicated and costly equipment is essential to radiological practice, and the adaptation of computer techniques and clinical investigation will be major areas of interest. Scarcity of essential materials could force development of alternative techniques.

Administration and manpower training problems will increase, and the recruitment and training of future generations of radiologists and allied health personnel must receive high priority. Development of radiological services for underdeveloped countries will become increasingly important. Research will demand investment of thought and energy with adequate financial support. Cooperative efforts of the profession and manufacturers will continue and become more frequent.

Finally, the continued provision of excellent health care in all of its aspects remains our primary responsibility.

REFERENCES

1. KRABBENHOFT, K., History of Radiological Journals, in BRUWER, A. J., *Classic Descriptions in Diagnostic Roentgenology*, pp. 1991–2029. Charles C Thomas, Publisher, Springfield, Illinois, 1964.

Index of Persons